Progress in Preventing Childhood Obesity

How Do We Measure Up?

Committee on Progress in Preventing Childhood Obesity

Jeffrey P. Koplan, Catharyn T. Liverman, Vivica I. Kraak, Shannon L. Wisham, *Editors*

Food and Nutrition Board

INSTITUTE OF MEDICINE
OF THE NATIONAL ACADEMIES

THE NATIONAL ACADEMIES PRESS
Washington, D.C.
www.nap.edu

THE NATIONAL ACADEMIES PRESS • 500 Fifth Street, N.W. • Washington, DC 20001

NOTICE: The project that is the subject of this report was approved by the Governing Board of the National Research Council, whose members are drawn from the councils of the National Academy of Sciences, the National Academy of Engineering, and the Institute of Medicine. The members of the committee responsible for the report were chosen for their special competences and with regard for appropriate balance.

The study was supported by Grant Nos. 052339 and 56982 between the National Academy of Sciences and the Robert Wood Johnson Foundation. Any opinions, findings, conclusions, or recommendations expressed in this publication are those of the authors and do not necessarily reflect the views of the organizations or agencies that provided support for the project.

Library of Congress Cataloging-in-Publication Data

Progress in preventing childhood obesity : how do we measure up? / Committee on Progress in Preventing Childhood Obesity ; Jeffrey P. Koplan ... [et al.], editors.
   p. ; cm.
  Includes bibliographical references and index.
  ISBN-13: 978-0-309-10208-7 (hbk.)
  ISBN-10: 0-309-10208-1 (hbk.)
  1. Obesity in children—United States—Prevention. 2. Child health services—United States—Evaluation. 3. Nutrition policy—United States—Evaluation. I. Koplan, Jeffrey. II. Institute of Medicine (U.S.). Committee on Progress in Preventing Childhood Obesity.
  [DNLM: 1. Child. 2. Obesity—prevention & control. WD 210 P964 2007]
  RJ399.C6P77 2007
  618.92'398—dc22

2006037547

Additional copies of this report are available from the National Academies Press, 500 Fifth Street, N.W., Box 285, Washington, DC 20055. Call (800) 624-6242 or (202) 334-3313 (in the Washington metropolitan area), Internet, http://www.nap.edu.

For more information about the Institute of Medicine, visit the IOM home page at: **www.iom.edu.**

Cover design by Samantha Razook Murphy.
Cover photograph by Harrison Eastwood.

Printed in the United States of America.

The serpent has been a symbol of long life, healing, and knowledge among almost all cultures and religions since the beginning of recorded history. The serpent adopted as a logotype by the Institute of Medicine is a relief carving from ancient Greece, now held by the Staatliche Museen in Berlin.

"Knowing is not enough; we must apply.
Willing is not enough; we must do."
—Goethe

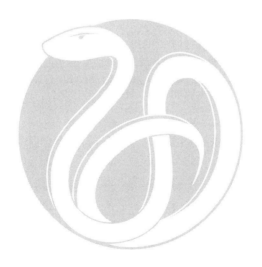

INSTITUTE OF MEDICINE
OF THE NATIONAL ACADEMIES

Advising the Nation. Improving Health.

THE NATIONAL ACADEMIES
Advisers to the Nation on Science, Engineering, and Medicine

The **National Academy of Sciences** is a private, nonprofit, self-perpetuating society of distinguished scholars engaged in scientific and engineering research, dedicated to the furtherance of science and technology and to their use for the general welfare. Upon the authority of the charter granted to it by the Congress in 1863, the Academy has a mandate that requires it to advise the federal government on scientific and technical matters. Dr. Ralph J. Cicerone is president of the National Academy of Sciences.

The **National Academy of Engineering** was established in 1964, under the charter of the National Academy of Sciences, as a parallel organization of outstanding engineers. It is autonomous in its administration and in the selection of its members, sharing with the National Academy of Sciences the responsibility for advising the federal government. The National Academy of Engineering also sponsors engineering programs aimed at meeting national needs, encourages education and research, and recognizes the superior achievements of engineers. Dr. Wm. A. Wulf is president of the National Academy of Engineering.

The **Institute of Medicine** was established in 1970 by the National Academy of Sciences to secure the services of eminent members of appropriate professions in the examination of policy matters pertaining to the health of the public. The Institute acts under the responsibility given to the National Academy of Sciences by its congressional charter to be an adviser to the federal government and, upon its own initiative, to identify issues of medical care, research, and education. Dr. Harvey V. Fineberg is president of the Institute of Medicine.

The **National Research Council** was organized by the National Academy of Sciences in 1916 to associate the broad community of science and technology with the Academy's purposes of furthering knowledge and advising the federal government. Functioning in accordance with general policies determined by the Academy, the Council has become the principal operating agency of both the National Academy of Sciences and the National Academy of Engineering in providing services to the government, the public, and the scientific and engineering communities. The Council is administered jointly by both Academies and the Institute of Medicine. Dr. Ralph J. Cicerone and Dr. Wm. A. Wulf are chair and vice chair, respectively, of the National Research Council.

www.national-academies.org

Staff

VIVICA I. KRAAK, Co-Study Director
CATHARYN T. LIVERMAN, Co-Study Director
LINDA D. MEYERS, Director, Food and Nutrition Board
SHANNON L. WISHAM, Research Associate
JON Q. SANDERS, Senior Program Assistant (until June 2006)
JESSICA COHEN, Christine Mirzayan Science and Technology Policy
    Graduate Fellow (June to August 2006)

Independent Report Reviewers

This report has been reviewed in draft form by individuals chosen for their diverse perspectives and technical expertise, in accordance with procedures approved by the National Research Council's Report Review Committee. The purpose of this independent review is to provide candid and critical comments that will assist the institution in making its published report as sound as possible and to ensure that the report meets institutional standards for objectivity, evidence, and responsiveness to the study charge. The review comments and draft manuscript remain confidential to protect the integrity of the deliberative process. We wish to thank the following individuals for their review of this report:

HEIDI ARTHUR, The Ad Council, New York, NY

BILL BEERY, Group Health Community Foundation, Seattle, WA

LORELEI DISOGRA, Nutrition and Health, United Fresh Fruit and Vegetable Association, Washington, DC

STEPHEN B. FAWCETT, Work Group for Community Health and Development/World Health Organization (WHO), University of Kansas, Lawrence

VANESSA NORTHINGTON GAMBLE, National Center for Bioethics in Research and Health Care, Tuskegee University, AL

DEBRA HAIRE-JOSHU, Department of Community Health, Saint Louis University School of Public Health, St. Louis, MO

SUSAN L. HANDY, Department of Environmental Science and Policy, University of California, Davis

CATHY KAPICA, former Global Director of Nutrition, McDonald's
  Corporation, Oakbrook, IL
JOE THOMPSON, Surgeon General, State of Arkansas and Arkansas
  Center for Health Improvement, Little Rock
BRIAN WANSINK, Department of Applied Economics and
  Management, Cornell University, Ithaca, NY

Although the reviewers listed above have provided many constructive
comments and suggestions, they were not asked to endorse the conclusions
or recommendations nor did they see the final draft of the report before
its release. The review of this report was overseen by **CUTBERTO GARZA,**
Boston College. Appointed by the National Research Council, he was responsible for making certain that an independent examination of this report was carried out in accordance with institutional procedures and that
all review comments were carefully considered. Responsibility for the final
content of this report rests entirely with the authoring committee and the
institution.

Preface

The remarkable growth of obesity in the young population in many parts of the world in a relatively short time span represents one of the defining public health challenges of the 21st century. At this early phase in addressing childhood obesity, action has begun on a number of levels to improve dietary patterns and increase physical activity in children and youth throughout the United States and in other countries. Schools, corporations, youth-related organizations, families, communities, foundations, and government agencies are working to implement a variety of policy changes, new programs, and other interventions. There is a great deal yet to be learned about how to evaluate these efforts and disseminate information on effective interventions. Additionally, lessons learned from other public health concerns such as the prevention of youth tobacco use and alcohol consumption can provide insights and directions for further efforts. However, the solutions to tobacco and alcohol consumption among our young people cannot be fully replicated due to the complexity of obesity and the ubiquity of food, sedentary habits, and familiar routines in our culture that contribute to the problem. A comprehensive response to the obesity epidemic requires connectivity, consistency, and continuity across multiple programs and sectors. Preventing childhood obesity will involve changes in social norms and the demand by the general public for healthier lifestyles and the products and opportunities that support physical activity and healthful diets. Innovations are needed that accelerate the pace of change that will move us toward these goals.

In 2002, the Institute of Medicine (IOM) responded to a congressional mandate by developing an action plan for preventing childhood obesity. The IOM report *Preventing Childhood Obesity: Health in the Balance* provided recommendations for further action by multiple stakeholders. As a natural outcome of that report, IOM established the Committee on Progress in Preventing Childhood Obesity in 2005 with support from the Robert Wood Johnson Foundation. The IOM committee was charged with undertaking a study to assess the nation's progress in preventing childhood obesity. It was also asked to engage in a dissemination effort promoting the implementation of the report's findings and recommendations through three symposia that were held in Atlanta, Georgia; Irvine, California; and Wichita, Kansas.

This report, *Progress in Preventing Childhood Obesity: How Do We Measure Up?*, places a specific focus on the evaluation of actions taken by all sectors of society and describes progress made toward the first report's recommendations. Evaluation is vital to identify effective interventions that can be scaled up to statewide or nationwide efforts, while ineffective interventions can be replaced with more promising evidence-based efforts. As the *Health in the Balance* report acknowledged, we must draw from the best available evidence rather than waiting for the best possible evidence to mount an effective and sustained response. Along the way, we must ask whether the interventions to promote healthful eating and increase physical activity are reaching enough people to make a substantial difference, and whether the breadth of interventions are adequate to address the scope of the problem.

An expanded and diverse evidence base will provide the foundation for a sustained effort toward reversing the current childhood obesity trends and improving the health and well-being of America's children and youth. We have made considerable progress in five years since the release of the Surgeon General's *Call to Action*. However, there is a great deal more work that all of us collectively need to undertake in order to adequately address the impending obesity crisis and thereby chart a healthier course for our future generations.

Jeffrey P. Koplan, *Chair*
Committee on Progress in
Preventing Childhood Obesity

Acknowledgments

I t was a great pleasure to chair the Institute of Medicine (IOM) Committee on Progress in Preventing Childhood Obesity. The 13-member committee brought tremendous expertise to this important topic from a variety of perspectives and was actively engaged in the committee's work. This report represents the result of six meetings, two public workshops, three regional symposia, and ongoing communication throughout the course of the study. It is also the result of a thoughtful analysis and interdisciplinary collaboration among the committee members who volunteered countless hours of their valuable time to complete this study. I would like to extend my sincere thanks to each of the committee members for their commitment to work through the issues addressed in this report.

This study was sponsored by the Robert Wood Johnson Foundation (RWJF). The committee and staff wish to thank RWJF staff including Risa Lavizzo-Mourey, James Marks, Kathryn Thomas, and Laura Leviton for their support and guidance on the committee's task during the course of the study. The committee also benefited from discussions with individuals who presented at or attended the committee's workshops, symposia, and meetings. We especially appreciate the contributions of Loel Solomon and Scott Gee from Kaiser Permanente; Susan Yanovski from the National Institute of Diabetes & Digestive & Kidney Diseases; Janet Collins from the Centers for Disease Control and Prevention (CDC); Penelope Royall from the U.S. Department of Health and Human Services (DHHS) Office of Disease Prevention and Health Promotion; Richard Kelly from the Federal Trade Commission; Eric Hentges from the U.S. Department of Agriculture; and Dana Carr from the U.S. Department of Education. I would especially like to thank Kathryn Thomas at the RWJF; Marni Vliet, Steve Coen, and Deanna Van Hersh at the Kansas Health Foundation; Gary Nelson, Martha Katz, Meg Watson, and Allison Maiuri at the Healthcare Georgia Foundation; and Robert Ross, George Flores, and Marion Standish at The California Endowment for collaborating with the committee and staff to organize and co-host the regional symposia. The symposia agendas and speakers are listed in Appendixes F, G, and H.

Many individuals were instrumental in providing useful data to the committee that was included in the report. We greatly appreciate the work and insights of Shiriki Kumanyika and Donna Nichols who served as consultants to the committee. We thank Bill Dietz, Edward Hunter, and Lynda Williams from CDC. We also thank Alison Kretser and Marjorie Goldstein for providing useful information used in the report. We would like to especially thank Tim Lobstein from the International Obesity Taskforce in London for sharing information about other country strategies and action plans to promote healthful eating, physical activity, and prevent obesity. Enrique Jacoby, Juan Rivera, Carlos Monteiro, and Fernando Vio were helpful in guiding the committee to obesity prevention activities and strategies in Latin America. Francesco Branca, Elina Hirvikallio, Raija Kara, Tim Lang, Wolf-Martin Maier, Canice Nolan, Philippe Roux, and Alberto Galvão A. A. Teles provided useful information about obesity prevention activities, strategies, and action plans in Europe.

We appreciate the constructive input offered by the reviewers of this report who provided a technical review of sections of the report. Special thanks are extended to Michael McGinnis and Rosemary Dederichs for their technical review of selected chapters. We also acknowledge the financial oversight of Anton Bandy and Gary Walker. The committee benefited greatly from the skillful copyediting of the report by Michael Hayes, cover design by Samantha Razook Murphy, and chapter illustrations by Becky Heavner. Finally, a study of this scope is only possible with the assistance of the IOM staff. I would like to thank co-study directors, Cathy Liverman and Vivica Kraak, research associate Shannon Wisham, board director Linda Meyers, policy fellow Jessica Cohen, and senior program assistant Jon Sanders for their steadfast devotion to the study process and final report.

Progress in Preventing Childhood Obesity: How Do We Measure Up? presents recommendations relevant to implementing and evaluating obesity prevention interventions within and across many sectors—government, industry, communities, schools, and home—and urges all sectors and invested stakeholders to take the collective actions needed to improve the health and well-being of children and youth.

Jeffrey P. Koplan, *Chair*
Committee on Progress in
Preventing Childhood Obesity

Contents

APPENDIXES*

*The complete symposia summaries for Appendixes F through H (pages 424–436) are not printed in this report. They are included on a CD-ROM attached to the inside back cover.

Progress in Preventing Childhood Obesity

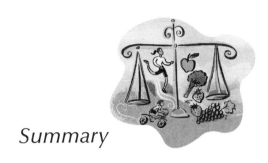

Summary

T he nation's growing recognition of the obesity crisis as a major public health concern for our children and youth has led to an array of diverse efforts aimed at increasing physical activity and promoting healthful eating. These efforts, however, generally remain fragmented and small-scale. Furthermore, there is a lack of systematic tracking and evaluation of childhood obesity prevention interventions. When compared to the strong commitment and heavy infusion of governmental and private-sector resources devoted to other possible major public health concerns, such as infectious disease outbreaks or bioterrorism events, there is a marked underinvestment in the prevention of childhood obesity and related chronic diseases.

Addressing the childhood obesity epidemic is a collective responsibility involving multiple stakeholders and different sectors—including the federal government, state and local governments, communities, schools, industry, media, and families. This was a clear message from the 2005 Institute of Medicine (IOM) report, *Preventing Childhood Obesity: Health in the Balance*.

Following the release of the *Health in the Balance* report, the Robert Wood Johnson Foundation asked the IOM to assess progress in childhood obesity prevention actions across a variety of sectors and also to engage in a dissemination effort that would promote the implementation of the 2005 report's findings and recommendations through three regional symposia. The dual purpose of convening each symposium was to galvanize childhood obesity prevention efforts among local, state, and national decision makers, community and school leaders, health care providers, public health professionals, and grassroots community-based organizations, as well as to apprise the committee of the experiences and insights of the broad variety of partnerships and activities related to preventing childhood obesity throughout the nation.

To respond to this task, the IOM appointed the Committee on Progress in Preventing Childhood Obesity, comprised of 13 experts in diverse disciplines including nutrition, physical activity, obesity prevention, pediatrics, family medicine, public health, public policy, health education and promotion, community development and mobilization, private-sector initiatives, behavioral epidemiology, and program evaluation. The committee obtained information through a comprehensive literature review, three regional symposia, and two public workshops.

The three regional symposia were held in Wichita, Kansas; Atlanta, Georgia; and Irvine, California; and served to inform the committee about ongoing and innovative promising practices and evaluation approaches that are being used to address the problem and assess the effectiveness of childhood obesity prevention efforts. The crosscutting themes that emerged from all three symposia to support childhood obesity prevention efforts were to forge strategic partnerships, educate stakeholders, increase resources, and empower local schools, communities, and neighborhoods.

This report, *Progress in Preventing Childhood Obesity: How Do We Measure Up?*, offers four distinct contributions to the childhood obesity discourse. It summarizes the findings of the three regional symposia; provides an evaluation framework that stakeholders can use to assess progress for a range of childhood obesity prevention efforts across different sectors and settings; measures progress for specific recommendations in the *Health in the Balance* report; and offers new recommendations for leadership and commitment to childhood obesity prevention efforts including an expansion of the nation's capacity and action in implementing, evaluating, and monitoring childhood obesity prevention initiatives and interventions.

The challenge presented in this report is to take the next steps toward developing a robust evidence base for effective childhood obesity prevention interventions and practices. Given the numerous changes being implemented throughout the nation to improve the dietary quality and extent of physical activity for children and youth, an overarching assessment of progress in preventing childhood obesity necessitates both the tracking of trends across the nation and a more detailed examination of lessons learned through the evaluations of relevant interventions, policies, and programs. Evaluations produce information or evidence that can be used to improve a policy, program, or an intervention in its original setting; refine those that need restructuring and adaptation to different settings and contexts; and revise or discontinue those efforts found to be ineffective. Evaluation is central to identifying and disseminating effective initiatives—whether they are national or local programs, large- or small-scale efforts.

EVALUATION FRAMEWORK

The committee uses the term *evaluation* to represent the systematic assessment of the quality and effectiveness of a policy, program, or initiative. It is an effort to determine whether and how an intervention has important and consequential outcomes. Many types of evaluations can contribute to the knowledge base by identifying promising practices and helping to establish causal relationships between interventions and various outcomes. Evaluation can also enhance our understanding of the intrinsic quality of the intervention and of the critical context where factors can moderate or mediate an intervention's effect in particular ways. The committee emphasizes that program evaluations of varying scope and size, at all levels and within and across all sectors, play a vital role in addressing the childhood obesity epidemic. Evaluation fosters collective learning, supports accountability and responsibility, reduces uncertainty, guides improvements and innovations in policies and programs, determines cost-effectiveness, and helps to leverage change in society.

Evaluations are conducted for multiple stakeholders and the findings broadly shared and disseminated. These audiences include policy makers, funders, and other elected and appointed decision makers; program developers and administrators; program managers and staff; and program participants, their families, and communities. Moreover, these diverse evaluation audiences tend to value evaluation for different reasons. The committee emphasizes the need for a collective commitment to evaluation by those responsible for funding, planning, implementing, and monitoring childhood obesity prevention efforts.

Although resources are limited, evaluation should be incorporated as an essential component of the program planning and implementation process rather than as an optional activity. Government agencies, foundations, and other funders of childhood obesity programs and interventions should incorporate evaluation requirements, as is current practice by many agencies and organizations. Similarly, program planners and those who implement policy changes should view evaluation as an integral part of their efforts. If something is valuable enough to invest time, energy, and resources, then it is also worthy of the investment necessary to carefully document the success of the effort.

All childhood obesity prevention policies and interventions deserve some type of evaluation. Evaluations can range in scope and complexity from comparisons of pre- and post-intervention counts of the number of individuals participating in a program to methodologically sophisticated evaluations with comparison groups and research designs. All types of evaluation can make an important contribution to the evidence base upon which to design policies, programs, and interventions.

The translation of evaluation and research findings into promising practices constitutes the primary means for accelerating national efforts to reverse the childhood obesity epidemic. Since the need for effective evaluation is ongoing, both the capacity and quality of evaluation will be positively influenced by a steadfast national commitment to support obesity prevention efforts and the rapid translation and dissemination of evaluation and research findings—across the geographical landscape—to stakeholders involved in obesity prevention efforts in states and communities. Furthermore, the social and cultural diversity within the United States precludes assumptions about the transferability of interventions from one sub-population to another and should therefore be assessed.

Changing stakeholder perceptions about evaluation—from considering it a daunting task of questionable value to a manageable and highly useful endeavor to inform their efforts—can be facilitated by considering four key evaluation questions to guide childhood obesity prevention policies, programs, and interventions (Box S-1). Although these questions are relevant to obesity prevention strategies and actions across all sectors, not every evaluation can be expected to address all of the questions. Rather, the relevance of the four evaluation questions depends on the type of obesity prevention intervention and the available evaluation resources and technical expertise.

BOX S-1
Questions to Guide Childhood Obesity
Prevention Policies and Interventions

1. How does the action contribute to preventing childhood obesity? What are the rationale and supporting evidence for this particular action as a viable obesity prevention strategy, particularly in a specific context? How well is the planned action or intervention matched to the specific setting or population being served?
2. What are the quality and reach or power of the action *as designed*?
3. How well is the action carried out? What are the quality and the reach or power of the action *as implemented*?
4. What difference did the action make in terms of increasing the availability of foods and beverages that contribute to a healthful diet, opportunities for physical activity, other indicators of a healthful diet and physical activity, and improving health outcomes for children and youth?

Experienced evaluators have long acknowledged the importance of identifying and understanding the key contextual factors (e.g., environmental, cultural, normative, and behavioral) that influence the potential impact of an intervention. The evaluation framework that the committee developed offers a depiction of the resources and inputs, strategies and actions, and a range of outcomes that are important to childhood obesity prevention. All are amenable to documentation, measurement, and evaluation (Figure S-1).

The evaluation outcomes selected will depend on the nature of the intervention, the timeline of the program or intervention, and the resources available to program implementers to collect, analyze, and interpret outcomes data. The timeline of the intervention often determines whether the evaluation can assess progress toward a short-term outcome (e.g., increasing participation in an after-school intramural sports team), an intermediate-term outcome (e.g., changes to the built environment that promote regular physical activity for children and youth) or a long-term outcome (e.g., a reduction in BMI levels of children participating in a new program). Outcomes can also be categorized based on the nature of the change: (1) structural, institutional, and systemic outcomes; (2) environmental outcomes; (3) population or individual-level cognitive and social outcomes; (4) behavioral outcomes (e.g., dietary and physical activity behaviors); and (5) health outcomes (Figure S-1).

The evaluation framework also illustrates the range of inputs and outcomes while giving careful consideration to the following factors:

- The interconnections and quality of interactions within and among the multiple sectors involved in childhood obesity prevention initiatives.
- The adequacy of support and resources for policies and programs.
- The contextual appropriateness, relevance, and potential power of the planned policy, intervention, or action.
- The multiple outcomes (e.g., structural, institutional, systemic, environmental, behavioral for individuals and the population, and health outcomes).
- The potential impact of interventions on adverse or unanticipated outcomes, such as stigmatization.
- The indicators used to assess progress made toward each outcome. Selecting the best indicators will depend on the purpose for which they are intended and the resources available to program staff to collect, analyze, and interpret relevant data.

A variety of crosscutting factors influence program experiences and the evaluation process, thereby requiring consideration at every stage of the evaluation framework for both individuals and populations. These include

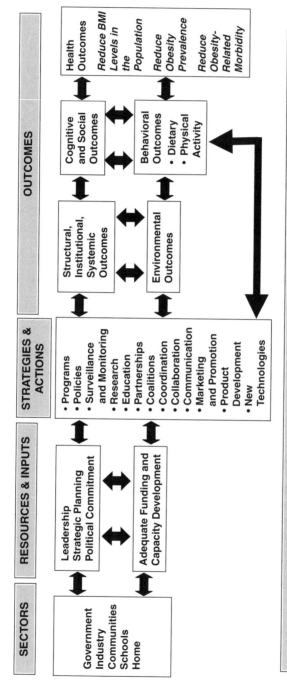

FIGURE S-1 Evaluation framework for childhood obesity prevention policies and interventions.

age, sex, socioeconomic status, and race/ethnicity; culture, immigration status and acculturation; bio-behavioral and gene-environment interactions; psychosocial status; and social, political, and historical contexts. Context refers to the set of factors or circumstances that surround a situation or event and give meaning to its interpretation. All of these factors should be taken into account when designing, monitoring, and evaluating obesity prevention initiatives as depicted in Figure S-1.

The committee has identified several relevant criteria that can be used to judge the design and quality of interventions and encourages funders and program planners to consider the following actions:

- Include diverse perspectives and attend to the sub-populations in the greatest need of prevention actions—particularly underserved, low-income, and high-risk populations that experience health disparities;
- Use relevant empirical evidence relevant to the specific context when designing and implementing the intervention;
- Identify similar or potentially synergistic efforts and make important cross-sectoral linkages and sustained collaborations; and
- Link structural, environmental, and behavioral changes in individuals and populations relevant to childhood obesity prevention.

CONCLUSIONS

The committee developed five broad conclusions (Box S-2) based on its assessment of progress in preventing childhood obesity that serve as the foundation for the report's recommendations and implementation actions discussed in the report.

RECOMMENDATIONS FOR ASSESSING PROGRESS

Reflective of the collective and interrelated responsibility of multiple sectors and stakeholders to create a healthy marketplace and media environment, healthy communities, healthy school environments, and healthy home environments, the committee developed four recommendations for this report. The committee's recommendations are relevant across five major sectors—government, industry, communities, schools, and home. The first recommendation underscores the importance of promoting leadership and commitment to treat childhood obesity prevention as an urgent national priority. The remaining three recommendations serve as the basis for evaluation activities within and across the sectors, accounting for interdependencies and dynamic changes that will affect obesity prevention actions. More details about the implementation of the recommendations for each sector are discussed throughout the report and collated in Appendix E.

BOX S-2
Conclusions

1. The country is beginning to recognize that childhood obesity is a serious public health problem that increases morbidity and mortality and that has substantial economic and social costs. However, the current level of investment by the public and private sectors still does not match the extent of the problem.

2. Government, industry, communities, schools, and families are responding to the childhood obesity epidemic by implementing a variety of policies, programs, and other interventions. All of these stakeholders bring strong values and beliefs to obesity-related issues, but evidence-based approaches are needed to guide the nation's collective actions in the response.

3. Current data and evidence are inadequate for a comprehensive assessment of the progress that has been made in preventing childhood obesity across the United States. Although the best available evidence should be used to develop an immediate response to the childhood obesity epidemic, a more robust evidence base that identifies promising practices must be developed so that these interventions can be scaled-up and supported in diverse settings.

4. Evaluation serves to foster collective learning, accountability, responsibility, and cost-effectiveness to guide improvements in childhood obesity prevention policies and programs. Multiple sectors and stakeholders should commit adequate resources to conduct these evaluations. Surveillance, monitoring, and research are fundamental components of childhood obesity prevention evaluation efforts.

5. Multiple sectors and stakeholders should conduct evaluations of different types and at different levels to assess and stimulate progress over the short term, intermediate term, and long term to reverse the childhood obesity trend and improve the health of the nation's children and youth.

These recommendations collectively call our attention to the urgent need to provide more and better information to improve peoples' lives through evaluation. Stakeholders in each sector are urged to identify and mobilize adequate resources for the evaluation of obesity prevention interventions for children and youth. The recommendations also advance an evaluation process that meaningfully engages diverse stakeholders in the evaluation design and process and that legitimizes the multiplicity of stakeholder perspectives, notably including program recipients along with funders, administrators, and professional staff.

There will be a greater likelihood of success when public, private, and voluntary organizations purposefully combine their respective resources, strengths, and comparative advantages to ensure a coordinated and sustained long-term effort. Evaluations will contribute to building a strong and diverse evidence base upon which promising and best practices can be identified, scaled up, and institutionalized across different settings and sectors.

Recommendation 1: Government, industry, communities, schools, and families should demonstrate leadership and commitment by mobilizing the resources required to identify, implement, evaluate, and disseminate effective policies and interventions that support childhood obesity prevention goals.

- Federal, state, and local governments should each establish a high-level task force to identify priorities for action, coordinate public-sector efforts, and establish effective interdepartmental collaborations.
- Industry should use the full range of available resources and tools to create, support, and sustain consumer demand for products and opportunities that support healthy lifestyles including healthful diets and regular physical activity.
- Community stakeholders should establish and strengthen the local policies, coalitions, and collaborations needed to create and sustain healthy communities.
- School boards, administrators, and staff should elevate the priority that is placed on creating and sustaining a healthy school environment and advance school policies and programs that support this priority.
- Families, parents, and caregivers should commit to promoting healthful eating and regular physical activity to create a healthy home environment.

Recommendation 2: Policy makers, program planners, program implementers, and other interested stakeholders—within and across relevant sectors—should evaluate all childhood obesity prevention efforts, strengthen the evaluation capacity, and develop quality interventions that take into account diverse perspectives, that use culturally relevant approaches, and that meet the needs of diverse populations and contexts.

- Federal and state government departments and agencies should consistently evaluate the effects of all actions taken to prevent childhood obesity and strengthen the evaluation capacity, paying particular attention to culturally relevant evaluation approaches.
- Industry should partner with government, academic institutions, and other interested stakeholders to undertake evaluations to assess its progress in preventing childhood obesity and promoting healthy lifestyles.
- Community stakeholders should strengthen evaluation efforts at the local level by partnering with government agencies, foundations, and academic institutions to develop, implement, and

support evaluation opportunities and community-academic partnerships.

- Schools and school districts should strengthen evaluation efforts by partnering with state and federal agencies, foundations, and academic institutions to develop, implement, and support evaluations of all relevant school-based programs.
- Parents and caregivers, as the policy makers in the household, should assess their family's progress in achieving positive lifestyle changes.

Recommendation 3: Government, industry, communities, and schools should expand or develop relevant surveillance and monitoring systems and, as applicable, should engage in research to examine the impact of childhood obesity prevention policies, interventions, and actions on relevant outcomes, paying particular attention to the unique needs of diverse groups and high-risk populations. Additionally, parents and caregivers should monitor changes in their family's food, beverage, and physical activity choices and their progress toward healthier lifestyles.

- Government at all levels should develop new surveillance systems or enhance existing surveillance systems to monitor relevant outcomes and trends and should increase funding for obesity prevention research.
- The U.S. Congress, in consultation with industry and other relevant stakeholders, should appropriate adequate funds to support independent and periodic evaluations of industry's efforts to promote healthier lifestyles.
- Community stakeholders and relevant partners should expand the capacity for local-level surveillance and applied research and should develop tools for community self-assessment to support childhood obesity prevention efforts.
- Schools and school districts should conduct self-assessments to enhance and sustain a healthy school environment, and mechanisms for examining links between changes in the school environment and behavioral and health outcomes should be explored.
- Parents and caregivers should monitor their families' lifestyle changes; and government, foundations, and industry should support applied research that examines family interventions in real-world settings.

Recommendation 4: Government, industry, communities, schools, and families should foster information-sharing activities and disseminate evaluation and research findings through diverse communication channels and media to actively promote the use and scaling up of effective childhood obesity prevention policies and interventions.

- Government at all levels should commit to the long-term support and dissemination of childhood obesity prevention policies and interventions that have been proven to be effective.
- Industry should collaborate with the public sector and other relevant stakeholders to develop a mechanism for sharing proprietary data and a sustainable funding strategy that can inform and support childhood obesity prevention interventions.
- Community stakeholders should partner with foundations, government agencies, faith-based organizations, and youth-related organizations to publish and widely disseminate the evaluation results of community-based childhood obesity prevention efforts.
- Schools should partner with government, professional associations, academic institutions, parent-teacher organizations, foundations, communities, and the media to publish and widely disseminate the evaluation results of school-based childhood obesity prevention efforts and related materials and methods.
- Government (federal, state, and local), communities, families, and the media should disseminate and widely promote the evaluation results of effective family- and home-based childhood obesity prevention efforts.

NEXT STEPS

Each of the recommendations is further expanded in the report, in which the committee recommends specific implementation actions that should be taken by government, industry, communities, schools, and parents and caregivers at home to ensure that there are adequate resources and a focus on strengthening the evaluation of childhood obesity prevention policies and interventions. Given the range of actions that are needed to move forward in preventing childhood obesity, the committee has identified immediate next steps that it deems essential priority actions in the near future.

Government

The federal, state, and local governments are actively engaged in childhood obesity prevention efforts. However, as noted above, the levels of funding and resources invested in these efforts and their evaluation are not commensurate with the seriousness of this public health problem. Government at all levels should provide coordinated leadership for the prevention of obesity in children and youth.

A critical next step for the federal government is to establish a high-level task force on childhood obesity prevention, as recommended in the *Health in the Balance* report (IOM, 2005), and underscored in this report. The committee recommends that the president request that the secretary of the U.S. Department of Health and Human Services (DHHS) to convene this high-level task force and the task force include as members the secretaries or senior officials of DHHS and the U.S. Departments of Agriculture, Education, Transportation, Housing and Urban Development, Interior, Defense, and other relevant departments and agencies. The purpose of the task force would be to ensure coordinated budgets, policies, and requirements for obesity prevention programs and to establish effective interdepartmental collaboration and priorities for action.

Furthermore, the federal government should provide a sustained commitment and long-term investment in childhood obesity prevention initiatives found to be effective (such as the VERB™ campaign) and those that are vital to measuring progress (such as national surveillance efforts to track trends in the obesity epidemic).

Surveillance systems—such as the National Health and Nutrition Examination Survey, the School Health Policies and Programs Study, the Youth Media Campaign Longitudinal Survey, the Youth Risk Behavior Surveillance System, and the National Household Transportation Survey—should be expanded to include relevant obesity-related outcomes. Surveillance systems that monitor the precursors of dietary and physical activity behaviors, such as changes in policies and the built environment, need to be expanded or developed.

Additionally, monitoring systems for USDA programs such as the Special Supplemental Nutrition Program for Women, Infants, and Children, the Food Stamp Program, and the school meals programs should be developed that assess a range of obesity-related outcomes for children and youth.

State and local governments should also demonstrate leadership on this issue and commit resources and policies that lead to actions that implement and evaluate changes in schools and communities.

Industry

Certain segments of relevant industries, including the food, beverage, restaurant, food retail, leisure and recreation, physical activity and fitness, and entertainment industries have responded constructively to the childhood obesity epidemic. However, other corporations in these industries are not yet engaged in obesity prevention; and other segments of the industry, such as the fitness, spectator sports, and transportation sectors, have not shown adequate involvement in obesity prevention actions. Nevertheless, careful and independent evaluations are needed to determine if industry is making a sufficient investment, sustained commitment, and whether those initiatives proposed by industry will be effective and contribute to desirable outcomes.

Industry and the public health community should work toward nurturing and strengthening partnerships that support obesity prevention efforts. To expand the federal research capacity to study the ways in which marketing influences children's and adolescents' attitudes and behaviors, industry is encouraged to provide data on pricing strategies, consumer food purchases, and consumption trends from proprietary retail scanner systems, household scanner panels, household consumption surveys, and marketing research. The collaborative work should examine the quality of the data, consider reducing the cost to make the data accessible, and establish priorities for applying the information to promote healthful diets and physical activity.

Corporate responsibility can be demonstrated by sharing marketing research findings, to the greatest extent possible, which will assist the public health sector to develop, implement, and evaluate more effective childhood obesity prevention policies, programs, and interventions. Data sharing will need to balance many considerations including transparency, public accessibility, the demands of the competitive marketplace, and legal issues. In certain cases, it may be appropriate for the data to be released after a time lag to keep the public informed with relatively recent data. The committee recommends that the public and private sectors engage in a collaborative process that will assist relevant stakeholders to share proprietary data for the public good.

Communities

Communities vary widely in the extent and nature of the resources available to be used in changing the built and social environments to facilitate physical activity and access to foods and beverages that contribute to a healthful diet. A number of state and local governments, foundations, nonprofit and youth-related organizations, faith-based organizations, and community coalitions are demonstrating innovative and collaborative approaches to childhood obesity prevention. However, there is much that remains to be learned, translated, and disseminated, particularly from effective evidence-based interventions that continue even when seed funding and external resources are no longer available.

The committee identified two immediate next steps for communities. The development of a validated community self-assessment tool, such as a community health index, will help communities identify their strengths and gaps in designing and evaluating childhood obesity-prevention efforts, ranging from local programs and evaluation capacity to the local physical and built environments, and the extent of community involvement.

Congress should appropriate funds for CDC, in partnership with the Department of Transportation, the Department of the Interior, and other relevant federal agencies, private-sector and nonprofit organizations, and community stakeholders to develop this type of well-validated tool that can be used in economically and culturally diverse communities. Additionally, the National Association of County and City Health Officials, in partnership with government agencies and other nonprofit and voluntary health organizations, should develop a means of compiling and sharing community-based evaluation results, lessons learned, and community action plans as well as provide links to resources, templates, and evaluation tools. A web-based database or repository of published and unpublished literature, case studies, and promising intervention websites is needed.

Schools

Schools are the current focus of many childhood obesity prevention efforts, particularly changes to the school food and beverage environment. Less attention has been paid to increasing physical activity in schools, although this issue seems to be gaining momentum. As is true for community efforts, wide variations in the extent of the efforts and resources available for investment in obesity prevention by individual schools, school districts, and state agencies are observed. Federal law requires that schools receiving federal funds for school meals must develop school wellness policies by the fall of 2006, which has stimulated school-based health promotion and obesity prevention efforts across the country. Additionally, teachers, food service personnel, school administrators, and state and federal agency staff have developed many creative and innovative approaches to improve students' diets and to increase physical activity, but these need to be evaluated. The committee encourages states and school districts to bolster their physical education and physical activity requirements and standards, as should preschool, child-care, and after-school programs. Accountability mechanisms are needed for state school nutrition and physical activity standards that include increased transparency and dissemination of school-by-school reports on success in meeting these standards. Furthermore, federal and state leadership is needed to provide adequate and sustained resources to implement changes relevant to obesity prevention in the school environment. Not only are political will and leadership needed to improve school nutrition and physical activity opportunities, but it is critically important that adequate and sustained funding be provided to reinforce these priorities so that attention to this issue does not result in unfunded mandates.

Home

Many families across the country are aware of their role in preventing childhood obesity and are actively making changes towards a healthier lifestyle, while others are not yet engaged in change. A next step for parents, caregivers, children, and adolescents is to periodically assess the home environment and ask the following questions: Are the foods and beverages that are available and prepared in the home healthful and served in reasonable portions? Is physical activity emphasized and a family priority? Do families have established rules or guidelines limiting leisure screen time? Incremental changes are valuable and signal that progress is occurring.

Conclusion

A succinct assessment of the nation's progress in preventing childhood obesity is not feasible given the diverse and varied nature of America's communities and population. However, it can be said that awareness of obesity has been raised, actions have begun, coordination and prioritization of limited resources are critical, and evaluation of interventions within and across all sectors is essential. A long-term commitment to create a healthy environment for our children and youth is urgently needed. This commitment will require widespread changes in social norms, institutions, and practices beyond those that directly involve children and youth.

1

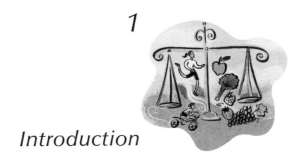

Introduction

In 2004, the Institute of Medicine (IOM) released the report, *Preventing Childhood Obesity: Health in the Balance,* which provided a blueprint for a comprehensive action plan to prevent childhood obesity[1] in the United States (IOM, 2005). The report emphasized an urgent need for collective responsibility and concerted actions to be undertaken by multiple stakeholders across different sectors—including the federal government, state and local governments, communities, schools, industry, media, and families—to address the evolving childhood obesity epidemic by preventing children and youth who are currently at a healthy weight[2] from developing a body mass index (BMI) at or above the sex-specific 95th percentile that defines obesity. Even as that report was being prepared, many childhood obesity prevention programs and policies were being initiated or already underway around the nation.

---

[1]Reflecting a classification based on the readily available measures of height and weight, this report uses the term *obesity* to refer to children and adolescents who have a body mass index (BMI) for age at or above the sex-specific 95th percentile of the BMI charts developed by the Centers for Disease Control and Prevention (CDC) in 2000. At risk for obesity is defined as a BMI for age at or above the sex-specific 85th percentile but less than the 95th percentile of the CDC BMI charts. In most children and youth, a BMI level at or above the 95th percentile indicates elevated body fat and reflects the presence or risk of related chronic disease. This report focuses on the primary prevention of childhood obesity.

[2]Healthy weight in children and youth is defined as a level of body fat that supports normal growth and development and at which there are no observed comorbidities.

In the two years since the release of the *Health in the Balance* report, childhood obesity prevention efforts have become the topic of discussion and the focus of action in homes, schools, communities, corporations, state legislatures, and federal agencies across the nation. Unfortunately, few of these new or ongoing efforts are being systematically documented or evaluated, thereby limiting the potential to learn from these efforts and to use the results in further developing and refining population-based approaches to prevent childhood obesity.

This subsequent IOM report, *Progress in Preventing Childhood Obesity: How Do We Measure Up?*, assesses progress made on the first report's recommendations by focusing on the evaluation of actions taken by all sectors of society. Given the numerous changes being implemented throughout the nation to improve the dietary quality and extent of physical activity for children and youth, an overarching assessment of progress in preventing childhood obesity necessitates both the tracking of trends across the nation and a more detailed examination of lessons learned through the evaluations of relevant interventions, policies, and programs. Evaluation is the basis for identifying effective interventions that can then be scaled up to statewide or nationwide efforts as well as ineffective interventions that can be refined or replaced with efforts that are shown to be more promising as a result of evidence-based analyses. A complementary set of efforts is needed—population-based public health interventions coupled with individual-level and institutional interventions—and these efforts should be collectively monitored and evaluated. The childhood obesity epidemic is at the point where it is time to move beyond a reactive small-scale approach and toward a proactive, coordinated, and sustained response.

As the previous report acknowledged, there is an urgent need for action on this public health concern—action requiring the use of the best available evidence. Now that numerous changes are underway to increase physical activity and improve dietary intake it is time to bolster the evidence base. Key questions to consider include the following: Are interventions to promote a healthful diet and to increase physical activity reaching enough people to make a difference? Is the breadth of interventions sufficiently adequate to address the scope of the problem? Much remains to be learned about how to effectively increase physical activity, improve dietary quality, and decrease sedentary lifestyles in America's children and youth.

HEALTH IN THE BALANCE REPORT

The *Health in the Balance* report acknowledged the many transformations in U.S. society over the past 30 years—including changes in the physical and built environments, social and cultural environments, and commercial and media environments—that have contributed to the energy imbalance and rising prevalence of obesity among America's children and youth. Using an ecological approach to identify leverage points for designing effective interventions to promote energy balance, the report addressed the range of factors that influence diet and physical activity: individual factors, behavioral settings, sectors of society, and the social norms and values that reinforce healthful eating and regular physical activity as the accepted and encouraged standard (Figure 1-1) (IOM, 2005).

The report concluded that childhood obesity is a nationwide health crisis requiring a population-based prevention approach and a substantial and comprehensive response. Key recommendations of that report include: the federal government should make childhood obesity prevention a national priority; industry and media should develop a healthy marketplace and media environment; community stakeholders and health care providers should work toward building healthy communities and improving access to obesity prevention services in primary-care settings; schools should develop healthier environments that promote both a healthful diet and regular physical activity; and parents and caregivers should foster a healthy family and home environment (IOM, 2005). All of these supportive environments have the potential to collectively promote energy balance—healthful eating behaviors, regular physical activity, and decreased sedentary behaviors—to help children and adolescents achieve a healthy weight while protecting their normal growth and development. One of the fundamental findings identified in the *Health in the Balance* report was the need to develop a stronger evidence base to more efficiently and effectively guide childhood obesity prevention interventions (IOM, 2005). This report focuses on the continued development of that evidence base through targeted research, ongoing surveillance and monitoring, and widespread evaluation.

STUDY BACKGROUND AND RATIONALE

Subsequent to the release of the *Health in the Balance* report, the Robert Wood Johnson Foundation requested that IOM conduct a study to assess the nation's progress in preventing childhood obesity and to engage in a dissemination effort promoting the implementation of the report's findings and recommendations through three symposia held in different regions of the country. The dual purpose of convening each symposium was to begin to galvanize obesity prevention efforts among local, state, and national decision makers; community and school leaders; health care providers; public health professionals; corporate leaders; and grassroots community-based organizations, as well as to apprise the committee of the experiences and insights of the broad variety of partnerships and activities related to preventing childhood obesity throughout the nation.

20

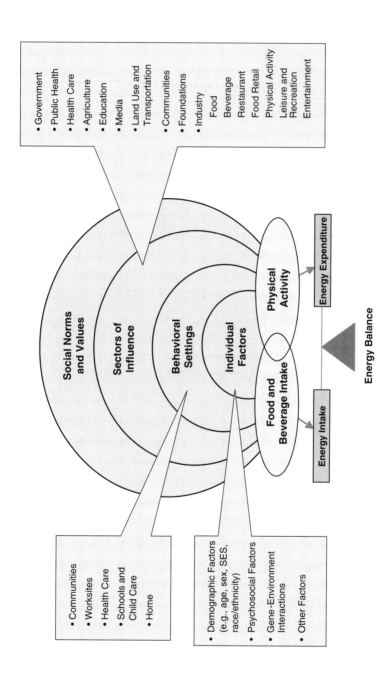

FIGURE 1-1 Comprehensive approach for preventing and addressing childhood obesity.
NOTE: Other relevant factors that influence obesity prevention interventions are culture and acculturation; biobehavioral interactions; and social, political, and historical contexts. See Figure 2-1 in Chapter 2.
SOURCES: Adapted from IOM (2005); CDC (2006a).

To respond to this task, IOM appointed the Committee on Progress in Preventing Childhood Obesity, which comprised 13 experts in diverse disciplines including nutrition, physical activity, obesity prevention, pediatrics, family medicine, public health, public policy, health education and promotion, community development and mobilization, private-sector initiatives, behavioral epidemiology, and program evaluation. The IOM committee held six meetings during the course of the study and a variety of sources informed its work. The committee obtained information through a comprehensive literature review, three regional symposia, and two public workshops.

Regional Symposia

The three regional symposia provided an opportunity for the committee to become informed about the numerous ongoing and innovative programs and policy changes being implemented throughout the nation. The symposia provided valuable insights into the challenges, barriers, and facilitating factors that may either hinder or promote the implementation and evaluation of a range of school-, community-, public-sector-, and industry-based efforts. Several crosscutting themes emerged from all three symposia: forge strategic partnerships; educate stakeholders; increase resources; and empower local schools, communities, and neighborhoods (Box 1-1).

In collaboration with the Kansas Health Foundation, the committee held its first symposium, *Progress in Preventing Childhood Obesity: Focus on Schools*, June 27 and 28, 2005 in Wichita, Kansas. Approximately 90 individuals who are active in childhood obesity prevention efforts in the Midwest and who represented a range of stakeholder perspectives and innovative practices in the school setting participated in the symposium, including teachers, students, principals, health educators, dietitians, state and federal health and education officials, food service providers, community leaders, industry representatives, and academic researchers. The discussion at the symposium focused on exploring the barriers and opportunities for sustaining and evaluating promising practices for creating a healthy school environment (Appendix F).

In partnership with Healthcare Georgia Foundation, the committee held its second symposium, *Progress in Preventing Childhood Obesity: Focus on Communities*, October 6 and 7, 2005, in Atlanta, Georgia. The symposium brought together a broad range of individuals and organizations involved in community-based efforts in the southeastern United States and included federal, state, and local health officials; students and teachers; community leaders; faith-based partners; and representatives of nonprofit youth-related organizations. The symposium focused on obtaining an understanding of how neighborhood and community grassroots efforts are mobilized; exploring the roles of city, county, and state agencies; and iden-

---

BOX 1-1
Discussion Themes from the Institute of Medicine
Regional Symposia

June 27–28, 2005, Wichita, Kansas, Focus on Schools
October 6–7, 2005, Atlanta, Georgia, Focus on Communities
December 1, 2005, Irvine, California, Focus on Industry

- Forge strategic partnerships
- Empower local schools, communities, and neighborhoods
- Educate stakeholders
- Increase resources for evaluation
- Evaluate obesity prevention programs and initiatives
- Document the benefits of obesity prevention
- Use a systems approach
- Develop a long-term strategic plan
- Collect and disseminate local data
- Identify leaders and build on cultural assets
- Collect, disseminate, and share data from industry
- Garner political support to ally public health and industry
- Market health and nutrition
- Make a business commitment to health

SOURCES: Appendixes F, G, and H.

---

tifying additional steps that stakeholders can take to overcome barriers to evaluation efforts (Appendix G).

In collaboration with The California Endowment, the committee held its third regional symposium on December 1, 2005, in Irvine, California. Recognizing that the health of individuals is closely linked to the consumer marketplace and the messages disseminated by the media, this symposium focused on the specific IOM report recommendations for stakeholders within industry and the media to explore the roles and responsibilities of the many relevant industries in encouraging and promoting healthy lifestyles for children, youth, and their families. Approximately 90 individuals active in childhood obesity prevention efforts and representing a range of stakeholder perspectives—representatives from food, beverage, and restaurant companies; marketing firms; physical activity and entertainment companies; the media; community leaders; health care professionals; public health educators; foundation leaders; state and federal government officials; researchers; and consumer advocates—participated in the symposium (Appendix H).

Additional Resources

Two additional public sessions provided input from federal government representatives, community-based organizations, and other interested stakeholders. The committee also sought information from a broad array of print and electronic sources, including peer-reviewed published research in public health, medicine, allied health, psychology, sociology, education, evaluation, and transportation; reports, background papers, position statements, and other resources (e.g., legal briefs and websites) from the federal government, state and local governments, professional societies and organizations, health advocacy groups, interest groups and trade organizations, and international health agencies; textbooks and other scientific reviews; federal and state legislation; and news releases on relevant topics.

The committee and IOM staff performed searches of relevant bibliographic databases including MEDLINE, AGRICOLA, CINAHL (Cumulative Index to Nursing and Allied Health Literature), Cochrane Database, EconLit, ERIC (Educational Resources Information Center), PsycINFO, Sociological Abstracts, EMBASE (Excerpta Medica), TRIS (Transportation Research Information Services), and LexisNexis. The results of these searches were limited to sources published from 2004 to 2006, to supplement the 2005 IOM report. Additional references were identified from the reference lists found in major review articles, key reports, websites, and relevant textbooks. The committee members, workshop presenters, consultants, and IOM staff also supplied references that were considered for this report.

Scope of the Report

This report summarizes the findings of the regional meetings; provides an evaluation framework for assessing progress in childhood obesity prevention efforts for different sectors, settings, and contexts; assesses progress on the specific recommendations presented in the *Health in the Balance* report; and offers recommendations on expanding evaluation efforts and utilizing evaluation results to support and inform future childhood obesity prevention efforts in the United States. It is beyond the scope of this report, however, to comprehensively examine progress in childhood obesity prevention across a variety of sectors. Rather, the committee's approach was to provide an overview of progress in different sectors and contexts, combined with an examination of evaluation approaches that could further progress. The report has undergone an independent and comprehensive peer-review process that is a hallmark of the National Academies before it was published by the National Academies Press.

OBESITY-RELATED TRENDS

Obesity Trends in U.S. Children and Youth

Since the 1970s there has been a steady and dramatic increase in overweight and obesity in the entire U.S. population. In 1991, the Centers for Disease Control and Prevention (CDC) had documented through the Behavioral Risk Factor Surveillance System (BRFSS) that four states had adult obesity prevalence rates of 15 to 19 percent and that no states had rates at or above 20 percent. By 2004, seven states had adult obesity prevalence rates of 15 to 19 percent, 33 states had adult obesity rates of 20 to 24 percent, and nine states had adult obesity rates of 25 percent or greater (CDC, 2005a).

Obesity rates among American children and youth have also increased significantly. Between 1963 and 2004, obesity rates quadrupled for older children, ages 6 to 11 years (from 4 to 19 percent), and tripled for adolescents, ages 12 to 19 years (from 5 to 17 percent) (Figure 1-2) (CDC, 2005b; Ogden et al., 2002, 2006). Between 1971 and 2004, obesity rates increased from 5 to 14 percent in 2- to 5-year-olds (Figure 1-2) (Ogden et al., 2006).[3] Given these trends, it does not appear that the *Healthy People 2010* target of reducing childhood obesity to 5 percent of the population (DHHS, 2000, 2004) will be reached by 2010.

At present, one-third (33.6 percent) of American children and adolescents are either obese or at risk of becoming obese (Ogden et al., 2006). National Health and Nutrition Examination Survey (NHANES) data show that the national obesity prevalence for 2- to 19-year olds was 13.9 percent in 1999–2000, which increased to 15.4 percent in 2001–2002 and to 17.1 percent in 2003–2004. In 2003–2004, 16.5 percent of 2- to 10-year olds were at risk of becoming obese (Ogden et al., 2006).

Between 1999–2000 and 2003–2004, the prevalence of obesity among girls increased from 13.8 to 16.0 percent and among boys increased from 14.0 to 18.2 percent (Ogden et al., 2006). Obesity prevalence rates in children and youth reveal significant differences by sex and between racial/ethnic and socioeconomic groups (Chapter 3) (Ogden et al., 2006). By 2010, it is projected that an estimated 20 percent of children and youth in the United States will be obese if the current trajectory continues (Sondik, 2004).

---

[3]Although surveillance systems have tracked children's and adolescents' weight trends since the 1960s for those ages 6 years and older, a rise in obesity prevalence was not observed until the late 1970s. Obesity prevalence estimates are often averaged across a span of years. The prevalence was estimated at 16 percent for 1999–2002 (CDC, 2005b).

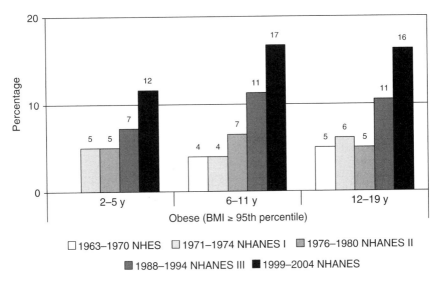

FIGURE 1-2 Obesity prevalence among U.S. children and adolescents by age and time frame, 1963 to 2004.

NOTE: Data for 1963 to 1965 are for children ages 6 to 11 years; data for 1966 to 1970 are for adolescents 12 to 17 years of age instead of 12 to 19 years. In this report, children with BMI levels at or above the 95th percentile of the CDC age- and sex-specific BMI curves for 2000 are referred to as *obese*, and children with BMI levels at or greater than the 85th percentile but less than the 95th percentile are referred to as being *at risk for obesity*. These cutoff points correspond to the terms *overweight* and *at risk for overweight*, respectively, that CDC uses for children and youth.

NHES=National Health Examination Survey; NHANES=National Health and Nutrition Examination Survey.

SOURCES: CDC (2005b); Ogden et al. (2002, 2006).

Economic Costs

In 2004, health care spending in the United States represented an estimated 16 percent of the U.S. gross domestic product (GDP), or $1.9 trillion, which translates to $6,280 per person (Smith et al., 2006). By 2015, the U.S. government forecasts that health care expenditures will reach $4 trillion, or nearly 20 percent of the nation's GDP (Borger et al., 2006). Thorpe and colleagues (2004) estimated the increases in obesity-attributable health care spending from 1987 to 2001 and found that increases in obesity prevalence alone accounted for 12 percent of the growth in health care spending. Increases in the proportion of and spending for obese adults relative to the proportion of and spending for normal weight adults accounted for 27 percent of the rise in inflation-adjusted per-capita health care spending during that time period, of which spending for diabetes accounted for 38 percent of the increase; spending for hyperlipidemia accounted for 22 percent; and spending for heart disease accounted for 41 percent.

Based on 1998 to 2000 data from BRFSS, an estimated 5.7 percent of medical expenditures were attributable to obesity (Finkelstein et al., 2003, 2004). For the Medicare and Medicaid populations, the expenditure percentages were higher: 6.8 and 10.6 percent, respectively. The higher percentage for Medicaid recipients reflects the higher prevalence of obesity among individuals of lower socioeconomic status (SES). Among the states, the percentage of medical expenditures attributable to obesity ranged from 4.0 percent in Arizona to 6.7 percent in Alaska and the District of Columbia. In ten states, the percentage of Medicaid spending attributable to obesity was equal to or greater than 12 percent (Finkelstein et al., 2003, 2004).

Total health care spending for children who receive a diagnosis of obesity (a small subset of the 17.1 percent of U.S. children considered to be obese) is approximately $280 million per year for those with private insurance and $470 million per year for those covered by Medicaid. The national costs for childhood-related obesity (including those who do not receive a diagnosis) are estimated to be $11 billion for private insurance and $3 billion for those with Medicaid. The medical costs for a child who is treated for obesity are approximately three times higher than those for the average insured child (Thomson Medstat, 2006).

ISSUES IN ASSESSING PROGRESS

In response to the rising prevalence and economic costs of childhood obesity, efforts are increasingly being initiated to address this public health concern. However, these efforts are not being consistently evaluated thereby limiting the opportunity to learn from them. The opportunity and the responsibility at hand are the development of a robust evidence base that can be used to deepen and broaden childhood obesity prevention efforts.

Evaluation serves to foster collective learning, accountability, and responsibility, and to guide improvements in obesity prevention policies and programs. As further discussed in Chapter 2, the committee uses the term *evaluation* to denote a systematic assessment of the quality and effectiveness of an initiative, program, or policy. Evaluation results can be used to identify and scale up those efforts that are successful in achieving desirable outcomes (e.g., improving diets, increasing physical activity, reducing sedentary behaviors, and numerous other intermediate outcomes), refine those that need restructuring and adaptation to different contexts, and revamp or discontinue those found to be ineffective. Harnessing the resources needed to support evaluation involves a commitment by many sectors and stake-holders to work toward the goal of improving population health.[4]

Two reviews of childhood obesity prevention interventions and activities indicate that far too few programs are being evaluated. Shaping America's Youth—a public-private partnership formed in 2003 in cooperation with the Office of the Surgeon General, the American Academy of Pediatrics, the American Diabetes Association, the Nutrition Department of the University of California at Davis, and numerous sponsoring private-sector companies—released a summary report of the first national registry of programs addressing childhood physical inactivity and excess weight (Academic Network, 2004). The report is based on the information provided by the 1,090 programs in the registry serving an estimated 4.6 million children. Even though funders stated that the availability of outcome measures was the primary criterion for funding awards, only one-half (53 percent) of the programs indicated that they had quantifiable outcome measures (Academic Network, 2004).

A similar pattern was observed in a recent review of the childhood obesity prevention literature by Flynn and colleagues (2006). Of 13,000 reports that described programs to promote healthy weight in children, only 500 provided adequate information about their implementation to identify promising practices. That review highlighted a large number of potentially useful interventions that are not being properly evaluated (Lobstein, 2006).

To encourage and expand evaluation efforts, it is important to take into consideration some of the issues that will need to be addressed. A further analysis of and additional detail about these considerations and other challenges is provided in Chapter 2:

- Evaluation is often not a priority for individuals and organizations that are developing a new policy, program, or intervention. With a focus on making changes, many programs do not take the time to assess the baseline status or measure outcomes[5] that could provide insights into whether the particular mechanism of change is effective. Often, evaluation is viewed as labor-intensive, expensive, and

---

[4]Population health is concerned with the state of health of an entire community or population as opposed to that of an individual and focuses on the interrelated factors that affect the health of populations over the life course, and the distribution of the patterns of health outcomes (Health Canada, 2001; IOM, 2003).

[5]An *outcome* is the extent of change in targeted policies, institutions, environments, knowledge, attitudes, values, dietary and physical activity behaviors, BMI, and other conditions between the baseline measurement and subsequent points of measurement over time (Chapter 2).

technically complex and is not perceived as a responsibility for a small-scale program in a school or community setting.

- Realistic outcomes need to be assessed. Not every new program or policy should be expected to achieve significant changes in BMI levels, particularly within the short time period in which outcome data are usually collected. Short-term and intermediate outcomes should be realistic and easy to measure and should be targeted to the specific intervention (Chapter 2). Examples of intermediate outcomes include increased time spent in physical activities, reduced time spent in sedentary activities such as viewing television or playing videogames, and increased physical fitness levels (Box 1-2).

- Resources for evaluation are often scarce. Programs and initiatives frequently exist on minimal funding, particularly at the local level. Technical assistance and resources designated for evaluation efforts are needed with an emphasis on practical and less costly methods of evaluation.

- Collaborative efforts need to be strengthened and a systems approach needs to be used to support obesity prevention. Frequently, efforts are focused on a single program or intervention and do not examine links to other interventions within the same school or community. A systems approach to health promotion and childhood obesity prevention offers the opportunity to develop and evaluate interventions in the context of the multiple ongoing efforts (Green and Glasgow, 2006; Midgley, 2006). Systems thinking among key stakeholders is needed to promote and sustain meaningful and enduring changes (Best et al., 2003a). However, evaluation methods for a systems approach are currently not well developed (Best et al., 2003b) and deserve further attention.

OVERVIEW OF THE REPORT

This report examines progress in preventing childhood obesity with an emphasis on the surveillance, monitoring, and evaluation of all programs, policies, and interventions used to prevent childhood obesity. The committee introduces an evaluation framework for childhood obesity prevention in Chapter 2 and provides a detailed examination of the key issues relevant to assessing the broad range of pertinent short-term, intermediate, and long-term outcomes. Chapter 2 also provides the committee's recommendations, which are further discussed with specific details on implementation steps in the remainder of the chapters. Chapter 3 focuses on issues relevant to diverse populations particularly those that are salient for high-risk groups, individuals of low SES, and racial/ethnic minority populations. The concepts introduced in Chapter 3 are carried through into the subsequent

BOX 1-2
Obesity Prevention Goals for Children and Youth

The goal of obesity prevention in children and youth is to create—through directed social change—an environmental-behavioral synergy that promotes the following:

For the *population* of children and youth

- Reduction in the incidence of childhood and adolescent obesity
- Reduction in the prevalence of childhood and adolescent obesity
- Reduction of mean population body mass index (BMI) levels
- Improvement in the proportion of children meeting the recommendations of the Dietary Guidelines for Americans 2005
- Improvement in the proportion of children meeting physical activity guidelines
- Achieving physical, psychological, and cognitive growth and developmental goals

For *individual* children and youth

- A healthy weight trajectory, as defined by the CDC BMI charts
- A healthful diet (consistent with the recommendations of the Dietary Guidelines for Americans 2005 in terms of quality and quantity)
- Appropriate amounts and types of physical activity
- Achieving physical, psychosocial, and cognitive growth and developmental goals

Because it may take a number of years to achieve and sustain these goals, intermediate goals are needed to assess progress toward reducing the rates of obesity through policy and system changes. Examples include:

- Increased numbers of children who safely walk and bike to school
- Improved access to and affordability of fruits and vegetables for low-income populations
- Increased availability and use of community recreational facilities
- Increased play and physical activity opportunities
- Increased numbers of new industry products and advertising messages that promote energy balance at a healthy weight
- Increased availability and affordability of healthful foods and beverages at supermarkets, grocery stores, and farmers' markets located within walking distance of the communities that they serve
- Changes in institutional and environmental policies that promote energy balance

SOURCE: IOM (2005).

chapters, which also focus on examples of progress in obesity prevention across specific sectors of activity: federal, state, and local governments (Chapter 4); a range of private-sector industries (Chapter 5); communities, including foundations, nonprofit and voluntary organizations, and health care professionals (Chapter 6); schools (Chapter 7); and families at home (Chapter 8). These chapters also provide recommendations for next steps in developing and enhancing data sources, evaluation measures, and other assessment tools. The report concludes in Chapter 9, with a focus on the actions that can assist the nation with moving forward in achieving rapid, effective, and meaningful progress to reduce obesity and improve the health status of children and youth.

REFERENCES

Academic Network. 2004. *Shaping America's Youth. Summary Report 2004*. Portland, OR. [Online]. Available: http://www.shapingamericasyouth.org/summaryreportKMD_PDFhr.pdf? cid=101 [accessed February 10, 2005].

Best A, Moor G, Holmes B, Clark PI, Bruce T, Leischow S, Buchholz K, Krajnak J. 2003a. An integrative framework for community partnering to translate theory into effective health promotion strategy. *Am J Health Behav* 18(2):168–176.

Best A, Moor G, Holmes B, Clark PI, Bruce T, Leischow S, Buchholz K, Krajnak J. 2003b. Health promotion dissemination and systems thinking: Towards an integrative model. *Am J Health Behav* 27(Suppl 3):S206–S216.

Borger C, Smith S, Truffer C, Keehan S, Sisko A, Poisal J, Clemens MK. 2006. Health spending projections through 2015: Changes on the horizon. *Health Aff* 25(2): w61–w73.

CDC (Centers for Disease Control and Prevention). 2005a. *Obesity Trends: U.S. Obesity Trends 1985–2004*. [Online]. Available: http://www.cdc.gov/nccdphp/dnpa/obesity/trend/maps/index.htm [accessed March 6, 2006].

CDC. 2005b. QuickStats: Prevalence of overweight among children and teenagers, by age group and selected period—United States, 1963–2002. *MMWR* 54(8):203. [Online]. Available: http://www.cdc.gov/mmwr/preview/mmwrhtml/mm5408a6.htm [accessed February 11, 2006].

CDC. 2006a. *A Public Health Framework to Prevent and Control Overweight and Obesity*. Atlanta, GA: CDC.

CDC. 2006b. *Overweight and Obesity: State-Based Programs*. [Online]. Available: http://www.cdc.gov/nccdphp/dnpa/obesity/state_programs/index.htm [accessed May 17, 2006].

DHHS (U.S. Department of Health and Human Services). 2000. Nutrition and overweight. Focus area 19. In: *Healthy People 2010*, Volume II, 2nd ed. [Online]. Available: http://www.healthypeople.gov/Document/pdf/Volume2/19Nutrition.pdf [accessed February 7, 2006].

DHHS. 2004. *Nutrition and Overweight. Progress Review*. [Online]. Available: http://www.healthypeople.gov/data/2010prog/focus19/Nutrition_Overweight.pdf [accessed February 6, 2006].

Finkelstein EA, Fiebelkorn IC, Wang G. 2003. National medical spending attributable to overweight and obesity: How much, and who's paying? *Health Aff* W3(Suppl):219–226.

Finkelstein EA, Fiebelkorn IC, Wang G. 2004. State-level estimates of annual medical expenditures attributable to obesity. *Obes Res* 12(1):18–24.

Flynn MA, McNeil DA, Maloff B, Mutasingwa D, Wu M, Ford C, Tough SC. 2006. Reducing obesity and related chronic disease risk in children and youth: A synthesis of evidence with "best practice" recommendations. *Obes Rev* 7(Suppl 1):7–66.

Green LW, Glasgow RE. 2006. Evaluating the relevance, generalization, and applicability of research: Issues in external validation and translation methodology. *Eval Health Prof* 29(1):126–153.

Health Canada. 2001. *The Population Health Template: Key Elements and Actions that Define a Population Health Approach.* [Online]. Available: http://www.phac-aspc.gc.ca/ph-sp/phdd/pdf/discussion_paper.pdf [accessed April 17, 2006].

IOM (Institute of Medicine). 2003. *The Future of the Public's Health in the 21st Century.* Washington, DC: The National Academies Press.

IOM. 2005. *Preventing Childhood Obesity: Health in the Balance.* Washington, DC: The National Academies Press.

Lobstein T. 2006. Comment: Preventing child obesity—An art and a science. *Obes Rev* 7(Suppl 1):1–5.

Midgley G. 2006. Systemic intervention for public health. *Am J Public Health* 96(3):466–472.

Ogden CL, Flegal KM, Carroll MD, Johnson CL. 2002. Prevalence and trends in overweight among US children and adolescents, 1999–2000. *J Am Med Assoc* 288(14):1728–1732.

Ogden CL, Carroll MD, Curtin LR, McDowell MA, Tabak CJ, Flegal KM. 2006. Prevalence of overweight and obesity in the United States, 1999–2004. *J Am Med Assoc* 295(13):1549–1555.

Smith C, Cowan C, Heffler S, Catlin A, National Health Accounts Team. 2006. National health spending in 2004: Recent slowdown led by prescription drug spending. *Health Aff* 25(1):186–196.

Sondik E. 2004 (January 21). *Data Presentation. Healthy People 2010 Focus Area Progress Review: Nutrition and Overweight.* U.S. Department of Health and Human Services.

Thomson Medstat. 2006. *Childhood Obesity: Costs, Treatment Patterns, Disparities in Care, and Prevalent Medical Conditions.* Research Brief. [Online]. Available: http://www.medstat.com/pdfs/childhood_obesity.pdf [accessed February 2, 2006].

Thorpe KE, Florence CS, Howard DH, Joski P. 2004. The impact of obesity on rising medical spending. *Health Aff* W4(Suppl):480–486.

2

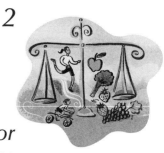

Framework for Evaluating Progress

The nation is in the midst of initiating changes in policies and actions that are intended to combat the childhood obesity epidemic across many sectors, including government, relevant private-sector industries, communities, schools, work sites, families, and the health care sector. Active evaluation of these efforts is needed. The *Health in the Balance* report (IOM, 2005) noted that

> As childhood obesity is a serious public health problem calling for immediate reductions in obesity prevalence and in its health and social consequences, the committee strongly believed that actions should be based on the best *available* evidence—as opposed to waiting for the best *possible* evidence (p. 111).

The challenge presented in this report is to take the next step toward developing a robust evidence base of effective obesity prevention interventions and practices. Evaluation is central to identifying and disseminating effective initiatives—whether they are national or local programs or large-scale or small-scale efforts. Once effective interventions are identified, they can be replicated or adapted to specific contexts[1] and circumstances, scaled up, and widely disseminated (IOM, 2005).

This chapter discusses the challenges and opportunities for evaluating childhood obesity prevention efforts. Key questions and principles designed to direct and guide evaluation efforts are presented. Furthermore, the com-

---

[1]In this report, *context* refers to the set of factors or circumstances that surround a situation or event and give meaning to its interpretation.

mittee introduces an evaluation framework that can be used by multiple stakeholders to identify the necessary resources and inputs, strategies and actions, and range of outcomes that are important for assessing progress toward childhood obesity prevention. Subsequent chapters provide specific examples to illustrate the use of the framework in conducting program evaluations in a variety of settings. The chapter concludes with the committee's recommendations that establish the foundation for the implementation actions discussed in subsequent chapters of the report.

OVERVIEW OF EVALUATION

Evaluation is an important component of public health interventions because it helps decision makers make informed judgments about the effectiveness, progress, or impact of a planned program. The committee defines *evaluation* as the systematic assessment of the quality and effectiveness of a policy,[2] program,[3] initiative, or other action to prevent childhood obesity. It is an effort to determine whether and how an intervention meets its intended goals and outcomes. Evaluations produce information or evidence that can be used to improve a policy, a program, or an initiative in its original setting; refine those that need restructuring and adaptation to different contexts; and revamp or discontinue those found to be ineffective. Evaluation fosters collective learning, supports accountability, reduces uncertainty, guides improvements and innovations in policies and programs, may stimulate advocacy, and helps to leverage change in society.

Many types of evaluations can contribute to the knowledge base by identifying promising practices and helping to establish causal relationships between interventions and various types of indicators and outcomes. Evaluations can also enhance understanding of the intrinsic quality of the intervention and of the critical context in which factors can moderate[4] or mediate[5] the interventions' effect in particular ways. Evaluations are needed to demonstrate how well different indicators predict short-term, intermediate-term, and long-term outcomes. An *indicator* (or set of indicators) helps provide an understanding of the current effect of an intervention, future

---

[2]*Policy* is used to refer to a written plan or a stated course of action taken by government, businesses, communities, or institutions that is intended to influence and guide present and future decisions.

[3]*Program* is used to refer to what is being evaluated and is defined as "an integrated set of planned strategies and activities that support clearly stated goals and objectives that lead to desirable changes and improvements in the well-being of people, institutions, environments, or all of these factors." See the glossary in Appendix B for additional definitions.

[4]A *moderator* is a variable that changes the impact of one variable on another.

[5]A *mediator* is the mechanism by which one variable affects another variable.

prospects from the use of the intervention, and how far the intervention is from achieving a goal or an objective. Indicators are used to assess whether progress has been made toward achieving specific outcomes. An *outcome* is the extent of change in targeted policies, institutions, environments, knowledge, attitudes, values, dietary and physical activity behaviors, and other conditions between the baseline measurement and measurements at subsequent points over time.

Evaluations can range in scope and complexity from comparisons of pre- and postintervention counts of the number of individuals participating in a program to methodologically sophisticated evaluations with comparison groups and research designs. All types of evaluations can make an important contribution to the evidence used as the basis on which policies, programs, and interventions are designed. A major purpose of this Institute of Medicine (IOM) report is to encourage and demonstrate the value for conducting an evaluation of all childhood obesity prevention interventions. The committee strongly encourages stakeholders responsible for childhood obesity prevention policies, programs, and initiatives to view evaluation as an essential component of the program planning and implementation process rather than as an optional activity. If something is considered valuable enough to invest the time, energy, and resources of a group or organization, then it is also worthy of the investment necessary to carefully document the success of the effort. The committee emphasizes the need for a collective commitment to evaluation by those responsible for funding, planning, implementing, and monitoring obesity prevention efforts.

Evaluation is the critical step in the identification of both successful and ineffective policies and interventions, thus allowing resources to be invested in the most effective manner. Because sufficient outcomes data are not yet available in most cases to evaluate the efficacy, effectiveness, sustainability, scaling up, and systemwide sustainability of policy and programmatic interventions, the committee uses the term *promising practices* in this report to refer to efforts that are likely to reduce childhood obesity and that have been reasonably well evaluated but that lack sufficient evidence to directly link the effort with reducing the incidence or prevalence of childhood obesity and related comorbidities. They are not characterized as *best practices*, as they have not yet been fully evaluated. Furthermore, the term *best practices* has inherent limitations in the conceptualization and application to health promotion and health behavior research. Green (2001) suggests that clinical interventions are typically implemented in settings with a great deal of control over the dose, context, and circumstances. The expectation that health promotion research will produce interventions that can be identified as best practices in the same way that medical research has done with efficacy trials should be replaced with the concept of best practices for the most appropriate interventions for the setting and population. Thus, best practices resulting from health promotion research focus on effective processes for implementing action and achieving positive change. These may include effective ways of engaging communities; assessing the needs and circumstances of communities and populations; assessing resources and planning programs; or connecting needs, resources, and circumstances with appropriate interventions (Green, 2001).

As described throughout this report, childhood obesity prevention efforts involve a variety of different interventions and policy changes occurring in multiple settings (e.g., in the home, school, community, and media). This "portfolio approach" to health promotion planning may be compared with financial investments in a diversified portfolio of short-term, intermediate-term, and long-term investments with different levels of risk and reward. This type of approach encourages the classification of obesity prevention interventions on the basis of their estimated population impact and the level of promise or evidence-based certainty around these estimates (Gill et al., 2005; Swinburn et al., 2005).

Evaluations are conducted for multiple stakeholders and the findings are broadly shared and disseminated (Guba and Lincoln, 1989). These audiences include policy makers, funders, and other elected and appointed decision makers; program developers and administrators; program managers and staff; and program participants, their families, and communities. Moreover, these diverse evaluation audiences tend to value evaluations for different reasons (Greene, 2000) (Table 2-1). Evaluations inform decision-

TABLE 2-1 Purposes of Evaluation for Different Audiences

Purpose	Audience
Inform decision-making and provide accountability	Policy makers, funders, and other elected and appointed decision makers
Understand how a program or policy worked as implemented in particular contexts and the relative contribution of each component to improve the intervention for replication, expansion, or dissemination or to advance scientific knowledge	Program developers, researchers, and administrators
Improve the program, enhance the daily program operations, or contribute to the development of the organization	Program managers and staff
Promote social justice and equity in the program	Program participants, their families, and communities

SOURCE: Greene (2000).

making, provide accountability for policy formulation and reassessment, and enhance understanding of the effectiveness of a program or policy change. Evaluations are also used to improve or enhance programs and promote the principles of social justice and equity in the program. Encouraging the dissemination of the evaluation results to a broad audience is an important element of developing a "policy-shaping community" that serves as a critical constituency for further implementation and evaluation efforts (Cronbach and Associates, 1980).

Evaluation should also be conducted with appropriate respect for diverse cultural practices, traditions, values, and beliefs (Pyramid Communications, 2003; Thompson-Robinson et al., 2004; WHO, 1998). As discussed further below and in Chapter 3, it is important to be particularly attentive to existing health and economic disparities in conducting evaluations of childhood obesity prevention actions and programs as reflected in the type of evaluation questions asked and the criteria used to make judgments about program quality and effectiveness.

Different types of evaluations (e.g., formative, process, and outcome evaluations) (Box 2-1) relevant to the stage of the intervention and the purpose of the evaluation are conducted. In addition, impact evaluation may be conducted to examine effects that extend beyond specific health outcomes and may include economic savings and benefits, cost-utility, and improved quality of life (CGD, 2006).

Large-scale interventions often build on multiple evaluations from the outset of the project so that at each step along the development and implementation of the project, data are collected and analyzed to assess the best use of resources and to make refinements as needed.

Evaluations provide data that are interpreted to generate judgments about the quality and the impact of the program experience for its participants and about the planned and desirable outcomes that have been achieved. These judgments often rest on established standards and criteria about educational quality and nutritional, dietary, or physical activity requirements, among other criteria. Too often an evaluation is focused on a narrow set of objectives or criteria and the broader policy or program goals may not be adequately considered. Additionally, stakeholders may vary in their judgments about how much improvement is sufficient for a program to be viewed as high quality and effective (Shadish, 2006). A comprehensive review of childhood obesity prevention interventions examined a variety of selection criteria for interventions including methodological quality, outcome measures, robustness in generalizability, and adherence to the principles of population health (e.g., assessments of the upstream determinants of health, multiple levels of intervention, multiple areas of action, and the use of participatory approaches). Of 13,000 programs that promote a healthy weight in children and that were recently reviewed, only 500 pro-

---

BOX 2-1
Types of Program Evaluations

The following are different types of evaluations that are conducted. A large-scale and more complex or sophisticated evaluation may conduct all types of these evaluations and assess a variety of multiple outcomes, as well as explain how they were achieved.

Formative Evaluation: A method of assessing the value of a program and shaping the features of an intervention at an early stage of development before the program or intervention is implemented. A formative evaluation focuses on issues such as understanding how a program works or whether a target audience understands messages or to test the feasibility of implementing an intervention in a new setting or context.

Process Evaluation: A means of assessing strategies and actions to reveal insights about the extent to which implementation is being carried out in accordance with expected standards and the extent to which a given action or strategy is working as planned.

Outcome Evaluation: An approach for assessing whether or not anticipated changes or differences occur as a result of an intervention. This type of evaluation assesses the extent of change in targeted attitudes, values, behaviors, policies, environments, or conditions between baseline measurement and subsequent points of measurement over time.

Time Course of a Program or Intervention

Formative Evaluation *What is needed?*	**Process Evaluation** *Is the program or intervention working as planned?*	**Outcome Evaluation** *Did the program or intervention achieve its objectives?*

---

vided adequate information about their implementation that could be used to identify promising practices for childhood obesity prevention based on chosen criteria (Flynn et al., 2006).

The committee has identified several relevant criteria that can be used to judge the design and quality of interventions and encourages funders and program planners to consider the following actions:

- Include diverse perspectives (House and Howe, 1999) and attend to the subpopulations in the greatest need of prevention actions—particularly underserved, low-income, and high-risk populations that experience health disparities;

- The use of relevant empirical evidence related to the specific context when an intervention is designed and implemented;
- The development of connections of program efforts with the efforts of similar or potentially synergistic programs, including a concerted effort to develop cross-sectoral connections and sustained collaborations; and
- The linkage of interventions that aim to produce structural, environmental, and behavioral changes in individuals and populations relevant to childhood obesity prevention.

The committee developed six overriding principles to guide the approach to program evaluation. First, evaluations of all types—no matter the scale or the level of complexity—can contribute to a better understanding of effective actions and strategies. Localized and small-scale obesity prevention efforts can be considered pilot projects, and their evaluation can be modest in scope. Second, defensible and useful evaluations require adequate and sustained resources and should be a required component of budget allocations for obesity prevention efforts—for both small local projects and large extensive projects. The scope and scale of evaluation efforts should be appropriately matched to the obesity prevention action. Third, evaluation is valuable in all sectors of obesity prevention actions. It is important to recognize that effective action for obesity prevention will not be achieved by a single intervention. However, an intervention or a set of interventions that produces a modest or preliminary change may contribute importantly to a larger program or effort. Multisectoral evaluations that assess the combined power of multiple actions can be especially valuable for informing what might work in other settings. Fourth, evaluation is valuable at all phases of childhood obesity prevention actions, including program development, program implementation, and assessment of a wide range of outcomes. In particular, evaluation can contribute to an improved understanding of the effects of different types of strategies and actions—leadership actions, augmented economic and human resources, partnerships, and coalitions—on the short-term, intermediate-term, and long-term outcomes. Fifth, useful evaluations are contextually relevant, are culturally responsive, and make use of the full repertoire of methodologies and methods (Chapter 3). Evaluations may need to be modified, depending on how programs evolve, the evidence collected, and shifts in stakeholder interests. Sixth, evaluation should be a fundamental component of meaningful and effective social change achieved by stakeholders engaging in a range of dissemination and information-sharing activities through diverse communications channels to promote the use and scaling up of effective policies and interventions. Because evaluation offers opportunities for collective learning and accountability, widespread dissemination of evaluation findings can lead to policy refinements, program improvements, community advocacy, and the strategic redirection of investments in human and financial resources.

EVALUATION CAPACITY

Insights obtained during the committee's three regional symposia suggest that there is a substantial gap between the opportunity for state and local agencies and organizations to implement obesity prevention activities and programs and their capacity to evaluate them (Figure 2-1). It was not surprising to find that at the community level, where the great majority of obesity prevention strategies are expected to be carried out, the capacity for conducting comprehensive program evaluations is limited. Research conducted in academic settings is the principal source of in-depth scientific evidence for specific intervention strategies. Existing public sector surveillance systems and special surveys serve as critical components for the ongoing monitoring and tracking of a wide range of childhood obesity-related indicators. Although more comprehensive evaluations are needed and surveillance systems need to be expanded or enhanced, especially for the monitoring of policy, system, and environmental changes, the gap between the opportunity for evaluations and the capacity to conduct evaluations at the local level appears to be a significant impediment to the identification and widespread adoption of effective childhood obesity prevention programs.

Three strategies might be helpful in addressing the opportunity-capacity evaluation gap. First, and most important, local program managers should be encouraged to conduct for every activity and program an evaluation that is of a reasonable scale and that is commensurate with the existing local resources. The evaluation should be sufficient to determine whether the program was implemented as intended and to what extent the expected changes actually occurred. For most programs for which strategies and desired outcomes are adequately described, careful assessment of how well those strategies are carried out (also called *fidelity*) and modest assessments of outcomes after the program is implemented compared with the situation at the baseline are sufficient. In these contexts, obtaining baseline measures at the outset of programs is critical. As noted above, every program deserves an evaluation but not every intervention program needs to or has the capacity to undertake a full-scale and comprehensive evaluation. Second, government and academic centers can increase the amount of guidance and technical assistance concerning intervention evaluations that they provide to local agencies (Chapter 4). Third, government and academic agencies and centers conducting comprehensive evaluations can more quickly identify activities and programs that deserve more

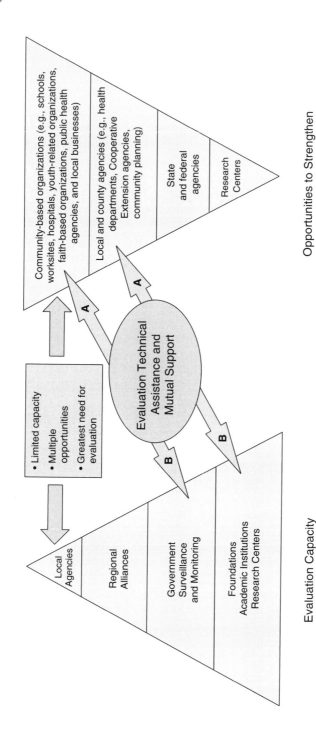

FIGURE 2-1 Closing the evaluation gap at the local level.

extensive evaluation if they communicate frequently with local agencies and each other about their interventions.

The two-way arrows highlighted in Figure 2-1 symbolize the dual benefit that is likely to result when the academic and governmental sectors partner with local programs to enhance evaluation capacity at the local level. The arrow tips marked "A" connote the delivery of local-level evaluation capacity building through the planned efforts of the academic and the governmental sectors. The arrow tips marked "B" reflect the opportunities for those in the academic and governmental sectors to work with and expand upon local pilot programs that show promise for attaining measurable health benefits and merit consideration for diffusion and replication.

Although it may be unrealistic to expect local-level program personnel to have the capacity to conduct full-scale comprehensive evaluations, it is not at all unreasonable for local-level programs to have in place practical mechanisms that will enable them to detect, record, and report on reasonable indicators of the progress and the impact of a program. Issues and examples related to who will pay for the evaluation efforts and the role of government and foundations are discussed throughout the report.

Training opportunities to enhance the ability of stakeholders to conduct evaluations are needed. As indicated above, evaluation is often viewed as primarily being within the purview of foundations, government, and academic institutions. Evaluation is a basic function and integral element of public health programs. However, the core competencies related to conducting community evaluations should be widely disseminated to staff members of nonprofit organizations, schools, preschools, after-school programs, faith-based organizations, child-care programs, and many others. The full utilization of the expertise of academic institutions, foundations, and public health departments in partnership with community and school groups will provide the knowledge base for well-designed evaluation strategies. Tools such as distance learning can take further advantage of disseminating this information. As discussed in Chapter 4, the Centers for Disease Control and Prevention (CDC)'s Nutrition and Physical Activity Program to Prevent Obesity and Other Chronic Diseases is focused on state capacity building, implementation, and enhanced training opportunities. Several practitioner-focused training programs have been developed through the CDC Prevention Research Centers (Chapters 4 and 6). Further, evaluation training for teachers and school staff can be included as a component of school wellness plans and will provide another opportunity to enhance evaluation capacity.

EVALUATION FRAMEWORK

Children and youth live in environments that are substantially different from those of a few decades ago. Many environmental factors substantially increase their risk for obesity. Efforts to evaluate obesity prevention programs should take into account the interconnected factors that shape the fabric of the daily lives of children and youth. Experienced evaluators have long acknowledged the importance of identifying and understanding the key contextual factors (e.g., the environmental, cultural, normative, and behavioral factors) that influence the potential impact of an intervention (Tucker et al., 2006). The evaluation framework that the committee developed offers a depiction of the resources, strategies and actions, and outcomes that are important to childhood obesity prevention. All are amenable to documentation, measurement, and evaluation (Figure 2-2). The evaluation framework also illustrates the range of important inputs and outcomes while giving careful consideration to the following factors:

- The interconnections and quality of interactions within and among the multiple sectors involved in childhood obesity prevention initiatives;
- The adequacy of support and resources for policies and programs;
- The contextual appropriateness, relevance, and potential power of the planned policy, intervention, or action;
- The relevance of multiple levels and types of outcomes (e.g., structural, institutional, systemic, environmental, and behavioral for individuals and the population and health outcomes);
- The potential impact of interventions on adverse or unanticipated outcomes, such as stigmatization or eating disorders (Doak et al., 2006); and
- The indicators used to assess progress made toward each outcome; selection of the best indicators will depend on the purpose for which they are intended (Habicht and Pelletier, 1990; Hancock et al., 1999) and the resources available to program staff to collect, analyze, and interpret relevant data.

CDC has developed three guides for evaluating public health and other programs relevant to obesity prevention, including: *Framework for Program Evaluation in Public Health* (CDC, 1999), *Introduction to Program Evaluation for Public Health Programs* (CDC, 2005a), and *Physical Activity Evaluation Handbook* (DHHS, 2002). The guides offer six steps for evaluating programs: (1) engage stakeholders, (2) describe the plan or program, (3) focus the evaluation design, (4) gather credible evidence, (5) justify conclusions, and (6) share lessons learned. Other important elements for program development and evaluation emphasized by the guides include the documentation of alliances, partnerships, and collaborations with those in other sectors; the establishment of program goals and objectives; the assessment of the available human and economic resources; and the selection of specific

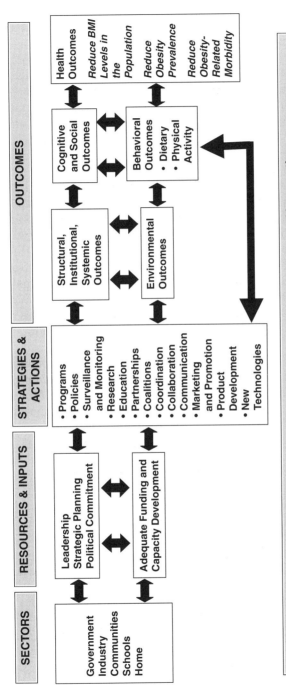

FIGURE 2-2 Evaluation framework for childhood obesity prevention policies and interventions.

intervention strategies that are appropriate for different settings and contexts. In addition to these evaluation steps, the framework described in this chapter: (1) encourages the evaluation of a range of outcomes—structural, institutional, systemic, environmental, cognitive, social, behavioral and health; (2) emphasizes the importance of crosscutting factors that influence the evaluation of policies and interventions; and (3) further elaborates the committee's ideas about relevant criteria for judging the design and quality of interventions. These features are discussed in the next section.

Components of the Evaluation Framework

Actions that prevent childhood obesity are expected to proceed through stages similar to those for other public health interventions. Progress in this field depends on consistent and sustained action as indicated in the left-to-right flow across the columns of the evaluation framework (Figure 2-2). The interchange and feedback that will nurture and contribute to this effort are indicated by the double-headed arrows throughout the framework diagram. Once a problem is identified, strategies are formulated to obtain funding and develop institutional and community capacity to address the problem. In some circumstances, the process begins when committed leaders seek to strengthen human and economic resources in multiple sectors through which a variety of actions and programmatic efforts will be implemented. Strategies and actions are tailored to address the known determinants and precursors of the health problem. From the outset, efforts are made to ensure that systems are in place to evaluate the process and generate the information used to inform midcourse corrections in the intervention and ascertain the extent to which important outcomes are achieved. Evaluation should also provide a better understanding of the problem and meaningful, effective, and sustainable ways to address it.

Sectors

The first column in the framework delineates the specific sectors in which childhood obesity prevention actions can be undertaken and evaluated—government, industry, communities, schools, and home. Sub-sectors are covered under the main sectors; for example, media is discussed under the industry sector (Chapter 5), foundations and health care are discussed under the communities sector (Chapter 6), and child-care and after-school are discussed under the school sector (Chapter 7). The activities of these sectors are interdependent; and prevention actions will have a higher likelihood of success when the public-sector, private-sector, and voluntary or nonprofit organizations purposefully combine their respective resources, strengths, and comparative advantages to ensure a coordinated effort over the long term.

Resources and Inputs

Key resources and inputs include leadership, political commitment, and strategic planning that elevate childhood obesity prevention to a high priority. Adequate and sustained funding through government appropriations and philanthropic funding and capacity development are needed to initiate and sustain effective obesity prevention efforts. Evaluation of these two sets of factors can provide information about the adequacy of the leadership and the resources committed to a specific childhood obesity prevention initiative (Chapter 4). An essential implication of this framework is that rhetoric is an inadequate response. Announcements or statements made by leaders in all sectors should be accompanied by resource allocation and policy and programmatic actions committed to reversing the childhood obesity epidemic. Evidence of planning and adequate resource allocation and appropriations by government leaders, philanthropic boards, senior corporate managers, and shareholders is needed.

At the national level, an example of both resource allocation and leadership is the Alliance for a Healthier Generation, a joint initiative of the William J. Clinton Foundation and the American Heart Association, which established the Healthy Schools Program[6] in 2006 with funding from the Robert Wood Johnson Foundation (RWJF). The purpose of this program is to foster healthy environments that support efforts to reduce obesity in school-aged children and youth (Alliance for a Healthier Generation, 2006a). In May 2006, the Alliance announced a new initiative in collaboration with industry representatives—including Cadbury Schweppes, The Coca-Cola Company, PepsiCo, and the major trade association that represents these companies, the American Beverage Association—to establish new guidelines to limit portion sizes; prohibit the sale of sweetened beverages and high-calorie, low-nutrient foods; and offer calorie-controlled servings of beverages to children and adolescents in the school environment. This is the Alliance's first industry agreement as part of the Healthy Schools Program and has the potential to affect an estimated 35 million students across the nation (Alliance for a Healthier Generation, 2006b) (Chapters 5 and 7).

From the outset of this effort, the Alliance stated two measurable objectives that can be used as outcome indicators to assess the program's

---

[6]The Healthy Schools Program is one of four initiatives of the Alliance for a Healthier Generation, which has set the goal to halt the increase in childhood obesity within 5 years and reverse the trend within 10 years in the United States.

progress: companies will work to implement changes to promote the availability of healthful beverages and foods in 75 percent of the public and private schools that they serve before the start of the 2008–2009 school year and in all U.S. schools by 2010 (Alliance for a Healthier Generation, 2006b) (Chapter 5). These objectives are both quantifiable and measurable, thus making it feasible to track progress.

However, the complexity of evaluating multiple ongoing initiatives is acknowledged. In contexts such as these, in which local programs are implemented while a larger-scale nationwide intervention is occurring, there may be parallel and reinforcing activities that present challenges in assessing the relative contribution of each intervention. A systems approach to health promotion and childhood obesity prevention offers the opportunity to develop and evaluate interventions in the context of the multiple ongoing efforts (Green and Glasgow, 2006; Midgley, 2006). However, evaluation methods of this approach are currently not well developed (Best et al., 2003) and further research is needed in this area. Methodological work in the evaluation of systemic initiatives in public education may offer some good starting points (for example, Ruiz-Primo et al., 2002).

Nevertheless, national leadership and support should be acknowledged and documented as a strategy that can support and reinforce the goals of local efforts.

Another example of leadership and resource allocation is the Healthy Carolinians Microgrants program. The program provided small support grants to each of 199 communities in North Carolina (up to $2,010) to increase local awareness of the objectives described in *Healthy People 2010*, mobilize resources, and create new partnerships in community health improvement (Bobbitt-Cooke, 2005).

Fawcett and colleagues (1995) have created a simple procedure that assists local program evaluators in documenting changes in programs, policies, and practices that are stimulated in part by organized community-based prevention strategies. The ability to document these events, the methods of which are accessible online (Fawcett et al., 2002), enables evaluators to share the relevant short-term indicators and outcomes of a program's progress while awaiting the long-term population health outcomes. Once the relevant events and accomplishments are documented, they can be plotted on a timeline to demonstrate the progress of the overall effort. It should be noted, however, that these events related to the observed changes in communities are associative rather than causative (Figure 2-3).

Strategies and Actions

As depicted in Figure 2-2, a variety of strategies and actions are needed to effectively use the resources and inputs for childhood obesity prevention

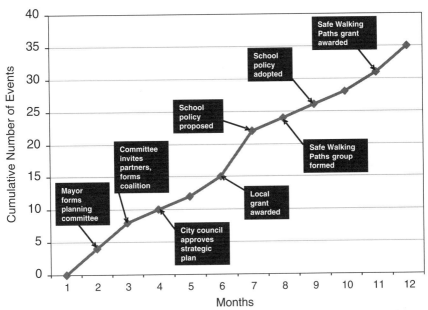

FIGURE 2-3 Hypothetical trends in the rate of community and system changes (e.g., the implementation of new programs and policies) stimulated by obesity prevention efforts during the first year.

(e.g., leadership, political commitment, funding, and capacity development) to produce positive outcomes. Strategies are the concerted plans for action that when implemented through changes such as new product development or the enactment of legislation on nutritional standards for school foods and beverages result in outcomes that can be assessed. Evaluating the extent to which strategies are being developed (e.g., state action plans, federal agency coordination) and implemented through actions (e.g., enactment of new legislation, marketing of new products) is a necessary step in determining the extent of progress in childhood obesity prevention. The interactions among complex social, economic, and cultural factors, combined with the varying availability of resources, require that interventions should be adapted to meet the particular needs, circumstances, or contexts of a community or setting. In the absence of generalizable solutions, effective planned childhood obesity prevention efforts will consist of a variety of potential strategies and actions based on an assessment of local needs, assets, conditions, and available resources. On the basis of the results of these assessments, obesity prevention program planners can draw from an array of strategies and actions, as depicted in the evaluation framework (Figure 2-2). All elements of the framework are amenable to evaluation.

The Kansas Coordinated School Health Program illustrates how several key strategies and actions (e.g., programs, coalition, collaboration, and coordination)[7] can be used in combination to promote health outcomes for school-aged children and youth (Kansas State Department of Education, 2004). Through a grant awarded by the Kansas Coordinated School Health Program, the Goddard School District (which is located in West Wichita, Sedgwick County, and which includes three elementary schools, one intermediate school, two middle schools, and one high school) offered health promotion activities and resources (Kansas State Department of Education, 2004; Greg Kalina, Coordinator of the Goddard School District Nutrition Program, personal communication, April 24, 2006) with the dual goal of benefiting both students and school staff:

- A mapped walking course on elementary school playgrounds and inside school hallways;
- Monday morning stretch exercises led by trained teachers on closed-circuit television at the intermediate school;
- The provision of pedometers and walk-run and marathon events for students, faculty, staff, and community residents;
- Nutritious snack options at staff and district committee meetings and the introduction of low-calorie and high nutrient snack options in schools;
- Two annual teacher in-service programs on healthful nutrition choices and physical fitness;
- A fitness center for staff, established with equipment donated by staff members and expanded with locally raised funds; and
- Training for staff on the proper use of the fitness center equipment.

Both formative and process evaluations can assist with the assessment of the quality of the strategies and actions used at an early phase of the implementation of interventions. These types of evaluations can reveal in-

---

[7]A *coalition* is an organized group of people in a community working toward a common goal. A coalition can have individual, group, institutional, community, and public policy goals. *Coordination* refers to the process of seeking concurrence from one or more groups, organizations, or agencies regarding a proposal or an activity for which they share some responsibility and that may result in contributions from each of these entities. *Collaboration* is defined as a cooperative effort between and among groups of people (e.g., governmental entities as well as private partners) through which partners work together toward mutual advantage and the achievement of common goals. Collaboration can range from informal ad hoc activities to more planned, organized, and formalized ways of working together.

sights at three levels: (1) the strength of the underlying rationale for the program as a vehicle for addressing childhood obesity, (2) the ways in which the program is well matched to specific settings, and (3) the ways and extent to which program implementation is being carried out in accordance with expected standards and the program is working as planned. The results attained through process evaluation not only will provide information that enables program planners to make needed adjustments in the program during its formative stages but also will yield critical insights about the intervention after outcomes data are available. In the Kansas initiative described above, process evaluation data could include records of children and staff who use the fitness center and walking course and the proportion of students and staff participating in the stretching exercises, as well as findings from teacher and student surveys assessing the perceptions of the value of these additions to the school district's facilities.

An example from West Virginia illustrates how attention to strategies and actions (the third column of the evaluation framework in Figure 2-2) provides support to local-level obesity prevention program activities. The Partnership for a Healthy West Virginia consists of representatives from education, health care, nonprofit and faith-based organizations, business, and state government who developed a 3-year statewide action plan to address obesity. One key component of the action plan was to provide policy recommendations to the West Virginia governor and legislature. The proposal was strategically built on previously successful education and advocacy efforts under the leadership and organizational credibility of the West Virginia Action for Healthy Kids Team, the West Virginia State Medical Association, and the American Heart Association. Two key policy recommendations were proposed: (1) enhance and increase the amount of physical education in all public schools and (2) limit access to sweetened carbonated soft drinks and high-calorie foods and meals in public schools while offering increased access to foods and beverages that contribute to a healthful diet. On the basis of the efforts of this state coalition, the governor introduced and supported the Healthy West Virginia Act of 2005. Both policy recommendations (policy implementation is a structural outcome in the fourth column of the evaluation framework) have been included in the new law (HWVA, 2005).

The challenge of tracking the implementation of the policies is being addressed by one of the partners, the State Department of Education. The Department's Office of Child Nutrition has the responsibility for monitoring compliance with the competitive food sales policy which includes monitoring the sale of sweetened soft drinks and the availability of foods with low nutritional value at the elementary, middle, and high school levels. The Office of Healthy Schools has the responsibility for tracking three key areas: (1) fitness testing using the FITNESSGRAM®/

ACTIVITYGRAM®[8]; (2) representative sampling of the body mass index (BMI) levels of students; and (3) adherence to State Board of Education standards for specified hours that students must engage in physical activity at the elementary, middle, and high school levels. Through a legislative mandate, the Office of Healthy Schools also operates a statewide, online health education assessment system called the Health Education Assessment Project. This system annually reaches 65,000 students from selected grade levels and assesses a wide range of student health knowledge, including knowledge of the need for physical activity and good nutrition. West Virginia school officials use the results of this assessment to identify knowledge gaps and make curriculum recommendations.

The California Teen Eating, Exercise, and Nutrition Survey (CalTEENS) (Box 2-2) is an example of intersectoral collaboration among a variety of stakeholders in the government, education, and industry sectors to promote childhood obesity prevention strategies. CalTEENS is a comprehensive biennial survey conducted in 1998, 2000, and 2002, of the eating and physical activity behaviors of more than 2 million of California's adolescents ages 12 to 17 years (Public Health Institute, 2004).

Both the Partnership for a Healthy West Virginia and CalTEENS benefit from participation by a broad range of partner organization and agencies. Furthermore, obesity prevention activities are often consistent with the goals of a wide range of other health initiatives, including those concerned with supporting chronic disease prevention, school health, work site health promotion, and urban planning strategies such as Smart Growth.

Outcomes

The evaluation outcomes selected will depend on the nature of the intervention; the timeline of the program or intervention; and the resources available to program implementers and evaluators to collect, analyze, and interpret outcomes data. The timeline of the intervention often necessitates whether the evaluation can assess progress toward a short-term outcome (e.g., increasing participation in an after-school intramural sports team), an intermediate-term outcome (e.g., changes to the built environment that promote regular physical activity for children and youth), or a long-term outcome (e.g., a reduction in BMI levels of children participating in a new program). Outcomes can also be categorized on the basis of the nature of the change (Figure 2-2):

---

[8]The FITNESSGRAM®/ACTIVITYGRAM® is a computerized tool that schools use to assess children's fitness and physical activity performance and abilities. It is used to increase parental awareness of children's fitness and physical activity levels by providing a direct way for physical education teachers to report the results of physical fitness assessments.

BOX 2-2
Organizations Supporting CalTEENS

- American Cancer Society
- American Heart Association
- California Adolescent Nutrition and Fitness Program
- California Center for Public Health Advocacy
- Department of Education
- California Elected Women's Association for Education & Research
- California 5 a Day Campaign
- California Latino 5 a Day Campaign
- California State Parent Teachers' Association
- Los Angeles County Health Department
- American Academy of Pediatrics

- Structural, institutional, and systemic outcomes;
- Environmental outcomes;
- Population or individual-level cognitive and social outcomes;
- Behavioral outcomes (e.g., dietary and physical activity behaviors); and
- Health outcomes.

Examples of the range of outcomes across different sectors are summarized in Table 2-2. The committee emphasizes the need to develop programs and interventions that can effect changes in all types of outcomes.

Structural, institutional, systemic, and environmental factors can significantly influence access to and the availability of healthful choices and behaviors. Neither children and youth nor their parents can choose to eat fruits and vegetables unless these are available, affordable, and culturally acceptable in their own communities and in the settings where they spend time. Children and youth cannot choose to spend their after-school time engaged in physical activities if they do not have safe spaces to engage in those activities or places to play. Nor will they increase their in-school physical activity in the absence of school policies that mandate and monitor requirements that children and youth engage in a specified level of physical activity each school day or week. These structural and environmental factors both constrain and enable individual and family choices about food and physical activity.

The federal government launched the Safe Routes to School (SRTS) program in 2005 to address some of these issues. The SRTS program assists communities around the nation with making walking and bicycling to school a safe and routine activity for children and youth. The program provides funding to states to administer a variety of initiatives,

TABLE 2-2 Examples of Outcomes in the Evaluation Framework

Outcome	Examples
Structural, institutional, and systemic outcomes[a]	• Revise zoning and land use requirements to promote active transport to schools. • Develop and implement a local school wellness policy. • Implement a policy that mandates daily physical education in a public school district. • Develop and support company and industrywide policies for opportunities and products that promote physical activity. • Enact a state law that requires nutrition labeling in full serve and quick serve restaurants. • Establish policies on the type of foods and beverages that are advertised and marketed to children ages 12 years and younger during children's broadcast and cable television programming. • Revise the mission of a community health center or community coalition to include obesity prevention as an area of programmatic responsibilities and outreach. • Create or enhance a company's employee wellness program by incorporating obesity prevention into its activities. • Increase company sales and profits for low-calorie and non-caloric beverages.
Environmental outcomes[b]	• Complete needed capital improvements on sidewalks and street crossings in a community that allows children to walk and bicycle to school. • Increase the number of miles of walking and bicycle paths in the community. • Initiate and sustain farmers' markets and farm stands in low-income communities to increase the availability of fresh produce. • Increase the availability, affordability, and consumption of beverage products in smaller containers in retail outlets, restaurants, and schools. • Attract a new grocery store to the inner city or enhance a corner store to expand the availability and affordability of fruits, vegetables, and other foods and beverages that contribute to a healthful diet. • Increase the availability and affordability of physical activity opportunities in communities.
Cognitive and social outcomes[c]	• Increase student awareness about the importance of healthful diets and physical activity. • Enhance student knowledge about energy balance at a healthy weight.

TABLE 2-2 continued

Outcome	Examples
	• Improve the self-efficacy of adolescents in using the Nutrition Facts label to select healthier options at the grocery store and in quick serve restaurants. • Change the societal attitude about the appropriate portion size for a take-out meal at full serve and quick serve restaurants. • Adopt a social norm that encourages children and parents to consume water and non-caloric beverages instead of sweetened beverages with meals.
Behavioral outcomes[d] dietary and physical activity outcomes	• Reduce the amount of recreational screen time (e.g., television, DVDs, videogames, and computers). • Increase numbers of students walking or biking to school. • Increase fruit and vegetable consumption for children and youth. • Increase consumer knowledge of company icons to identify healthier food and beverage products. • Increase consumer use of products that encourage energy expenditure. • Improve physical fitness levels on standardized tests. • Increase and sustain breastfeeding rates among new mothers and their infants.
Health outcomes[e]	• Reduce BMI levels in the population. • Reduce obesity prevalence. • Reduce obesity-related morbidity.

[a]*Structural outcomes* represent the development, implementation, or revision of policies, laws, and resources affecting the dietary patterns and physical activity behaviors of children, youth, and their families. *Institutional outcomes* are changes in organizational cultures, norms, policies, and procedures related to dietary patterns and physical activity behaviors. *Systemic outcomes* are changes in the way that eating and physical activity environments and health systems are organized and delivered.

[b]*Environmental outcomes* are changes that create a health-promoting environment, including access to low-calorie and high nutrient foods and beverages and opportunities for regular physical activity.

[c]*Cognitive outcomes* are changes in an individual's knowledge, awareness, beliefs, and attitudes about the importance of healthful diets and regular physical activity to reduce the risk of obesity and related chronic diseases. *Social outcomes* are changes in social attitudes and norms related to dietary and physical activity behaviors that support healthy lifestyles.

[d]*Behavioral outcomes* are changes made by individuals or populations that affect their diet and physical activity levels and enhance health.

[e]*Health outcomes* are changes made by individuals or populations that either reduce or increase their risk of developing specific health conditions.

from building safer street crossings to establishing programs that encourage children and their parents to walk and bicycle safely to school (FHWA/DOT, 2006). The Marin County, California, SRTS program, for example, is focused on reducing local automobile congestion around schools while promoting students' healthy and sustainable habits. The program includes several components that have proven to be effective, including classroom education, special events, and incentives that encourage children and adolescents to choose alternative forms of transportation to schools, as well as technical assistance to identify and remove the barriers to walking, bicycling, carpooling, or taking transit to school. Evaluations of the SRTS program have demonstrated that making environmental changes can lead to increases in children's physical activity patterns (Parisi Associates, 2002; Staunton et al., 2003) (Chapters 4 and 7). The California Department of Health Services has replicated the SRTS program in other cities, which has led to outcomes such as community audits of street, sidewalk, and bikeway conditions; the improved mobility of pedestrians and bicyclists; reduced speed and volume of motor vehicles; and improved motor vehicle compliance with traffic laws (Parisi Associates, 2002). Results linking the SRTS program to health outcomes for children and youth have not yet been reported.

Behavioral outcomes are the population and individual mediators of behavior (e.g., awareness, knowledge, attitudes, beliefs, values, preferences, and skills) and actual behavioral and social changes that affect dietary patterns and physical activity, and thus, energy balance. These outcomes not only are important at the individual level (such as outcomes desired by a pediatrician, nurse, or teacher when he or she is counseling a child or adolescent and his or her parents about healthy dietary practices and physical activity) but also apply on a population level to those implementing large-scale campaigns or programs targeting communities, states, or regions. An outcome of concern has been the potential for stigmatization of children and youth who are obese. Ongoing efforts are examining stigmatization as well as normalization of obesity (i.e., larger sizes and portions becoming the accepted norm).

Behavioral outcomes include changes in dietary patterns and physical activity for children and adolescents to achieve energy balance at a healthy weight. Planet Health is an example of an efficacious school-based intervention designed to reduce BMI levels and obesity prevalence in a multiethnic group of middle-school-aged children in an affluent setting. The program provided evidence that a well-planned and well-evaluated intervention aimed at reducing television viewing time, increasing physical activity, and improving nutrition behaviors can make a difference in reducing obesity prevalence in girls (Gortmaker et al., 1999). It is one of the few childhood obesity prevention interventions that has conducted a cost-benefit and cost-effectiveness evaluation. The results of this evaluation found that the Planet Health program is likely to be cost-effective as it is currently implemented (Wang et al., 2003).

The end outcomes relate to promoting health—increasing the number of children and adolescents who are at a healthy weight, reducing the BMI levels in the population, reducing the number and prevalence of children and youth who are obese or at risk for obesity, and reducing the risks for obesity-related comorbidities such as type 2 diabetes and cardiovascular diseases (Chapter 3). These are the ultimate outcomes, but their achievement may require years of effort with sustained resources and societal change.

Crosscutting Factors

Certain programs, policies, strategies, or actions may be effective for some groups but not others. A variety of crosscutting factors influence program experiences and thus the evaluation process and will need to be considered at every stage of the evaluation framework for both individuals and populations. These include age, sex, socioeconomic status, race/ethnicity, culture, immigration status, acculturation, biobehavioral and gene-environment interactions, and psychosocial status, as well as social, political, and historical contexts. Context refers to the set of factors or circumstances that surround a situation or event and give meaning to its interpretation. All of these factors should be taken into account when obesity prevention initiatives are designed, monitored, and evaluated, as depicted in Figure 2-2 (Hopson, 2003) (Chapter 3).

A useful example of the important roles that are played by some of these crosscutting factors (e.g., age, sex, and race/ethnicity) can be drawn from the VERB™ social marketing campaign. The goal of the VERB campaign was to encourage more than 21 million multiethnic American tweens (i.e., ages 9 to 13 years) to become more physically active. (See Chapter 4 for a detailed description of the VERB campaign.) Before CDC launched the 5-year, VERB—*It's what you do.* campaign in 2002, it conducted a formative evaluation that used marketing research techniques to gain insights into a variety of relevant factors to assist in understanding how physical activity levels can be increased and maintained in the targeted age group. The formative research showed that tweens would respond positively to messages that promoted moderate physical activity in a socially inclusive environment and that emphasized self-efficacy, self-esteem, and belonging to their peer group (Potter et al., 2004).

Key Evaluation Questions and Approaches

Changing stakeholder perceptions about evaluation—from a daunting task of questionable value to a manageable and highly useful endeavor that informs future efforts—can be facilitated by considering four key evaluation questions to guide childhood obesity prevention policies and interventions. Although these questions are relevant to obesity prevention actions, strategies, and programs across all sectors, not every evaluation can be expected to address all of the questions.

The relevance of the four evaluation questions (Box 2-3) depends on the type of the obesity prevention action, policy, or program and the available evaluation capacity (e.g., resources and technical expertise). The majority of childhood obesity prevention interventions are implemented at the local level, where the resources, time, opportunities, skills, and capacity for conducting an evaluation are often limited compared with those available to academic institutions and state or federal governmental agencies. Although some of the evaluation capacity gap can be filled through collaborative partnerships between local agencies and academic institutions, a large portion of locally implemented interventions will occur with no opportunity for conducting a full-scale evaluation. Yet all promising childhood obesity prevention interventions deserve some level of evaluation. Small-scale, grassroots, and exploratory efforts can be evaluated inexpensively and modestly, and if deemed appropriate, subjected to a more sophisticated evaluation at a later stage.

CDC and RWJF are in an early stage of collaborating on a process called the Pre-Assessment of Community-Based Obesity Prevention Interventions Project to identify promising interventions that meet certain ob-

---

BOX 2-3
Questions to Guide Childhood Obesity
Prevention Policies and Interventions

1. How does the action contribute to preventing childhood obesity? What are the rationale and the supporting evidence for this particular action as a viable obesity prevention strategy, particularly in a specific context? How well is the planned action or intervention matched to the specific setting or population being served?
2. What are the quality and the reach or power of the action *as designed*?
3. How well is the action carried out? What are the quality and the reach or power of the action *as implemented*?
4. What difference did the action make in terms of increasing the availability of foods and beverages that contribute to a healthful diet, opportunities for physical activity, other indicators of a healthful diet and physical activity, and improving health outcomes for children and youth?

jective and minimum criteria to consider programs for an in-depth and rigorous evaluation of their effectiveness. The process is expected to be transparent and guided by expert peer reviewers. This evaluability assessment process would allow the selection of programs that are likely to produce the greatest magnitude of impact for the financial investment. The most promising initiatives would be presented to potential funders for more extensive evaluation funding (Laura Kettel-Khan, CDC, personal communication, May 27, 2006).

Evaluation involves multiple methodological approaches, all of which should be used to reach the goal of reducing and preventing childhood obesity. Various evaluation methods are likely to be relevant to each of the four questions as discussed below.

Question 1. How does the action contribute to preventing childhood obesity? What are the rationale and the supporting evidence for this particular action as a viable obesity prevention strategy, particularly in a specific context? How well is the planned action or intervention matched to the specific setting or population being served?

These are descriptive questions about the nature and extent of childhood obesity challenges and the responses in the relevant contexts and are likely to be well addressed by three sets of methods:

- Review of the existing literature and databases (e.g., the demographic, nutrition and dietary intake, physical activity, health promotion, urban planning and community design, transportation, social science, anthropology, food and beverage marketing, and entertainment literature databases) can serve to extract pertinent information about the nature and the extent of the childhood obesity epidemic in the settings and contexts to be served and may perhaps allow longitudinal monitoring of the epidemic.
- Use various methods to focus on specific characteristics of the settings and contexts to be served such as consumer focus groups, key informant interviews, community-based participatory research, needs assessments, and asset mapping (Goldman and Schmalz, 2005; Green and Mercer, 2001; Kretzmann and McKnight, 1993).
- Encourage networking to identify and describe the other childhood obesity prevention actions underway in these settings and contexts.

Question 2. What are the quality and reach or power of the action as designed?

This question calls for an in-depth description of the planned action, with special attention to its underlying logic and rationale, and for an assessment of its quality and viability as an approach to obesity prevention among children and youth in the settings and contexts being served. For example, are the objectives aligned with the recommendations for population-level change?

Two sets of parallel methods are likely to be relevant for this question:

- Qualitative methods may be useful for developing a sound and comprehensive description of the planned action, intervention, or program. These include document review and text analysis (e.g., of program or policy proposals, legislative initiatives, or media campaigns). Individual and group interviews with program planners, administrators, and implementers are also useful for the identification of critical components of and rationales for the intervention, program, or policy being planned.
- The quality of the theory or logic and rationale for the proposed intervention, program, or action can then be assessed by turning to relevant literature and to experts, as well as practitioners in the contexts being served. These assessments call for qualitative methods such as document review, interviews, and concept mapping, and can be supplemented by policy analysis.

Question 3. How well is the action carried out? What are the quality and reach or power of the action as implemented?

These implementation questions are far-reaching and their answers require the use of a variety of methods in combination. Evaluating the implementation of programs is often called *process evaluation*. A process evaluation is defined as the means of assessing strategies and actions to reveal insights about the extent to which implementation is being carried out with regard to expected standards, the "dose" of the intervention received, and the extent to which a given action or strategy is working as planned. For example, quantitative data on the level of program participation or the depth of the reach to target populations (e.g., changes in knowledge, attitudes, or beliefs) may be determined from administrative or program records or may be assessed by surveys. Observations and interviews—both structured (quantitative) and unstructured (qualitative)—can play a useful role in gathering data and evidence about the program's implementation and effectiveness. These data offer windows into how the participants experienced the action or the program. Furthermore, an analysis of the media coverage of an action, program, or policy can also yield valuable information about the quality of program implementation.

Question 4. What difference did the action make in terms of increasing the availability of foods and beverages that contribute to a healthful diet, opportunities for physical activity, other indicators of a healthful diet and physical activity, and improving health outcomes for children and youth?

Finally, the question of the consequences and changes that resulted from the action evaluated invokes a variety of evaluation strategies. At this point, expectations about evaluation designs are appropriately scaled to the scope and size of the intervention. In most local and community-based settings, relatively modest comparisons of pre- and postintervention counts or the preintervention–postintervention results for selected outcome measures will provide sufficient information. In tandem with other information on program quality, as available, and professional judgment, these preintervention–postintervention comparisons are likely to be sufficient to determine if the intervention deserves to be continued, needs improvement, or should be rejected.

More methodologically sophisticated methods relevant to larger-scale interventions may involve:

- A correlational methodology that seeks to establish associative relationships between participation in or exposure to an intervention and subsequent changes in structures or environments, attitudes, or behaviors;
- A case study approach, which seeks to provide an understanding in some depth of the dynamics of change in selected contexts, with special attention to important contextual influences; and
- Experimental and quasiexperimental methodologies that focus on establishing defensible causal relationships between an intervention, action, or program, on the one hand, and changes in structures and environmental factors or individual attitudes, knowledge, and behaviors, on the other hand.

The larger the scope and the higher the level of resources devoted to the initial intervention, the more important it is to consider the value of using more sophisticated evaluation methods at the outset. This is particularly true for interventions in which state or federal policies are involved because the entire target population is affected and, once implemented, adequate baseline measures of the preimplementation status may be impossible to obtain. The larger and more sophisticated correlational, case study, experimental or quasiexperimental evaluations should also include cost and benefit information to allow estimates of the cost-effectiveness and the cost-utility of interventions to be made (Siegel et al., 1996). Mixed-method

---

BOX 2-4
Applying the Evaluation Framework to
Childhood Obesity Prevention Interventions

Contexts and Sectors
How does the action contribute to preventing childhood obesity? What are
the rationale and the supporting evidence for this particular action as a via-
ble obesity prevention strategy, particularly in a specific context? How well
is the planned action or intervention matched to the specific setting or pop-
ulation being served?

- What are important descriptive demographic, sociocultural, and geographical characteristics of the contexts being served? What proportion of the population is at high risk for obesity in the various contexts and sectors being served?
- What is the present character and extent of the childhood obesity epidemic at this time in the contexts being served? What do children, caretakers, and intermediaries want and what are their barriers to change?
- What activities in other sectors are happening in the relevant contexts?

Resources and Inputs, Strategies, and Actions
What are the quality and reach or power of the action as designed? How well
is the action carried out? What are the quality and reach or power of the
action as implemented?

- To what extent and in what ways is the *program design*
  - Coherent, logical, comprehensive, and representative of a plausible idea?
  - Grounded in relevant theory and research about the actions observed?
  - Offering an intervention or experience of sufficient scope and magnitude ("dose") that changes could be expected from it?
  - Well matched to the relevant characteristics of the local context, including socioeconomic status and cultural diversity?

---

evaluation designs[9] can be useful for catalyzing thoughtful, creative, and innovative changes and identifying promising childhood obesity prevention interventions.

Connecting the Key Evaluation Questions to the Evaluation Framework

It is helpful to think about the components of the evaluation framework—sectors, resources and inputs, strategies and actions, and outcomes—in light of the four evaluation questions (Box 2-4). In planning an evalua-

---

[9]A mixed-method design involves methodologies drawn from a variety of disciplines and both qualitative and quantitative data gathering and analysis methods that combine extensive descriptions of context and the experiences of program participation with standardized assessments of changes in institutions or systems, the environment, and individual or population behaviors.

- Responsive to the needs of those affected by the program, policy, or intervention? Especially attentive to the needs of those at greatest risk?
- To what extent and in what ways does the *program implementation*
  - Include materials and activities of high quality and high relevance or meaningfulness to intended program participants?
  - Reach its target audience?
  - Have visibility and support?
- To what extent are program resources sufficient?
- To what extent and in what ways is the program connected or linked to other obesity prevention efforts in the contexts being served?

Outcomes
What difference did the action make in terms of increasing the availability of foods and beverages that contribute to a healthful diet, opportunities for physical activity, other indicators of a healthful diet and physical activity, and improving health outcomes for children and youth?

- To what extent did the program attain its intended outcomes—including structural, institutional, and systemic outcomes; environmental outcomes; population or individual-level cognitive and social outcomes; behavioral outcomes (e.g., dietary and physical activity); and health outcomes?
- What components of the program accounted for achieving the desired outcomes or help explain why outcomes were not attained?
- What other important effects did the program accomplish? What accounts for these effects? What are the impacts of the program on adverse or unanticipated outcomes?
- In what ways and to what extent did the program address the particular needs of populations most at risk for obesity?

tion, consideration should be given to the fact that the relevance of each set of evaluation questions will depend on the scope and maturity of the action or program undertaken. A new or modest initiative may be best evaluated by concentrating on evaluative questions related to the context or the sector and to program design and implementation. A more mature initiative should be evaluated in terms of its intermediate-term or long-term outcomes (e.g., behavioral or health outcomes), contextual relevance, and the quality of the implementation. A policy may be best evaluated by focusing on structural or environmental outcomes. An educational program may be best evaluated in terms of its impact on individual- or family-level changes in knowledge, attitudes, beliefs, and behaviors. Local or community-based actions may be able to monitor only selected indicators of knowledge or attitudinal or institutional change. Whatever the nature of the evaluation, it can make an important contribution to the overall knowledge base regarding childhood obesity prevention.

ISSUES AND CHALLENGES IN EVALUATING PROGRESS
FOR CHILDHOOD OBESITY PREVENTION

Several issues identified in Chapter 1 require attention in the early stages of an evaluation design. First, evaluation is often not a priority for the individuals or the organizations that are developing a new policy, program, or intervention. Second, realistic outcomes need to be selected to measure progress. It is often more realistic for programs to identify and examine short-term and intermediate-term outcomes than long-term health outcomes such as changes in BMI levels. Third, resources for evaluation are often scarce and should be optimally used and complemented with technical assistance and training. Fourth, the strengthening of collaborative efforts and the use of a systems approach to childhood obesity prevention are important and must be pursued, along with methodologies that can effectively assess the quality and effectiveness of collaborative and systemic initiatives.

Like many other public health crises, the current childhood obesity epidemic has multiple, concurrent, and interconnected causes. As articulated in the *Health in the Balance* report (IOM, 2005), these causes include the uneven distribution of low-calorie and high nutrient foods, and lack of affordable fresh fruits and vegetables in communities and schools; the easy availability and access to foods and beverages that are high in total calories, fat, saturated and *trans* fats, added sugars, and sodium; the marketing of products to children and youth that appeal to their tastes but that have limited nutritional value; community settings that do not naturally support and encourage children and youth to be physically active; school policies that do not support or enforce the requirements for adequate time for physical activity; and social norms that reinforce both a sedentary lifestyle and the consumption of high-calorie processed foods and beverages. These problems are related to the distribution, access, and costs of healthful diets and the availability of safe places for children to play. They are present throughout the nation but may have the most detrimental impact and reverberations in low-income and resource-constrained communities (Chapter 3). The complexity of the childhood obesity epidemic poses several challenges for the prevention effort and the evaluation approach that need to be acknowledged. The challenges can be grouped into issues of causation, the measurement of dietary patterns and physical activity behaviors, the development of interventions, surveillance and monitoring by use of different data sources and measurement tools, and the translation of findings to diverse settings and populations.

Attributing Causation and Effects to Interventions

Because of the numerous and intertwined determinants of changes in dietary intake and physical activity it is often difficult for a single intervention, especially if it is modest in scope, to have a measurable impact (Swinburn et al., 2005). In addition, the impact of targeted programmatic interventions is difficult to determine when other often broader population-level interventions, such as media campaigns or increases in opportunities for physical activity in the community, are going on at the same time. The effectiveness of targeted programmatic interventions may also be obscured by gaps or barriers elsewhere in the chain. For example, classroom instruction on the value of physical activity, even if it is effective, may be irrelevant to children or youth who do not have safe places to be active outside or who are more strongly attracted to new sedentary pursuits, such as watching television shows, playing sedentary DVDs and videogames, or using the Internet. Furthermore, behavioral improvements resulting from an intervention in one setting may be offset by compensation or regression in other settings. For example, an increase in activity level during a physical education class may be counterbalanced by a change in after-school activities that increase the time that a child or adolescent spends in sedentary activities, such as more recreational screen time. Similarly, reducing calorie intake with a more nutritious lunch purchased in the school cafeteria may be offset by the increased consumption of high-calorie snacks after school. Finally, interventions addressing systemic and environmental precursors of childhood obesity and other factors early in the causal chain cannot be expected to demonstrate changes in the prevalence of childhood obesity in the short term.

The difficulties inherent in assessing the contribution, if any, of a single intervention, plus the multiplicity of interventions currently being implemented at the individual, family, community, state, and national levels, elevate the need for summary evaluation methods. Thus, in addition to evaluations of specific policies and programs, there is a need for population-wide assessment that examines the overall progress of the prevention of childhood obesity. Surveillance and monitoring will provide the data needed for these types of assessments.

Measuring Dietary Patterns and Physical Activity Behaviors

Current methods of measuring dietary patterns and activity behaviors are insufficiently precise to accurately detect subtle changes in energy balance that can influence body weight (IOM, 2005, 2006; NRC, 2005). The difficulties lie in measuring the energy involved in a specific exposure (e.g., the number of calories consumed at lunch or expended in physical education class) and the full range of places, times, and ways in which energy expenditure occurs (e.g., at home or school, during or after school, or during free time or scheduled activities). All currently available measures of dietary and physical activity behaviors capture only a portion of daily behaviors and do so, at best, with only modest accuracy. Similar problems exist for the measurement of the determinants of excess energy consumption or insufficient energy expenditure. For example, accurate methods of measuring access to fruits, vegetables, and other low-calorie high nutrient foods and beverages or places for engaging in physical activity are still being developed. In addition, the specific characteristics of the built environment that are instrumental in making foods and beverages that contribute to a healthful diet accessible or that encourage play and physical activity on a regular basis are not known. Therefore, the evaluation tools, indicators, or performance measures[10] that are available may lack sufficient specificity (e.g., precision) or sensitivity (e.g., ability to measure incremental change at appropriate levels) to relate specific behaviors to specific outcomes. The task of evaluation will be greatly facilitated by research on and the development of more accurate measurement tools, indicators, and performance measures.

CDC is in an early phase of developing the Obesity Prevention Indicators Project, which will identify and select potential indicators and performance measures for the evaluation of obesity prevention programs and interventions. This process proposes to provide a forum for the sharing of information among funding agencies about current and future strategies and initiatives on program funding, monitoring, and evaluation; the development of criteria for the identification and the selection of common indicators that can be shared across national-, state-, and community-level programs; and the summary and dissemination of selected indicators for program evaluation by intervention setting and also according to recommendations presented in *Healthy People 2010* and the *Health in the Balance* report (IOM, 2005) (Laura Kettel-Khan, CDC, personal communication, May 27, 2006).

Developing Interventions

Interventions pertaining to the structural and systemic causes of childhood obesity, such as those focused on overcoming the paucity of public parks and playgrounds in high-risk neighborhoods or providing easy access

---

[10]A *performance measure* links the use of resources with health improvements and the accountability of programs or partners. Performance measures are used to ensure the efficient and effective use of resources, especially financial resources.

to fresh fruits and vegetables, are recognized as important contributors to the prevention of childhood obesity. However, there is limited empirical evidence to guide their development or their evaluation. Innovative approaches to evaluation design that measure the relative impact of multiple changes to the built environment on a population's behaviors are needed, for example, methods that assess the collective impact of designing sidewalks, walking trails, and public parks on physical activity levels (TRB and IOM, 2005). Analyses of the contribution of community change to population health outcomes that have been conducted in other areas of public health, such as automobile and highway safety, may offer insight into methods that can be used to assess the contribution of environmental changes (e.g., amount, intensity, duration, and level of exposure) to long-term population-level outcomes. Modifications of highways, intersections, and pedestrian crossings, in conjunction with changes in the use of seatbelts, child safety seats, and other interventions have been extensively evaluated (Economos et al., 2001; NTSB, 2005).

Translating and Transferring Findings to Diverse Settings and Populations

The social and cultural diversity within the United States precludes assumptions about the transferability of interventions from one subsector of the population to another. A program that succeeds in Oakland, California, may not do well in Birmingham, Alabama. This does not mean that interventions are not transferable, because despite the cultural and racial/ethnic diversity of the U.S. population, we share many common characteristics. However, it means that transferability is not assured and should be assessed. As new information is generated, it will be important to ensure that the new information and evidence is promptly incorporated into ongoing interventions (Chapter 3). Table 2-3 describes three main areas—knowledge generation, knowledge exchange, and knowledge uptake—and 12 in-

TABLE 2-3 Three Areas and 12 Components of Evidence-Based Policymaking

Knowledge Generation	Knowledge Exchange	Knowledge Uptake
Credible design	Relevant content	Accessible information
Accurate data	Appropriate translation	Readable message
Sound analysis	Timely dissemination	Motivated user
Comprehensive synthesis	Modulated release	Rewarding outcome

SOURCE: Choi (2005).

terdependent elements of evidence-based policymaking (Choi, 2005). The knowledge generation, exchange, and uptake sequence can be used to generate, translate, and transfer or adapt the results of obesity prevention research and program evaluations to present promising practices to different target audiences.

Surveillance and Monitoring: Data Sources and Measurement Tools

Surveillance and monitoring activities generally do not provide an adequate evaluation of any single intervention effort. They do, however, provide an essential assessment of the progress of the overall effort to the prevention of childhood obesity. Current surveillance systems are primarily designed to monitor the health and behavioral components of the obesity epidemic. Surveillance systems that monitor the precursors of changes in dietary and physical activity behaviors, such as policy change or alterations in the built environment, need to be expanded or developed.

A variety of surveillance systems are useful sources of data. Several types of measurement tools can be used to monitor and evaluate childhood obesity prevention policies and interventions. Appendix C provides a detailed summary of many available data sources and outcome indicators that may be used to assess progress by use of the evaluation framework for different sectors. A brief summary is provided below.

Several organizations monitor policies as well as proposed or enacted state legislation related to obesity prevention (Appendix C; Chapters 4 and 7). Examples include the CDC's Nutrition and Physical Activity Legislative Database (CDC, 2005b), the National Conference of State Legislatures' summary of childhood obesity policy options (NCSL, 2006), the Trust for America's Health annual report of federal and state policies and legislation (TFAH, 2004, 2005), and NetScan's Health Policy Tracking Service for state legislation on school nutrition and physical activity (NetScan, 2005). However, there is great variability within and across these legislative databases. The committee noted that a central database or information repository that tracks obesity-related legislation and that can be periodically updated is needed.

Several national and state cross-sectional and longitudinal surveys provide indicators and outcomes related to childhood obesity prevention surveillance and monitoring (Appendixes C and D). Different types of proprietary data sources could potentially be informative for the monitoring and evaluation of childhood obesity prevention policies and interventions. However, because proprietary data are collected for commercial purposes by private companies, either the data are not publicly available or the cost of obtaining the data is prohibitively expensive (IOM, 2006). Nevertheless, marketing research data about children and adolescents, trends in the marketing of consumer food and beverage products, and food retailer super-market scanner point-of-sale data (IOM, 2006; NRC and IOM, 2004) (Chapter 5) can be purchased from marketing and media companies and analyzed, and the results can be published in peer-reviewed publications. Moreover, because marketing data become less commercially useful over time, older data may be donated for public use purposes.

A comprehensive inventory of the available databases and measure-ment tools is beyond the scope of this study. However, programs may use different tools in various settings to obtain results about indicators and outcomes. These include the BMI report card and the FITNESSGRAM®/ ACTIVITYGRAM® used in the school setting (Chapter 7); health impact assessments used for environmental changes (Chapter 6); mobilizing action through community planning and partnerships (Chapter 6); and a system dynamics simulation modeling (Homer and Hirsch, 2006). This type of modeling can be used to understand a variety of factors—obesity trends in the United States, the types of interventions needed to alter obesity trends, the subpopulations that should be targeted by specific interventions, and the length of time needed for actions to generate effects (Laura Kettel-Khan, CDC, personal communication, May 27, 2006).

Support Needed from Research and Surveillance

The evaluation framework presented in this report is offered in direct support of the U.S. childhood obesity prevention efforts. As obesity preven-tion programs, strategies, and actions continue to be initiated around the country, evaluation can play a critical role in furthering our collective understanding of the complex character and contours of the obesity prob-lem and of meaningful and effective ways to address it. The committee emphasizes that program evaluations of varying scope and size at all levels and within all sectors have a vital role to play in addressing the childhood obesity epidemic. Evaluation can help to document progress, advance ac-countability, and marshal the national will to ensure good health for all of our children and youth.

In support of this commitment to evaluation, targeted research is also needed to

- Develop better methods to measure all components of the evaluation framework and to strengthen available data sources so that more complete and accurate information is available for the components; this is especially relevant for methods to accurately assess the eating patterns and physical activity behaviors of children and youth.
- Enable the ongoing assessment and research into the complex dy-namics of childhood obesity, especially those that cross disciplinary

boundaries such as marketing and community change, policy analysis, or economics and education; and

- Sustain efforts in this area so that long-term health outcomes can be achieved; these include reducing the BMI levels in the population, reducing obesity prevalence and at-risk obesity prevalence, and reducing obesity-related morbidity in children and youth.

The translation of evaluation and research findings into promising and best practices constitute the primary means for accelerating national efforts to reverse the epidemic of childhood obesity. Since the need for effective evaluation is ongoing, both the capacity and quality of evaluation will be positively influenced by the presence of a national commitment to support obesity prevention research and the rapid dissemination of research findings—across the geographical landscape—to stakeholders involved in prevention efforts in states and communities.

The health outcomes will not be achieved by any single obesity prevention program or action and, consequently, fall outside the boundaries of most program and policy evaluations. This is true for certain behavioral outcomes as well. At the same time, vigilant and credible monitoring of these population-level indicators and indices is critical to the overall national plan to prevent childhood obesity, and is a responsibility that should be assumed by the health agencies of the government (Chapter 4). Vertically integrated surveillance systems that offer usable data at local, state, and national levels are particularly important.

Implications of the Issues and Challenges

The comprehensive data needed to inform large and complex evaluations will come, in a large part, from more modest assessments. From these evaluations will flow the information required to improve knowledge about which activities and programs should be examined more fully and which should be recommended for more expansive implementation. Unfortunately, there has been limited recognition of the value of carefully designed but modest evaluations. This chapter has discussed issues that may be useful in guiding the design and implementation of practical evaluations. The evaluation framework portrays the wide range of strategies and outcomes that can be evaluated and the need for evaluations with various levels of methodological complexity. Much can be learned from more modest assessments that use quantitative and qualitative methods. The four key evaluation questions may also be useful in indicating innovative approaches, such as mixed-method approaches, to evaluation (Greene and Caracelli, 1997, 2003; Tashakkori and Teddlie, 2003).

SUMMARY AND RECOMMENDATIONS

A meaningful evaluation of a nationwide childhood obesity prevention effort is possible only through the collective commitment of the stakeholders responsible for planning, implementing, and monitoring prevention actions. The evaluation framework presented in this chapter will assist in identifying relevant contexts and sectors; necessary resources and inputs; effective strategies and actions; and explicit institutional, environmental, behavioral, and health outcomes that signify meaningful changes in obesity-related indicators. Evaluation efforts should focus on the specific characteristics of the contexts being served; the rationale and supporting evidence for a particular action that is matched to particular contexts; the quality and reach or power of the action implemented; and the difference that the action makes in preventing childhood obesity, especially for those most at risk.

The committee's four recommendations emphasize the need for leadership, evaluation, and dissemination across all relevant sectors—government, industry, communities, schools, and families. Each of these recommendations is further expanded upon in Chapters 4 through 8, in which the committee recommends specific implementation actions that should be taken to ensure the availability of adequate resources and a focus on strengthening childhood obesity prevention efforts and their evaluation. An exception is Chapter 3, which only includes recommendations 2 and 3 because they explicitly identify the need to account for diverse perspectives when designing culturally relevant interventions that address the special needs of diverse populations and high-risk groups. All the recommendations and implementation steps are summarized in Appendix E.

These recommendations are consistent with those of many other reports (CDC, 1999, 2005a; CGD, 2006; DHHS, 2002; WHO, 1998). They collectively call attention to the urgent need to provide more and better information to improve peoples' lives through evaluation. The recommendations emphasize the importance of dedicating significant resources to the evaluation of interventions. They also advance an evaluation process that meaningfully engages diverse stakeholders in the evaluation design and process and that legitimizes the multiplicity of stakeholder perspectives, notably, program recipients along with funders, administrators, and professional staff.

Recommendation 1: Government, industry, communities, schools, and families should demonstrate leadership and commitment by mobilizing the resources required to identify, implement, evaluate, and disseminate effective policies and interventions that support childhood obesity prevention goals.

Recommendation 2: Policy makers, program planners, program implementers, and other interested stakeholders—within and across relevant sectors—should evaluate all childhood obesity prevention efforts, strengthen the evaluation capacity, and develop quality interventions that take into account diverse perspectives, that use culturally relevant approaches, and that meet the needs of diverse populations and contexts.

Recommendation 3: Government, industry, communities, and schools should expand or develop relevant surveillance and monitoring systems and, as applicable, should engage in research to examine the impact of childhood obesity prevention policies, interventions, and actions on relevant outcomes, paying particular attention to the unique needs of diverse groups and high-risk populations. Additionally, parents and caregivers should monitor changes in their family's food, beverage, and physical activity choices and their progress toward healthier lifestyles.

Recommendation 4: Government, industry, communities, schools, and families should foster information-sharing activities and disseminate evaluation and research findings through diverse communication channels and media to actively promote the use and scaling up of effective childhood obesity prevention policies and interventions.

There will be a greater likelihood of success when public, private, and voluntary organizations purposefully combine their respective resources, strengths, and comparative advantages to ensure a coordinated effort over the long term. Evaluations will contribute to building a strong and diverse evidence base on which promising and best practices can be identified, scaled up, and institutionalized across different settings and sectors.

REFERENCES

Alliance for a Healthier Generation. 2006a. *What is the Healthy Schools Program?* [Online]. Available: http://www.healthiergeneration.org/ [accessed May 8, 2006].

Alliance for a Healthier Generation. 2006b. *Alliance for a Healthier Generation and Industry Leaders Set Healthy School Beverage Guidelines for U.S. Schools.* [Online]. Available: http://www.healthiergeneration.org/beverage.html [accessed May 8, 2006].

Best A, Moor G, Holmes B, Clark PI, Bruce T, Leischow S, Buchholz K, Krajnak J. 2003. Health promotion dissemination and systems thinking: Towards an integrative model. *Am J Health Behav* 27(Suppl 3):S206–S216.

Bobbitt-Cooke M. 2005. Energizing community health improvement: The promise of microgrants. *Prev Chronic Dis* [Online]. Available: http://www.cdc.gov/pcd/issues/2005/nov/05_0064.htm [accessed March 4, 2006].

CDC (Centers for Disease Control and Prevention). 1999. Framework for program evaluation in public health. *MMWR* 48(RR-11):1–42.

CDC. 2005a. *Introduction to Program Evaluation for Public Health Programs: A Self-Study Guide*. [Online]. Available: http://www.cdc.gov/eval/evalguide.pdf [accessed April 13, 2006].

CDC. 2005b. *State Legislative Information: Search for Bills*. [Online]. Available: http://apps.nccd.cdc.gov/DNPALeg/ [accessed April 24, 2006].

CGD (Center for Global Development). 2006. *When Will We Ever Learn? Improving Lives Through Impact Evaluation*. Washington, DC: CGD. [Online]. Available: http://www.cgdev.org/content/publications/detail/7973 [accessed June 6, 2006].

Choi BCK. 2005. Twelve essentials of science-based policy. *Prev Chronic Dis* [Online]. Available: http://www.cdc.gov/PCD/issues/2005/oct/05_0005.htm [accessed March 4, 2006].

Cronbach LJ and Associates. 1980. *Toward Reform of Program Evaluation*. San Francisco, CA: Jossey-Bass.

DHHS (U.S. Department of Health and Human Services). 2002. *Physical Activity Evaluation Handbook*. Atlanta, GA: CDC, DHHS. [Online]. Available: http://www.cdc.govnccdphp/dnpa/physical/handbook/pdf/handbook.pdf [accessed June 1, 2006].

Doak CM, Visscher TL, Renders CM, Seidell JC. 2006. The prevention of overweight and obesity in children and adolescents: A review of interventions and programmes. *Obes Rev* 7(1):111–136.

Economos CD, Brownson RC, DeAngelis MA, Foerster SB, Foreman CT, Gregson J, Kumanykia SK, Pate RR. 2001. What lessons have been learned from other attempts to guide social change? *Nutr Rev* 59(3):S40–S56.

Fawcett SB, Sterling TD, Paine-Andrews A, Harris KJ, Francisco VT, Richter KP, Lewis RK, Schmid TL. 1995. *Evaluating Community Efforts to Prevent Cardiovascular Disease*. Atlanta, GA: National Center for Chronic Disease Prevention and Health Promotion, Centers for Disease Control and Prevention.

Fawcett SB, Schultz J, Carson V, Renault V, Francisco V. 2002. Using Internet-based tools to build capacity for community based participatory research and other efforts to promote community health and development. In Minkler M, Wallerstein N, eds. *Community Based Participatory Research for Health*. San Francisco, CA: Jossey-Bass. Pp. 155–178.

FHWA/DoT (Federal Highway Administration/Department of Transportation). 2006. *Safe Routes to Schools*. [Online]. Available: http://safety.fhwa.dot.gov/saferoutes/ [accessed June 10, 2006].

Flynn MA, McNeil DA, Maloff B, Mutasingwa D, Wu M, Ford C, Tough SC. 2006. Reducing obesity and related chronic disease risk in children and youth: A synthesis of evidence with "best practice" recommendations. *Obes Rev* 7(Suppl 1):7–66.

Gill T, King L, Webb K. 2005. *Best Options for Promoting Healthy Weight and Preventing Weight Gain in NSW*. Sydney, Australia: NSW Centre for Public Health Nutrition and NSW Department of Health. [Online]. Available: http://www.cphn.biochem.usyd.edu.au/resources/FinalHealthyWeightreport160305.pdf [accessed May 23, 2006].

Goldman KD, Schmalz KJ. 2005. "Accentuate the positive!": Using an asset-mapping tool as part of a community-health needs assessment. *Health Promot Pract* 6(2):125–128.

Gortmaker SL, Peterson K, Wiecha J, Sobol AM, Dixit S, Fox MK, Laird N. 1999. Reducing obesity via a school-based interdisciplinary intervention among youth: Planet Health. *Arch Pediatr Adolesc Med* 153(4):409–418.

Green L. 2001. From research to "best practices" in other settings and populations. *Am J Health Behav* 25(3):165–179.

Green LW, Glasgow RE. 2006. Evaluating the relevance, generalization, and applicability of research: Issues in external validation and translation methodology. *Eval Health Prof* 29(1):126–153.

Green LW, Mercer SL. 2001. Can public health researchers and agencies reconcile the push from funding bodies and the pull from communities? *Am J Public Health* 91(12):1926–1943.

Greene, JC. 2000. Understanding social programs through evaluation. In: Denzin NK, Lincoln YS, eds. *Handbook of Qualitative Research*, 2nd ed. Thousand Oaks, CA: Sage Publications. Pp. 981–999.

Greene JC, Caracelli VJ. eds. 1997. *Advances in Mixed-Method Evaluation: The Challenges and Benefits of Integrating Diverse Paradigms. New Directions for Evaluation No. 74.* San Francisco, CA: Jossey-Bass.

Greene JC, Caracelli, VJ. 2003. Making paradigmatic sense of mixed methods practice. In: Tashakkori A, Teddlie C, eds. *Handbook of Mixed Methods in Social and Behavioral Research.* Thousand Oaks, CA: Sage Publications. Pp. 91–110.

Guba EG, Lincoln YS. 1989. *Fourth Generation Evaluation.* Thousand Oaks, CA: Sage Publications.

Habicht JP, Pelletier DL. 1990. The importance of context in choosing nutritional indicators. *J Nutr* 120(Suppl 11):1519–1524.

Hancock T, Labonte R, Edwards R. 1999. Indicators that Count! Measuring population health at the community level. *Can J Public Health* 90(Suppl 1):S22–S26.

Homer JB, Hirsch GB. 2006. System dynamics modeling for public health: Background and opportunities. *Am J Public Health* 96(3):452–458.

Hopson R. 2003. *Overview of Multicultural and Culturally Competent Program Evaluation. Oakland, CA: Social Policy Research Associates.* [Online]. Available: http://www.calendow.org/reference/publications/pdf/evaluations/TCE0509-2004_Overview_of_Mu.pdf [accessed April 18, 2006].

House ER, Howe KR. 1999. *Values in Evaluation and Social Research.* Thousand Oaks, CA: Sage Publications.

HWVA (Healthy West Virginia Act). 2005. *Partnership for a Healthy West Virginia.* [Online]. Available: http://www.healthywv.com/ [accessed April 13, 2006].

IOM (Institute of Medicine). 2005. *Preventing Childhood Obesity: Health in the Balance.* Washington, DC: The National Academies Press.

IOM. 2006. *Food Marketing to Children and Youth: Threat or Opportunity?* Washington, DC: The National Academies Press.

Kansas State Department of Education. 2004. *Kansas Coordinated School Health.* [Online]. Available: http://www.kshealthykids.org/ [accessed February 12, 2006].

Kretzmann JP, McKnight JL. 1993. *Building Communities from the Inside Out.* Chicago, IL: ACTA Publications.

Midgley G. 2006. Systemic intervention for public health. *Am J Public Health* 96(3):466–472.

NCSL (National Conference of State Legislatures). 2006. *Childhood Obesity—2005 Update and Overview of Policy Options.* [Online]. Available: http://www.ncsl.org/programs/health/ChildhoodObesity-2005.htm [accessed April 24, 2006].

NetScan. 2005. *School Nutrition & Physical Education Legislation: An Overview of 2005 State Activity.* [Online]. Available: http://www.rwjf.org/files/research/NCSL%20-%20April%202005%20Quarterly%20Report.pdf [accessed April 24, 2006.

NRC (National Research Council). 2005. *Improving Data to Analyze Food and Nutrition Policies.* Washington, DC: The National Academies Press.

NRC and IOM. 2004. *Children's Health, The Nation's Wealth.* Washington, DC: The National Academies Press.

NTSB (National Transportation Safety Board). 2005. *We Are All Safer: Lessons Learned and Lives Saved, 1975–2005.* 3rd edition. Safety Report NTSB/SR-05/01. Washington, DC: NTSB [Online]. Available: http://www.ntsb.gov/publictn/2005/SR0501.pdf [accessed August 14, 2006].

Parisi Associates. 2002. *Transportation Tools to Improve Children's Health and Mobility.* California Office of Traffic Safety; Safe Routes to School Initiative, California Department of Health Services; Local Government Commission. [Online]. Available: http://www.dot.ca.gov/hq/LocalPrograms/SafeRTS2School/TransportationToolsforSR2S.pdf [accessed June 3, 2006].

Potter LD, Duke JC, Nolin MJ, Judkins D, Huhman M. 2004. *Evaluation of the CDC VERB Campaign: Findings from the Youth Media Campaign Longitudinal Survey, 2002–2003.* Rockville, MD: WESTAT.

Public Health Institute. 2004. *Fact Sheet.* [Online]. Available: http://www.calendow.org/news/press_releases/2004/03/CalTEENSpresskit.pdf [accessed June 3, 2006].

Pyramid Communications. 2003. Communities Helping Children Be Healthy: A Guide to Reducing Childhood Obesity in Low-Income African-American, Latino and Native American Communities. [Online]. Available: http://www.rwjf.org/files/publications/HealthyChildren.pdf [accessed February 20, 2006].

Ruiz-Primo MA, Shavelson RJ, Hamilton L, Klein S. 2002. On the evaluation of systemic science education reform: Searching for instructional sensitivity. *J Res Sci Teach* 39(5):369–393.

Shadish WR. 2006. The common threads in program evaluation. *Prev Chronic Dis* [Online]. Available: http://www.cdc.gov/Pcd/issues/2006/jan/05_0166.htm [accessed August 7, 2006].

Siegel JE, Weinstein MC, Russell LB, Gold MR. 1996. Recommendations for reporting cost-effectiveness analyses. Panel on Cost-Effectiveness in Health and Medicine. *J Am Med Assoc* 276(16):1339–1341.

Staunton CE, Hubsmith D, Kallins W. 2003. Promoting safe walking and biking to school: The Marin County success story. *Am J Public Health* 93(9):1431–1434.

Swinburn B, Gill T, Kumanyika S. 2005. Obesity prevention: A proposed framework for translating evidence into action. *Obes Rev* 6(1):23–33.

Tashakkori A, Teddlie C. eds. 2003. *Handbook of Mixed Methods in Social and Behavioral Research.* Thousand Oaks, CA: Sage Publications.

TFAH (Trust for America's Health). 2004. *F as in Fat: How Obesity Policies are Failing America.* Washington, DC: The Trust for America's Health. [Online]. Available: http://healthyamericans.org/reports/obesity/ObesityReport.pdf [accessed July 23, 2006].

TFAH. 2005. *F as in Fat: How Obesity Policies are Failing America 2005.* Washington, DC: The Trust for America's Health. [Online]. Available: http://healthyamericans.org/reports/obesity2005/Obesity2005Report.pdf [accessed July 23, 2006].

Thompson-Robinson M, Hopson RK, SenGupta S. eds. 2004. *In Search of Cultural Competence in Evaluation: Towards Principles and Practices.* New Directions for Evaluation #102. San Francisco, CA: Jossey-Bass.

TRB (Transportation Research Board) and IOM. 2005. *Does the Built Environment Influence Physical Activity? Examining the Evidence.* TRB Special Report 282. Washington, DC: The National Academies Press. [Online]. Available: http://books.nap.edu/html/SR282/SR282.pdf [accessed December 29, 2005].

Tucker P, Liao Y, Giles W, Liburd L. 2006. The REACH 2010 logic model: An illustration of expected performance. *Prev Chronic Dis* [Online]. Available: http://www.cdc.gov/pcd/issues/2006/jan/05_0131.htm [accessed March 4, 2006].

Wang LY, Yang Q, Lowry R, Wechsler H. 2003. Economic analysis of a school-based obesity prevention program. *Obes Res* 11(11):1313–1324.

WHO (World Health Organization). 1998. *Health Promotion Evaluation: Recommendations to Policy-Makers. Report of the WHO European Working Group on Health Promotion Evaluation.* Copenhagen, Denmark: WHO.

3

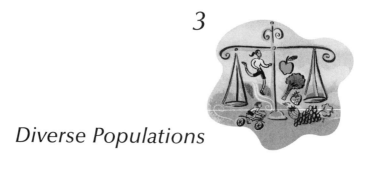

Diverse Populations

The obesity epidemic is occurring among boys and girls throughout the United States, among younger children and adolescents, across all socioeconomic groups and among all racial/ethnic subpopulations. However, in several racial/ethnic groups, in low-income populations, and among recent immigrants to the United States, the rates of obesity among children and youth are alarmingly high or are increasing faster than average. The children and youth who are at the highest risk for obesity often experience other social, economic, and health disparities concurrently and do not live in environments that inherently support health-promoting behaviors. In addition, although some of the risk factors for obesity are relatively ubiquitous in settings where American children and youth spend their time (e.g., communities, schools, shopping malls, retail stores, and home), epidemiologic evidence shows that African-American, Hispanic/Latino, American Indian/Alaska Native, and Pacific Islander populations and children experiencing poverty are more likely to live in environments with inadequate support for health-promoting behaviors. Assessing the impact of these different environments presents an enormous challenge for tracking progress against obesity in diverse populations. On the other hand, the diversity of the U.S. population and the variation in patterns of obesity-related risks also provide opportunities to expand our understanding of how trends, patterns, and risk factors manifest in certain environments and to identify the types of interventions that are likely to be effective when they are tailored specifically to build on a population's characteristics, perspectives, and social and cultural assets.

Much remains to be learned about the role of race/ethnicity, socioeconomic status (SES), and regional disparities in childhood obesity to build an evidence base that will support the most effective strategies and promising practices. Progress in preventing childhood obesity should include an examination of efforts to define and address the contexts and mechanisms that lead to and perpetuate childhood obesity in environments with excessive risks. Several recommendations in the *Health in the Balance* report (IOM, 2005) emphasized the need for prominent government leadership and community collaboration to develop and promote programs and policies that will collectively encourage healthful eating patterns and physical activity behaviors, particularly for young populations at the highest risk for obesity and related chronic diseases.

Helping at-risk children and youth balance their energy intakes and their energy expenditures requires an understanding of the complex and interacting influences of the social, economic, and built environments and the adverse environmental conditions that low-income and racially/ethnically diverse populations encounter as they regularly attempt to obtain affordable foods, beverages, and meals that contribute to a healthful diet and find opportunities to engage in recreational play and physical activity (Day, 2006; Glanz et al., 2005; Goodman, 2003; Gordon-Larsen et al., 2006; IOM, 2005; Jetter and Cassady, 2005; Powell et al., 2004). A multifaceted approach to address obesity and related health considerations is relevant to children and youth overall but leads to different perspectives on the appropriate solutions for specific populations, depending on their historical and sociopolitical contexts and the timing and rate of relevant economic and lifestyle transitions (Kumanyika, 1994; Kumanyika and Golden, 1991).

Because the focus of this report is on evaluation, this chapter provides only a brief overview of the context for these issues. The reader is referred to the extensive body of research regarding the interactions among societal, cultural, genetic, and biobehavioral risk and protective factors and their implications for promoting population health (Dabelea et al., 2000; Gillman et al., 2003; Halfon and Hochstein, 2002; Halfon and Inkelas, 2003; IOM, 2001, 2003; Krieger, 1994; Krieger and Davey Smith, 2004; McEwen, 2001; NRC and IOM, 2000, 2004; Reilly et al., 2005; Rosenbloom, 2002). The chapter focuses on the key issues relevant to improving the implementation and evaluation of obesity prevention efforts involving high-risk and culturally diverse populations.

UNDERSTANDING SPECIFIC CONTEXTS

Many aspects of society have changed concomitantly with the rise in childhood obesity. A broader understanding of the potential interplay among these societal changes and children's biological and behavioral re-sponses is needed. For the population subgroups most affected by obesity, the relevant adverse social and environmental factors may be concentrated or magnified. A variety of causal pathways are associated with many aspects of systemic disadvantage (e.g., poverty, substandard housing, limited educational opportunities, and low levels of social integration), which can lead to adverse health, social, and economic circumstances (Gostin and Powers, 2006). These factors have greater impacts on those with the fewest resources to buffer these influences. The subpopulations that have the highest prevalence of obesity are those considered to be socially, economically, and politically disadvantaged in other respects. Thus, although the determinants of obesity are generally of the same nature among all population groups, special considerations are needed to assess whether the pathways to progress in preventing childhood obesity in the entire population will also reach the subgroups who are the most affected. Long-term investments that support the development or adaptation and evaluation of childhood obesity prevention initiatives are needed. These initiatives also need to be adapted to various settings, contexts, and subpopulations for their dissemination if they are proven to be effective.

Obesity Prevalence

Obesity and its risk-behavior determinants (e.g., high levels of consumption of energy-dense and low-nutrient diets, physical inactivity, and sedentary behaviors) are major drivers of health disparities by race/ethnicity as they contribute to three of the disease categories responsible for the majority of excess mortality: type 2 diabetes, cardiovascular diseases (CVDs), and cancer (Wong et al., 2002). Obesity and at-risk obesity prevalence rates in American children and youth reveal significant differences by age and sex and between racial/ethnic groups (Freedman et al., 2006; Hedley et al., 2004; Ogden et al., 2006; Sherry et al., 2004). There does not appear to be a general excess risk in all age and gender groups, although the increases in obesity over the past 30 years have been especially pronounced at the upper part of the body mass index (BMI) distribution for children and youth. From 1971–1974 to 1999–2002, the prevalence of individuals in certain subgroups with BMI levels above the 99th percentile increased substantially. Additionally, African-American girls ages 6 to 17 years have experienced greater increases in obesity prevalence than white children and adolescents. These increases began in the 1970s, whereas the increases among individuals in other racial/ethnic groups were not observed until the 1980s (Freedman et al., 2006).

By tracking obesity prevalence rates in subpopulations and evaluating the progress achieved by obesity prevention interventions, it may be possible to reduce the risk of obesity in these groups and ensure that primary obesity prevention strategies are reaching the entire target population. It is also important to track increases in BMI levels and obesity prevalence because childhood obesity is associated with an increased risk of CVD and mortality in adulthood (Li et al., 2004; Srinivasan et al., 2002).

In 2003–2004, National Health and Nutrition Examination Survey (NHANES) data showed that 33.6 percent of U.S. children and adolescents were either obese (17.1 percent) or at risk of becoming obese (16.5 percent) (Ogden et al., 2006). The analysis of trends from NHANES data reveal that, when compared with non-Hispanic white cohorts, non-Hispanic black and Mexican-American children and adolescents, ages 2 to 19 years, have a greater prevalence of obesity.[1] Non-Hispanic African-Americans and Mexican-American children and adolescents are also at greater risk of becoming obese (Hedley et al., 2004; Ogden et al., 2006). The prevalence rates of obesity and at risk for obesity in children and adolescents by age, sex, and racial/ethnic group for 2003 and 2004 are shown in Figure 3-1.

State-specific prevalence and trends among 2- through 4-year-old children from low-income U.S. families were examined from 1989 to 2000. The results showed significant increases in obesity among low-income children in 30 states and significant decreases in childhood underweight in 26 states (Sherry et al., 2004). Although no geographic predominance was apparent, the number of states reporting obesity prevalence rates of more than 10 percent increased from 11 in 1989 to 28 in 2000. The number of states reporting decreased rates of underweight also rose during the same time frame, as reflected by 9 states in 1989 and 23 states in 2000 that had underweight prevalence rates equal to or less than 5 percent (Sherry et al., 2004).

National obesity prevalence data are limited for American Indian/ Alaska Native and Asian/Pacific Islander children and youth. Nevertheless, an analysis of data for 9,464 American Indian children and youth, ages 5 to 18 years, compared with NHANES II data (1976 to 1980) found that 39 percent had BMIs above the 85th percentile (Jackson, 1993). Another analysis estimated the prevalence of obesity in a sample of 1,704 7-year-old children from 7 American-Indian communities across the United States to be between 27 and 30 percent for boys and girls, and the at-risk obesity prevalence was estimated at 20 to 21 percent for boys and girls (Caballero et al., 2003). In 2002 and 2003, an analysis of 11,538 American Indians, ages 5 to 17 years, attending 55 schools on 12 reservations located in the

---

[1]Obesity is defined in this report as a BMI for age at or above the sex-specific 95th percentile of the Centers for Disease Control and Prevention (CDC) BMI charts developed in 2000. At risk for obesity is defined as a BMI for age at or above the sex-specific 85th percentile but less than the 95th percentile of the CDC BMI charts.

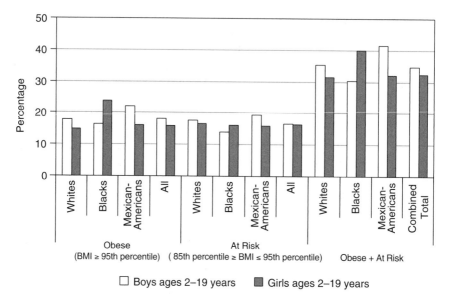

FIGURE 3-1 Percentage of U.S. children and adolescents ages 2 to 19 years who are obese or at risk for obesity by sex and race/ethnicity in 2003 to 2004.
SOURCE: Ogden et al. (2006).

Aberdeen Area of the Indian Health Service (North Dakota, South Dakota, Iowa, and Nebraska), found that both the obesity prevalence and the at-risk obesity prevalence rates exceeded the levels for all U.S. children at almost every age group. The obesity prevalence rate was 24 percent for 5-year-old American-Indian children. Nearly one half (47 percent) of 5-year-old boys and 41 percent of 5-year-old girls were at risk for obesity (Zephier et al., 2006).

There are limited data on the prevalence rates of obesity among Alaska-Native children and youth. One analysis examined the BMI levels of 1,632 students, ages 3 to 18 years, in 20 rural Alaskan communities. Results showed that nearly 50 percent were either obese (25 percent; n = 407) or at risk for obesity (24 percent; n = 392) (Dirks et al., 2006). National prevalence data for Asian/Pacific-Islander populations are not available. However, the obesity prevalence rate among a sample of low-income preschool children in Hawaii was 8.7 percent in 1997, whereas the national mean that year was 10.3 percent. However, the rate caught up to the national mean in 2002, with prevalence rates of 13.1 percent in Hawaii and 13.5 percent nationally (Baruffi et al., 2004). A cross-sectional study of 21,911 Samoan, Filipino, Hawaiian, Asian, Hispanic/Latino, African-American, and white toddlers ages 12 to 59 months participating in the Hawaii Special Supplemental Nutrition Program for Women, Infants, and Children (WIC) in 1997 and 1998 found a higher than expected prevalence of obesity among preschoolers ages 2 to 4 years. Samoan toddlers had the highest prevalence of obesity at 27 percent, followed by Filipinos (12.4 percent), Hawaiians (11.3 percent), Hispanics (10.1 percent), Asians (9.0 percent), whites (8.5 percent), and African Americans (7.3 percent) (Baruffi et al., 2004).

Health Effects of Childhood Obesity

Type 2 diabetes, which accounted for less than 3 percent of all cases of new-onset diabetes among children and adolescents two decades ago, today accounts for between 30 and 45 percent of new-onset cases among adolescences and young adults (ADA, 2000; Rosenbloom et al., 1999). An analysis of data from NHANES (1999–2000), representing 27 million U.S. adolescents, showed a higher prevalence of impaired fasting glucose levels (an indicator for type 2 diabetes risk) among obese adolescents (17.8 percent) that among adolescents of normal weight (7.0 percent). In addition, the data showed that the rate of impaired fasting glucose levels was most pronounced among Mexican-American adolescents (13.0 percent) compared with the rates among African-American (4.2 percent) and white adolescents (7.0 percent) (Williams et al., 2005). On the basis of an analysis of data from NHANES (1999 to 2002) with a sample of 4,370 adolescents ages 12 to 19 years, the prevalence of type 2 diabetes was substantial and was projected to affect more than 39,000 U.S. adolescents and 2.77 million adolescents with impaired fasting glucose levels. These estimates present important implications for public health because of the high level of conversion from an impaired fasting glucose level to type 2 diabetes in adults and the increased risk of CVD in individuals with type 2 diabetes (Duncan, 2006).

American-Indian/Alaska-Native, African-American, and Hispanic/ Latino adolescents have a higher prevalence of type 2 diabetes than white adolescents; and this rise has occurred in parallel with the obesity epidemic among both children and adults (Gahagan et al., 2003; Oeltmann et al., 2003; Pinhas-Hamiel and Zeitler, 2005). American Indians/Alaska Natives have the highest rates of type 2 diabetes of any racial/ethnic group in the United States (National Diabetes Information Clearinghouse, 2005) and significant rates of heritability of CVD (North et al., 2003). Type 2 diabetes is a major public health crisis among American Indian/Alaska Native adolescents. From 1990 to 1998, the total number of young American Indians/ Alaska Natives diagnosed with diabetes increased by 71 percent, and the prevalence increased by 46 percent (6.4 per 1,000 population to 9.3 per 1,000 population). An increase in prevalence was greater among adolescents ages 15 to 19 years and young adults (Acton et al., 2002). Between

1990 and 2001, the prevalence of type 2 diabetes increased by 106 percent among 15- to 19-year-old American-Indian youth and increased by 50 percent among American-Indian children and youth younger than 15 years of age (IHS National Diabetes Program, 2004).

Sociodemographic Profiles

Racial/Ethnic Diversity of the U.S. Population

According to the 2000 U.S. Census, approximately 30 percent of the U.S. population identified themselves as members of a racial or an ethnic minority group. The 2000 Census counted more than 36 million African Americans (12.9 percent of the population); more than 35 million Hispanics/Latinos (12.5 percent) who live in the United States and another 3.8 million who live in the Commonwealth of Puerto Rico; nearly 12 million Asians (4.2 percent); 874,000 Native Hawaiians and other Pacific Islanders; and 4.3 million people (1.5 percent of the total U.S. population) reported that they were American Indians/Alaska Natives (2.4 million or 1 percent reported only American Indian/Alaska Native as their race), of which 35.9 percent live in American Indian areas (which include reservations) or Alaska Native village areas (Hobbs and Stoops, 2002; Ogunwole, 2006). By 2050, it is projected that these groups will account for almost 50 percent of the U.S. population (MBDA, 1999). The ethnic minority population is expected to account for nearly 90 percent of the total growth in the U.S. population, from an ethnic/racial minority population of 69 million in 1995 to one of 186 million in 2050 (MBDA, 1999). Thus, the term "minority" is increasingly misleading as a descriptor for diverse racial/ethnic groups in the aggregate, at least with respect to the proportion of the multicultural U.S. population.

Geographic Variation in Population Diversity

Each of the 50 states throughout the nation has growing childhood, youth, and adult obesity burdens that are leading to overwhelming economic, health, and social challenges that will reverberate at the federal, state, and local levels. Certain issues for high-risk populations dominate in certain states and localities where racial and ethnic minority populations are a numerical majority. Currently, this is the case in California, given the higher proportion of Hispanics/Latinos and African Americans compared with the proportion of non-Hispanic whites.

Hispanics/Latinos, who represent 20 different nationalities, are the nation's largest and fastest-growing ethnic group as the result of ongoing immigration and natural increases in the birth rates of Hispanic/Latino citizens (NRC, 2006a). Given current demographic trends, nearly one in five U.S. residents will be of Hispanic/Latino origin by 2025 (NRC, 2006b).[2]

In addition to California, it is projected that by 2025, Texas, New Mexico, Hawaii, and the District of Columbia will also have population distributions in which non-Hispanic whites will be the minority (MBDA, 1999). Collectively, these four states and the District of Columbia represent 25 percent of the entire U.S. population. From this perspective on U.S. population demographics, finding ways to meet the challenges of addressing childhood obesity in racially, ethnically, and culturally diverse contexts becomes an urgent priority.

Socioeconomic Status, Poverty, Health Disparities, and Health Outcomes

Socioeconomic Status and Poverty

Patterns of disease are best understood within the context of social determinants of health, which represent the societal conditions that affect health and that can be changed by social and health policies and programs. Three categories of social determinants that potentially affect health include social institutions (e.g., cultural and faith-based organizations, political structures, and economic systems including availability and distribution of fresh fruits and vegetables), physical surroundings (e.g., neighborhoods, worksites, towns, and cities), and social relationships (e.g., social networks and the differential treatment of subpopulations) (Anderson et al., 2003b). The implications of social determinants of health for assessing and evaluating progress in obesity prevention are discussed at the end of this chapter and in Chapter 6.

Research has shown that the SES characteristics of the neighborhood in which individuals live (e.g., average income and percent unemployment) are better predictors than individual characteristics of morbidity and mortality (Diez-Roux et al., 1997; Finkelstein et al., 2004; Jargowsky, 1997), and that poverty is the most powerful single determinant of health (Lynch et al., 1997). Poverty causes poor health through its connection with reduced access to and use of health care services (with the quality of preventive, primary, and specialty health care services for this population often

---

[2]The terms *Hispanic* and *Latino* are used interchangeably in this report. Both terms are used in the U.S. census. The United States population includes individuals from 20 Spanish-speaking nationalities, of which nearly one-half are foreign born and 40 percent are undocumented immigrants. Immigrants from Mexico, Puerto Rico, and Cuba represent more than 75 percent of the Hispanic/Latino population in the United States (NRC, 2006a,b).

being lower), food insecurity[3] and low-quality diets, and behaviors that do not support healthy lifestyles (DHHS and AHRQ, 2005; NCHS, 2005). African-American, Hispanic/Latino, and American Indian/Alaska Native households are substantially overrepresented among all U.S. households with incomes below the poverty level (DeNavas-Walt et al., 2005; NRC, 2006b; Robert and House, 2000). Moreover, children and adults in families with incomes below or near the federal poverty level[4] have poorer health outcomes than those in families with higher incomes (DHHS and AHRQ, 2005; IOM, 2003).

In 2003, 11 percent of U.S. children had no health insurance (Annie E. Casey Foundation, 2006). Children in low-income families are substantially more likely than children in higher-income families to lack health care coverage (NCHS, 2005). In 2002 and 2003, uninsured children were three times more likely than their counterparts with insurance (32 percent versus 11 percent, respectively) to have not had a visit to a physician or health clinic for health care within the previous year (NCHS, 2005). Racial/ethnic minority children and youth face a number of barriers to receiving timely, appropriate, and high-quality health care services (NCHS, 2005; NRC, 2006a). Children covered by Medicaid are nearly six times more likely than children covered by private insurance to be treated for obesity. In addition, the treatment of obesity in children covered by Medicaid is more expensive (approximately $6,700/year) than the treatment of obesity for children covered by private insurance (approximately $3,700/year) (Thomson Medstat, 2006). Children with obesity experience higher rates of hospitalizations and greater use of physician services than their nonobese peers (Thomson Medstat, 2006).

The percentage of Americans living in poverty increased from 11.3 percent in 2000 to 12.5 percent in 2003. The 2004 poverty rate among children under 6 years of age was 21 percent (Annie E. Casey Foundation, 2006). In 2004, 38.2 million individuals (an estimated 11.9 percent of the total population), including 13.9 million children, lived in households with food insecurity (Nord et al., 2005). Several studies examining the relationships among food insecurity, SES, and obesity in children or youth have not been able to demonstrate a strong association or causal effect after adjustment for other factors (Hofferth and Curtin, 2005; Kaiser et al., 2002; Matheson et al., 2002; Whitaker and Orzol, 2006).

---

[3]*Food insecurity* describes households that have limited or an uncertain availability of nutritionally adequate and safe foods or that have the inability to acquire such foods in a socially acceptable way.

[4]Federal poverty guidelines are issued annually in the *Federal Register* by the U.S. Department of Health and Human Services and are used to determine the financial eligibility of individuals and households for federal assistance programs (DHHS, 2006a).

Many racial/ethnic minority subpopulations have experienced social, political, and historical contextual events that continue to have long-lasting effects on their physical health, psychosocial well-being, and economic livelihoods (Duran et al., 1998; NRC, 2006b; Williams and Collins, 1995). The challenges associated with understanding the relationship between SES and obesity risk are discussed in Box 3-1.

Immigration and Acculturation

Immigrants are the fastest-growing segment of the U.S. population. As a percentage of the total population, the foreign-born population increased

---

BOX 3-1
Challenges in Understanding the Relationship
Between Socioeconomic Status and Obesity Risk

Despite the substantial variation in BMI that exists as a function of both SES and race/ethnicity, uncertainties remain as to whether these rates can be attributed solely to SES, because obesity disparities are not the same across ethnic groups and they do not emerge at comparable times during childhood (Parsons et al., 1999). There is no consensus about the reasons for these disparities, although recent research provides certain insights. Variation in obesity risk by race/ethnicity and SES appears to occur early in life. An assessment of 16,000 preschool children, ages 2 to 4 years, enrolled in the Head Start Program in New York City found that 27 percent were obese and 15 percent were at risk for obesity. An estimated one in four Head Start children in that sample were found to be obese by the age of 2 years, and one in three children were obese by the age of 4 years. Although obesity was identified as a problem among all Head Start children in New York City, Hispanic/Latino and African-American preschoolers are disproportionately affected (New York City Department of Health and Mental Hygiene, 2006). Moreover, socioeconomic deprivation in childhood has been found to be both a strong predictor of obesity in adulthood for African-American adult women (James et al., 2006a) and adult hypertension in adulthood for African-American men (James et al., 2006b).

Mexican-American children and youth living along the U.S.-Mexico border experience higher levels of economic disadvantages and special challenges in accessing foods that contribute to a healthful diet, regular physical activity, and health care services (Abarca and Ramachandran, 2005; Ruiz-Beltran and Kamau, 2001). Low-SES Mexican school-aged children living along the U.S. border in Tijuana, adjacent to San Diego County in California, have been found to be at increased risk of obesity and related chronic diseases, which may be related to less healthful food choices for children attending schools in low-SES neighborhoods (Villa-Caballero et al., 2006). In contrast, among Mexican children and adolescents, particularly those living in urban areas, obesity is increasing among higher SES groups (IOM, 2007).

Analyses of nationally representative longitudinal data—the National Longitu-dinal Survey of Youth (Strauss and Knight, 1999; Strauss and Pollack, 2001) and the National Longitudinal Study of Adolescent Health (NLSAH) (Goodman, 1999)—have suggested that family SES is inversely related to obesity prevalence in children and that the effects of SES and race/ethnicity are independent of other variables. A more recent analysis of a nationally representative sample of adoles-cents enrolled in the NLSAH examined trends in racial/ethnic disparities for lead-ing health indicators from *Healthy People 2010* (Harris et al., 2006) across multiple domains from adolescence to young adulthood. The results revealed that the health risk increased for 15 of 20 indicators among racially/ethnically diverse ado-lescents. Access to health care decreased from the teen to the adult years for most U.S. racial/ethnic groups, and the disparity was particularly high for Ameri-can Indians (Harris et al., 2006).

Analyses of nationally representative cross-sectional data reveal additional findings that can help to provide an understanding of the relationship between SES and obesity. An examination of the 1988 to 1994 NHANES data showed that the prevalence of obesity in white adolescents was higher for those in low-income families, but there was no clear relationship between family income and obesity in individuals in other age or racial/ethnic subgroups (Ogden et al., 2003; Troiano and Flegal, 1998). A more recent analysis of trends in the association between poverty and adolescents' obesity risk was conducted for four cross-sectional NHANES surveys conducted from 1971 to 2004 (Miech et al., 2006). Although the obesity prevalence did not differ by SES or family poverty status for teens through age 14 years, a widening disparity was observed for 15- to 17-year-olds, especially boys, girls, non-Hispanic whites, and non-Hispanic African Americans. There was a 50 percent higher risk of obesity among adolescents in poor families compared with that among adolescents in non-poor families. Possible mechanisms that con-tributed to the obesity risk for adolescents were physical inactivity, higher levels of consumption of sweetened beverages, and skipping breakfast (Miech et al., 2006).

from 4.7 percent in 1970 to 11.5 percent in 2002 (Dey and Lucas, 2006). The children of immigrant families are thus among the fastest-growing and the most ethnically diverse segment of the American child population. The median age of the individuals who make up the Hispanic/Latino second generation, for example, is just over 12 years (NRC, 2006b). Significant differences in the physical health status exist among U.S.-born and foreign-born individuals. Differences in the lengths of stay of immigrants in the United States suggest that the role of acculturation on immigrant health is complex and differs for various racial/ethnic groups (Dey and Lucas, 2006; Goel et al., 2004; Gordon-Larsen et al., 2003). However, what is clear from the available evidence is that the acculturation of young and adult immi-grant populations is associated with the adoption of lifestyle behaviors and social norms that promote weight gain and obesity.

An analysis of a nationally representative sample of 13,783 adolescents from the National Longitudinal Study of Adolescent Health found that second- and third-generation adolescents of U.S. immigrant families, especially Asian-American and Hispanic/Latino adolescents born in the United States, are twice as likely to be obese than the first-generation residents (Popkin and Udry, 1998). In another study, acculturation to the United States was identified as a risk factor for obesity-related behaviors, such as increased television viewing and higher levels of consumption of energy-dense and low-nutrient foods among Asian-American and Hispanic/Latino adolescents (Unger et al., 2004).

The disparities in the rates of obesity for Hispanic/Latino adolescents have been attributed to environmental, contextual, biological, and socio-cultural factors, in addition to differences in income and education (NRC, 2006a,b). The families of foreign-born immigrant youth are more likely to have both lower family incomes and mothers with lower levels of education. They are also more likely than their American-born counterparts to live in communities with higher densities of immigrants and greater linguistic isolation (Gordon-Larsen et al., 2003). Additionally, children from immigrant families have more compromised physical health than children from nonimmigrant families and use health care services less frequently (Huang et al., 2006).

The deleterious effects of acculturation among Hispanic/Latino youth suggests that this ethnic population will be increasingly burdened by the complications of obesity, and the U.S. health care system will be faced with larger numbers of Hispanics/Latinos experiencing chronic diseases and their complications (NRC, 2006a).

These trends for immigrant youth parallel the observations for immigrant adults. Among the different immigrant subgroups, the number of years of residence in the United States is associated with higher BMI levels after 10 years, and the prevalence of obesity among immigrants who have lived in the United States for at least 15 years has been found to approach that of American-born adults (Goel et al., 2004).

Health Disparities and Health Outcomes

Health disparities are commonly defined as the population-specific differences in the presence of disease, health outcomes, or access to health care among racial, ethnic, and SES groups (Chen et al., 2006; Lavizzo-Mourey et al., 2005; Yancy et al., 2005). Because of the complexity of identifying, measuring, and monitoring health status and health determinants, it is challenging to reach a consensus about the dimensions of health disparities. Complicated relationships and interactions among race, ethnicity, gender, income, education, degree of acculturation, immigrant status, and place of residence have an impact on health disparities and health outcomes (IOM, 2006). Additionally, the lack of complete and accurate data examining health disparities among children between and within racial and ethnic groups and children living across a full spectrum of SES levels limits understanding of the relative contributions and moderators of these disparities (Chen et al., 2006).

Key influences on understanding the pathways to health include a more complete knowledge of prenatal and other vulnerable periods; predisease pathways, representing the early and long-term precursors to disease; cumulative health risks across time; gene-environment interactions; and the intergenerational transmission of behaviors (NRC, 2001). Exposure to life stressors and health status are inextricably connected. For example, the effects of adverse childhood experiences, especially during critical developmental periods in childhood, on obesity and the health risks of stress and depression are areas of ongoing research (Ackard et al., 2003).

Adverse childhood experiences are an example of a set of life contexts which are experienced early in life, yet have profound effects on health and obesity risks into adulthood, independent of SES, race, and ethnicity. The Adverse Childhood Experiences (ACE) Study explored the exposures of more than 13,000 adult enrollees in a health maintenance organization to eight categories of adverse childhood experiences (e.g., abuse). The risk for obesity increased with the number and the severity of each type of childhood abuse (Williamson et al., 2002). Although the ACE Study addressed adult health outcomes rather than childhood health outcomes, the results support the hypothesis that a variety of physical, mental health, and social problems have common roots and that negative health-related behaviors may serve as coping strategies to manage the long-term consequences of childhood stress. Difficult and stressful childhood circumstances may increase the risk for mental health problems in children, which may in turn increase the risk for behaviors that contribute to childhood obesity (Goodman and Whitaker, 2002; Lumeng et al., 2003; Williamson et al., 2002). Many of these responses decrease the ability of individuals to self-regulate both physiological and emotional responses (van der Kolk and Fisler, 1994).

An improved understanding of the complex interplay of the environmental and the biological factors that influence behaviors can be achieved only through the synthesis of the findings of many scientific disciplinary perspectives. Such a synthesis of findings will allow a greater understanding of the complex web of risk factors for childhood obesity, enhance the ability to design more effective interventions, and improve the ability to develop appropriate evaluation measures (Box 3-2). Additionally, further research is needed to clarify the vulnerable periods in childhood and adolescence with particular relevance to risks for obesity and to understand how best to apply this knowledge to preventive efforts.

BOX 3-2
The Life Course Approach to Health

A life course approach refers to how health status at any given age or for any given birth cohort reflects both contemporary conditions and prior living circumstances, from in utero through childhood, adolescence, and adulthood. This perspective views health as the product of these life experiences—both the risks and the protective experiences and environments—and acknowledges that life experiences have a cumulative impact. This approach also recognizes that individuals have developmental trajectories that are both biological and social over time and that they are shaped by the social, economic, political, technological, and ecological contexts of societies. A life course health development framework can be used to understand and address the complex web of interacting risk factors that place individuals and populations at higher risk for health disparities, including childhood obesity. This framework shows the close interaction of risk factors that may initially appear to be unrelated but that resonate across the web of health influences at multiple levels, from the societal level to the community and individual levels. Changes in any of these risks will have long-term effects and implications for the individual into adulthood. The development of health trajectories is characterized by the following features:

- The multiple determinants of health operate in genetic, biological, behavioral, social, and economic contexts that change throughout the life course.
- Health development is an adaptive process involving multiple interactions between these contexts and biobehavioral regulatory systems (e.g., the neuroendocrine system).
- Health trajectories are the cumulative result of risk and protective factors and other influences that can influence biobehavioral regulatory systems during critical periods of development.
- The timing and sequence of biological, psychological, cultural, and social experiences influence the health and development of children, youth, and populations.

SOURCES: Halfon and Hochstein (2002); Krieger (2001); Yu (2006).

INTERVENTIONS AND POLICY LEVERS
FOR HIGH-RISK POPULATIONS

Because the communities and populations that are at higher risk for childhood obesity are often those with larger numbers of ethnically diverse and lower-SES groups, it is important to take into account the collective contexts of these communities as interventions are developed or adapted. As important as the issue of obesity prevention may be, many of these communities are facing problems that have immediate consequences (e.g., unemployment, poor schools, and violence) leaving fewer resources available for obesity prevention. The barriers to the implementation of obesity prevention programs in these contexts should be acknowledged in designing and implementing interventions. For example, communities may be less receptive to people who do not live with them and who have limited experience with the daily realities of the communities. Additionally, there may be limited response to those who identify the priorities of the community without participatory input from community members. The short-term nature of research projects and grant funding can also be an impediment to community engagement if effective programs are dismantled before a problem is sufficiently addressed or before approaches are modified and institutionalized for long-term sustainability. Further, lifestyle change interventions may be perceived as a negative judgment of a community, which may increase the level of fatalism or sense of futility about whether a problem can be addressed, as well as create conflict between communities and external program staff. Careful attention to these issues can be instrumental in overcoming barriers. Seeking community involvement early on and throughout an intervention's development, implementation, and evaluation is particularly important.

Because many conditions and health outcomes share common underlying causes and affect individuals in the same families and communities, it will be necessary to address these problems in an integrated way as they are experienced in communities (Kumanyika, 2005). It must also be acknowledged that interventions that have worked in one community may not be effective or may need to be adapted to low-income and racially/ethnically diverse communities because of such factors as competing risks and threats, cost, an overwhelmed local infrastructure, or different cultural values and practices. An ecologic and culturally competent[5] paradigm is urgently needed to address the spectrum of barriers that racial/ethnic groups and low-income children and youth face to identify the most promising practices that will reduce the prevalence of obesity and promote healthy lifestyles.

Issues Related to Progress

Despite the multiple challenges that diverse communities experience, resources and assets exist that should be used to design, implement, and evaluate childhood obesity prevention interventions. Many communities have a strong sense of their cultural roots, including a deep connection to

---

[5]Culturally competent approaches provide culturally and linguistically appropriate services and have the potential to reduce health disparities among member of different racial and ethnic groups. Cultural competency is optimized when the target populations are involved in all phases of a program or intervention from planning to implementation, monitoring, and evaluation.

their families and histories of healthful traditional foods and physical activities. The translocation of cultural values onto these communities has proven to be less effective than the use of interventions that arise from community values. For example, many community interventions that promote the health of the family and community are more likely to be successful than those that promote actions intended to improve one's own health. This cultural belief in the value of working to enhance the common good may be a leverage point for interventions, especially given the powerful effect that collective efficacy[6] has on obesity risk in youth (Cohen et al., 2006). Other strengths often include a respect for elders, a network of an extended family with norms governing an individual's place within that structure, strong spiritual values, and the integral nature of movement to music (such as dance) as a celebratory activity throughout life.

Interventions that are designed and evaluated with meaningful input from a community and that reinforce the strengths and assets of the community members are more likely to be effective and sustainable. Actively involving key stakeholders, decision makers, or sectors of a community as integral components of an intervention team at all stages, from the initial conceptualization of the intervention to monitoring and evaluation, can enhance trust between the researchers and community members (DHHS, 2001; Pyramid Communications, 2003) (Appendix G). Researchers and funders are using community-based participatory research approaches that emphasize collaboration with communities to explore and act on local concerns. This research approach allows stakeholders to identify the key problems to be studied, formulate research questions in culturally sensitive ways, and use study results to support relevant program and policy development or social change. Every obesity prevention initiative does not require using participatory research methods. However, when the results of an initiative are to be used for and by communities, members of the community should collaborate in all stages, including generating the findings and determining the ways in which the evaluation results are formulated, interpreted, and applied (Green and Mercer, 2001).

The culture and beliefs held by a community may be a powerful tool that can be used to promote health beyond an intervention. For example, in a diabetes prevention study conducted in a Pima Indian community, the biological outcomes for the lifestyle intervention group were less positive than those for the control group whose activities emphasized Pima history and culture (Narayan et al., 1998). As efforts are made to evaluate the effectiveness of obesity prevention interventions nationwide, there is a need to standardize interventions for comparison purposes. However, this must

---

[6]*Collective efficacy* is the willingness of community members to look out for each other and intervene when problems arise.

be balanced with the adaptation of interventions to local cultures and worldviews (Yancey et al., 2006c).

A variety of opportunities exist for targeting, implementing, and evaluating policies and interventions reaching diverse populations of children and youth at the highest risk for obesity and related chronic diseases. For example, the Head Start Program delivers a range of services related to comprehensive nutrition and nutrition education to foster healthy development and school readiness in low-income preschool children ages 2 to 5 years throughout the nation. The U.S. Department of Agriculture (USDA) administers 15 federal food assistance and nutrition safety-net programs through the states to improve the nutritional well-being of low-income households with children and youth. (See Chapter 4 and Appendix D for information on the evaluation of these programs.)

Policy makers can reinforce current programs to foster food security and equity by adding a specific childhood obesity prevention component to the Head Start Program and the USDA-administered federal nutrition programs including the Food Stamp Program (FSP), the WIC program, and the school nutrition programs (Kumanyika and Grier, 2006). Other potential policy levers include Medicaid, the State Child Health Insurance Program (SCHIP) (Lurie et al., 2005), and the engagement and mobilization of faith-based communities to achieve childhood obesity prevention goals (Chapter 6).

As a means to improve existing evaluation and surveillance systems, federal and state initiatives—such as the Early and Periodic Screening, Diagnostic, and Treatment program, which provides comprehensive health care services for infants, children, and adolescents enrolled in Medicaid; the SCHIP; WIC; FSP; and the school nutrition programs—should measure the impact of the programs on obesity risk beyond outputs[7] in order to further document the structural, policy, behavioral, and health outcomes that are directly linked to childhood obesity rates.

Moreover, there will need to be a creative pursuit of innovative and cost-effective interventions such as the Farmer's Market Nutrition Program (USDA, 2006), and evaluating the effectiveness of interventions such as school health report cards in reaching low-income and uninsured children in states where children do not receive regular preventive health care services from a primary care provider.

Because fewer opportunities for physical activity are found, on average, in low-income communities and those with higher proportions of racially/ethnically diverse groups, innovative programs are needed that promote

---

[7]*Outputs* refer to the direct products of activities, usually a tangible deliverable produced as a result of an activity. Examples of outputs include the number of people reached, the number of sessions conducted, the number of volunteers engaged, or the amount of educational material distributed.

environmental justice—efforts that address the disproportionate exposures to harmful environmental conditions by low-income and minority communities—and opportunities for physical activity for populations at high risk for obesity (Day, 2006; Powell et al., 2004). Changes in the built environment are needed in many cities and communities to enhance opportunities for physical activity; however, environmental intervention approaches are less well developed, particularly in terms of legislative policy changes (Burdette and Whitaker, 2005; Sallis and Glanz, 2006; Sloane et al., 2006; Yancey et al., 2006c; Zimring et al., 2005).

The challenges presented by neighborhood violence, inadequate pedestrian safety accommodations (e.g., high-speed traffic, few signals or stop signs), the deterioration of parks and sidewalks, and dual working parents indicate that the school and after-school settings are critical venues for reaching children and youth. Increasing the amount of time in physical education and the quality of physical education in schools is an important step (Burgeson et al., 2001) (Chapter 7). For example, physical education has been demonstrated to result in a decrease in weight gain among elementary school girls (Datar and Sturm, 2004). However, this is as far as most states have pursued measures to increase childhood physical activity from a legislative perspective and many of these efforts have been limited (TFAH, 2005) (Chapter 7).

More collective efforts that have been evaluated and proven to be effective are needed to reintroduce vigorous physical activity across the entire school day to achieve increases in energy expenditure among children and youth (Kumanyika and Grier, 2006; Yancey et al., 2005). One example of an intervention approach developed in less affluent urban and suburban schools with substantial ethnic minority populations is Take 10!® (Lloyd et al., 2005; Stewart et al., 2004), described in Box 3-3.

BOX 3-3
Innovative Physical Activity Promotion Programs

Take 10!®
Take 10!® is a classroom-based program that integrates physical activity into the curriculum of kindergarten to fifth-grade elementary school students. Ten-minute physical activity sessions are linked to math, science, social studies, and language arts lessons to substitute for sedentary, didactic learning approaches. Early studies of Take 10!® by the International Life Sciences Institute (ILSI) Center for Health Promotion have demonstrated the feasibility and utility of this approach for regularly engaging students and teachers in physical activity at a moderate to vigorous intensity range for 10 minutes and found that it can count toward the minimum 30 minutes of moderate to vigorous physical activity per day in schools recommended by the Centers for Disease Control and Prevention. Evaluation results have

shown that 75 percent of teachers reported that they were able to do a Take 10![®] activity at least three times per week in the first two semesters, and the program was sustained by 60 to 80 percent of the teachers for three or more times per week after 1 year (ILSI, 2006; ILSI Center for Health Promotion, 2005; Lloyd et al., 2005; Stewart et al., 2004).

Physical Activity Across the Curriculum

The goals of the Physical Activity Across the Curriculum (PAAC) study were to incorporate physical activity into regular academic lessons and to assist students with accumulating each week 90 to 100 minutes of physical activity that they perform during the school day, in addition to physical education (PE) and recess. The evaluation methods included direct observation of weekly physical activity by using SOFIT,[a] the collection of annual BMI measurements, the performance of weekly and annual surveys and annual focus groups with teachers, and the collection of measures of health risk and academic achievement at the baseline and 3 years after the intervention (Donnelly, 2005). The results of the National Institutes of Health-funded study of PAAC/Take 10![®] conducted by researchers at the University of Kansas demonstrated that by the beginning of the third year of implementation, more than 70 percent of elementary school non-PE teachers had been conducting 10-minute physical activity breaks in 14 low-income intervention schools across 3 cities in which an estimated 75 percent of students qualified for free or reduced-cost lunches (ILSI Center for Health Promotion, 2005).

Moving School Project

The Moving School project, is another model that was developed in Germany. Moving School replaces the static sitting position, in which children in traditional schools spend the majority of their time (97 percent of lesson time) sitting, with dynamic sitting (53 percent), standing (31 percent), and walking (10 percent) during class time. The study evaluated the differences in physical activity between 22 second-grade students in a Moving School in Hannover, Germany, and 25 second-grade students in a traditional school in Flanders, Belgium. Accelerometer data revealed significantly greater levels of physical activity among the students of the Moving School than among those in the traditional school (Cardon et al., 2004).

[a]SOFIT is a comprehensive tool for assessing the quality of physical education instruction for children in schools. It provides a measure of student activity levels, lessons, and teachers' behaviors during class time.

Examples of Progress

Ongoing and new initiatives across the country provide examples of programs and policy changes focused on improving nutrition and increasing physical activity in populations at high risk for obesity. At the Institute of Medicine (IOM) committee's symposium focused on communities held in Atlanta, Georgia in October 2005, high school students from New York

City described their participation in the efforts of the TRUCE Fitness and Nutrition Center. The TRUCE Center endeavors to engage young people in proactive health initiatives that nurture social responsibility, promote investment in the community, and help to prevent adolescent obesity (Appendix G) (Box 3-4).

The Latino Childhood Obesity Prevention Initiative, administered through the nonprofit organization Latino Health Access, is a multiyear demonstration project that involves parents, students, teachers, principals, and other stakeholders in making changes relevant to increasing physical activity and improving nutrition in four schools in Orange County, California. The first phase of the program focused on building common ground and raising awareness of the issues through community and parent meetings, formation of an advisory group, exercise classes offered for parents, and use of assessment tools. The effectiveness of the program was evaluated through various indicators, such as the levels of parental participation,

---

BOX 3-4
Harlem Children's Zone

In New York City's Central Harlem neighborhood an extensive community development and enrichment initiative, The Harlem Children's Zone, offers a range of programs that have the potential to positively address childhood obesity. The TRUCE Fitness and Nutrition Center provides African-American and Hispanic/Latino adolescents with a safe space where they can participate in educational, physical activity, and social opportunities including health promotion and nutrition education. The project has demonstrated the importance of physical activity and nutrition in maintaining wellness and preventing disease, involving young people in developing public health strategies, promoting academic excellence, and providing a safe environment with opportunities for physical activity. In response to a community-mapping exercise that documented the lack of available fresh fruits and vegetables in Harlem, the TRUCE Center initiated the Garden Mosaic Project. The Center reclaimed an abandoned city-owned lot where students worked alongside other community members to transform the space into a community garden. To demonstrate their mission of social responsibility, the harvested food is donated to a local soup kitchen that serves homeless people within their community. A key element of the intervention—intergenerational role modeling and storytelling in accordance with African-American tradition—reinforced a positive ethnic identity and self-efficacy as students worked with elderly community members in all aspects of gardening. Evaluations have primarily focused on process and outputs such as monitoring the number of children and youth involved in the program and asking the youth to keep journals to reflect on their learning experiences.

SOURCES: Appendix G; Garden Mosaics (2006).

attendance at events, and parental involvement in physical activity. The second phase of the program focused on mobilizing action. The indicators used to assess this effort included the extent of parental recruitment of other parents to participate in healthful meal preparation classes, the extent of parental participation in school board and city council meetings, and the number of parents participating in physical activity with their children. Evaluation results for Phase I and II indicate that the desired outcomes were achieved. Phase III of the project is under way and will attempt to reduce barriers to incorporating healthy dietary habits and physical activity behaviors for the schools and families (DHHS, 2006b).

American Indian and Alaska Native communities have developed a number of initiatives to address the childhood obesity epidemic (Appendix D), including the development of partnerships with nonprofit organizations, state and local governments, and the federal government. In recognition of the high rates of type 2 diabetes among individuals in native communities described earlier in this chapter, the U.S. Congress established the Special Diabetes Program for Indians (SDPI) through the Indian Health Service (IHS) in 1997 (IHS National Diabetes Program, 2004). Annual SDPI allocations are distributed as ongoing grants to 318 different IHS, tribal, and urban Indian programs in 35 states to provide diabetes prevention and treatment programs (IHS National Diabetes Program, 2004). Each site designs and carries out its own diabetes intervention depending on local priorities. A 2002 survey of programs showed that after SDPI was initiated, 75 percent (compared with 13 percent before the initiation of SDPI) have community-based healthful eating programs for American Indian children, youth, and families; 50 percent (compared with 18 percent before the initiation of SDPI) have school-based healthful eating programs for children; 83 percent (compared with 41 percent before the initiation of SDPI) routinely screen for obesity in children and youth; 60 percent (compared with 18 percent before the initiation of SDPI) currently offer weight management programs for children and youth; 71 percent (compared with 10 percent before the initiation of SDPI) have community-based physical activity programs for children, youth, and families; and 53 percent (compared with 22 percent before the initiation of SDPI) provide school-based physical activity programs. In addition, a number of programs used SDPI funds to provide fitness classes for children and youth, build or improve playgrounds, initiate walking clubs, and provide aerobics classes (IHS National Diabetes Program, 2004).

Nome is a community of approximately 3,500 people situated on the Bering Sea in northwest Alaska. More than half of the city's population is Alaska Native, predominantly members of one of the several Eskimo groups who live in the Norton Sound Region. Summercise is a program sponsored by the Norton Sound Health Corporation; Kawerak, Inc.; the Nome Eskimo Community; the city of Nome; and the Nome Community Center. These sponsors work together to recruit health professionals and healthy role models from the community to provide classes for Nome children during the summer months. Class offerings include many activities drawn from the Eskimo traditions of the region, such as dances, games, and the collection and preparation of traditional subsistence foods. Children are asked to choose a health goal to work on over the summer, such as eliminating sweetened soda, candy, or chips, or being more physically active.

Another example of community action is provided by the Centers for Disease Control and Prevention's Racial and Ethnic Approaches to Community Health (REACH) 2010 demonstration grants. REACH 2010 grants directly support 40 community coalitions throughout the United States, of which 27 (70 percent) focus on CVD or diabetes prevention and management (Jenkins et al., 2004; Levy et al., 2004; Liburd et al., 2005; Ma'at et al., 2002; Tucker et al., 2006). These coalitions include traditional public health partners (e.g., local and state health departments, community-based organizations, universities, and safety-net programs) and nontraditional partners (e.g., boards of education, faith-based organizations, and city or county urban planning and redevelopment agencies).

Cherokee Choices, a program of the Eastern Band of Cherokee Indians in North Carolina, is funded by a REACH 2010 grant. One of its main components is an obesity and diabetes risk-reduction project located at the Cherokee Elementary School. The initiative uses American Indian mentors, who provide healthful eating and physical activity interventions. They also provide emotional support, teach emotional coping skills, assist with academic tutoring, organize trips to sites of cultural significance, and use other techniques to improve the overall health and self-esteem of the children and to decrease their perceived stress. Teachers have reported a variety of positive outcomes, such as a change in the school culture, with a greater emphasis on being healthier. Participants in the mentoring program report positive connections with their mentors, fewer conflicts and improved communication with friends, greater interest in school, fewer missed school days, and greater knowledge of healthful food and beverage choices. The Walk and Talk after-school program is a component of Cherokee Choices and attendance has grown over time (Jeff Bachar, Cherokee Choices program manager, personal communication, June 7, 2006).

Many of the REACH 2010 grants target African-American communities, each of which has a substantive focus on promoting physical activity and healthful eating by using a comprehensive community-wide approach to create systems changes at various levels and with the reinforcement of change at the individual level (Ma'at et al., 2002). Although these projects are not primarily aimed at reducing childhood obesity, a number of their features differentially influence the sociocultural, economic, and physical environments of children and youth (e.g., a focus on women as the family health and nutrition decision makers and caregivers). The programs also attempt to change the organizational practices of adults who are parents, teachers, religious leaders, and coaches and who serve other gatekeeper and decision-maker roles. The programs also pair the demand generation with the supply creation (e.g., the pairing of experiential learning, role modeling, and the provision of culturally relevant health data with healthier restaurant menu items, healthier products in food retail outlets, healthier snacks and refreshments at events and functions, and the incorporation of physical activity into meetings and events in a culturally relevant way such as low- to moderate-intensity movement to music). Project elements include the implementation of organizational wellness programs in local government offices, small businesses, and nonprofit agencies (Yancey et al., 2004, 2006a); the establishment of cardiovascular wellness centers at churches and other faith-based institutions, beauty salons, and barbershops (Ma'at et al., 2002); the organization of a coalition of black churches aimed at educating and supporting women to influence their churches to model healthy behavior change; and the hiring and training of lay health advisers to provide outreach and education in targeted neighborhoods, including the establishment of a farmers' market to link increased access to healthful foods with economic development for local and neighborhood businesses (Liburd et al., 2005).

EVALUATION APPROACHES FOR DIVERSE POPULATIONS

Multicultural and culturally competent approaches to evaluation have only recently emerged as important considerations in evaluating social and public health policies and programs. Applying a paradigm that acknowledges the differences in how people from various backgrounds experience life and view the world will assist and enrich the evaluation of obesity prevention initiatives across and within SES groups and ethnically and culturally diverse populations (Brach and Fraserirector, 2000; Hopson, 2003).

As discussed in Chapter 2, there are a variety of perspectives on what constitutes a high-quality program or effort to prevent childhood obesity. The committee encourages programs and interventions to address several program quality dimensions, including consideration of the needs of underserved and high-risk populations, the use of relevant empirical evidence when the program is designed and implemented, the identification of similar efforts and the establishment of important cross-sectoral connections and collaborations, and consideration of the spectrum of outcomes (e.g., structural, institutional, systemic, behavioral, and health). Programs and interventions should also be able to show how changes in short-term or intermediate outcomes relate to changes in long-term outcomes.

Interventions with evaluation components that target underserved populations and that also increase the level of engagement of these populations in communitywide approaches are urgently needed to effectively address childhood obesity in these diverse groups. Successful engagement will require the identification of the distributional equity and the differential effects of programs on underserved ethnically diverse groups and groups of various SES in order to inform "midcourse corrections" or the next generation of interventions. The capacity to reduce the obesity risk or disparities among certain subpopulations may be adopted as a selection criterion for intervention actions.

Behavioral interventions and evaluation approaches should be expanded into a variety of multicultural and resource-limited settings. The magnitude of the influence of any health promotion intervention will depend on the combination of its effectiveness, the extent and quality of its implementation, and its sustainability (Rogers, 2003). The active promulgation and the use of a variety of evidence-based programs and policies are needed to foster the societal uptake and institutionalization of obesity prevention interventions. Certain types of behavioral outcomes (e.g., tobacco use and immunization status) are easier to evaluate than other outcomes (e.g., cultural competency, social cohesion, civic engagement, and collective efficacy) (Anderson et al., 2003b, 2005).

Furthermore, it is challenging to accurately assess the intermediate outcomes of community interventions aimed at broad social determinants of health, such as community advocacy and economic and educational opportunities, that effect change across multiple intermediate and long-term outcomes because of the limitations in establishing links between upstream health promotion interventions and health outcomes (Anderson et al., 2005) (Chapter 6). The approaches taken must balance the trade-offs between initial selectivity, which improves retention and homogeneity (internal validity), and broader inclusiveness, which preserves relevance to the targeted population (external validity).

Important considerations for the design, implementation, monitoring, and evaluation of culturally competent obesity prevention interventions in diverse populations include the following:

- Build on cultural assets (e.g., the salience of dance as a common form of physical activity among African Americans and Hispanics/ Latinos) (Beech et al., 2003; Boon and Clydesdale, 2005; Day, 2006; Robinson et al., 2003; Yancey et al., 2006c), recognize the role of cultural influence on health, and integrate culturally competent approaches into the delivery of health care and social services (Anderson et al., 2003a; Andrulis, 2005).

- Address multiple health issues pertinent to a range of stakeholders in order to build momentum and community support for interventions (e.g., the Harlem Fitness Zone and the Cherokee Choices projects) and the Active Living by Design interventions (Sallis et al., 2006).
- Recognize that the use of nonintervention control groups may not be acceptable to ethnic minority communities; rather, delayed intervention designs may be more tenable (Boon and Clydesdale, 2005).
- Involve researchers who are knowledgeable about the racial/ethnic groups or cultures being studied or evaluated (American College of Epidemiology, 1995; Anderson et al., 2003a; Gil and Bob, 1999; Hopson, 2003; IOM, 1994; Kumanyika et al., 2005).
- Focus attention on the process of intervening in addition to achieving outcomes. This may include particular attention to delivery channels, messengers, materials and messages, and other cultural adaptations or targeting. Subgroup analyses are critical, and, when differences are found, further examination is needed to explore why the interventions are not effective for certain subgroups (e.g., characteristics of the intervention itself or how it was implemented) (Kreuter and McClure, 2004; Yancey et al., 2006b).

Expanding Surveillance to Identify Areas With High Obesity Burdens and Related Chronic Disease

Data collection and analyses for surveillance and monitoring are core functions of governmental public health practices. However, methodological limitations to the identification and documentation of health disparities must be addressed. The public health infrastructure has the capacity to monitor aggregate racial/ethnic groups (e.g., categories defined by the U.S. Bureau of the Census). However, some individuals in racially/ethnically diverse communities may not participate in formal national data-gathering efforts because of logistical issues and concerns about how the data might be used. These challenges may result in the underrepresentation of racial/ethnic minority populations in national surveillance systems. Representative surveillance and monitoring systems must be established to allow the monitoring of minority populations at potential health risk. The REACH 2010 Risk Factor Survey, for example, is conducted annually in African-American, Hispanic/Latino, Asian/Pacific Islander, and American Indian communities throughout the United States (CDC, 2004). Data from this survey demonstrate that residents in racial/ethnic minority communities experience greater disease risk and burden than individuals in the general population living in similar areas or states.

The continuous and expanded surveillance of health status in racial/ ethnic minority communities is an important measurement challenge for evaluators, yet it is needed to provide accurate disease prevalence estimates for evaluating culturally targeted prevention strategies for smaller geographic areas (e.g., for certain zip codes, school catchments areas, or census tracts). Expanding access to surveillance data would decrease the burden placed on community-based organizations, school districts, and other local government agencies to monitor and evaluate interventions, thereby allowing them to focus on the service delivery missions that motivate their activities (Yancey et al., 2005). The federal and state governments can expand their roles in collecting data by race/ethnicity and refining the definitions of race/ethnicity categories (Lurie et al., 2005).

Surveillance and monitoring systems may not provide the data needed for a comprehensive assessment of program quality. Community-based participatory research is one qualitative research approach to inquiry that emphasizes community partnerships and action for social change and the reduction of health disparities as an integral component of the research process (McAllister et al., 2003). Indeed, qualitative indicators require more precise definitions. Yet, effective programs and services will depend on the ability to measure and evaluate these indicators and integrate an understanding of the indicators into interventions. The ability to measure an array of indicators, both qualitative and quantitative, for a variety of diverse populations and outcomes is central to the elimination of health disparities and the prevention of childhood obesity in high-risk communities.

SUMMARY AND RECOMMENDATIONS

Quantitative assessment of progress over the past few years in preventing childhood obesity in diverse population groups is difficult. Examples are provided throughout the chapter of localized successes and innovative programs that are being implemented and evaluated across the nation. Large-scale initiatives focused on disproportionately affected groups are needed and should incorporate participatory approaches into their design, implementation, and evaluation.

Making progress toward closing the childhood obesity and health disparity gaps in high-risk racial/ethnic minority populations and diverse low-income populations will depend on several factors. These include a national commitment to substantially improve the social and built environments of high-risk communities; defining the contexts and mechanisms that lead to and perpetuate childhood obesity; and designing, implementing, and evaluating effective and culturally competent interventions, evaluation tools, and outcome measures.

Childhood obesity prevention efforts should creatively identify and build upon community assets, collective efficacy, and other leverage points where the needs of diverse populations are served, such as federal nutrition safety-net programs and shared cultural values and traditions. Attention to these factors will promote the implementation and evaluation of promising interventions that can help identify future best practices that support childhood obesity prevention efforts.

Recommendations 2 and 3 discussed in Chapter 2 explicitly propose further action focused on strengthening the implementation and the evaluation of obesity prevention interventions, policies, and initiatives relevant to culturally and ethnically diverse populations. This emphasis highlights the need to carefully consider and involve the people most affected in the policy change or intervention.

Recommendation 2: **Policy makers, program planners, program implementers, and other interested stakeholders—within and across relevant sectors—should evaluate all childhood obesity prevention efforts, strengthen the evaluation capacity, and develop quality interventions that take into account diverse perspectives, that use culturally relevant approaches, and that meet the needs of diverse populations and contexts.**

Recommendation 3: **Government, industry, communities, and schools should expand or develop relevant surveillance and monitoring systems and, as applicable, should engage in research to examine the impact of childhood obesity prevention policies, interventions, and actions on relevant outcomes, paying particular attention to the unique needs of diverse groups and high-risk populations. Additionally, parents and caregivers should monitor changes in their family's food, beverage, and physical activity choices and their progress toward healthier lifestyles.**

REFERENCES

Abarca J, Ramachandran S. 2005. Using community indicators to assess nutrition in Arizona-Mexico border communities. *Prev Chronic Dis* [Online]. Available: http://www.cdc.gov/Pcd/issues/2005/jan/04_0082.htm [accessed July 23, 2006].

Ackard DM, Neumark-Sztainer D, Story M, Perry C. 2003. Overweight among adolescents: Prevalence and associations with weight-related characteristics and psychological health. *Pediatrics* 111(1):67–74.

Acton KJ, Burrows NR, Moore K, Querec L, Geiss LS, Engelgau MM. 2002. Trends in diabetes prevalence among American Indian and Alaska Native children, adolescents, and young adults. *Am J Public Health* 92(9):1485–1490.

ADA (American Diabetes Association). 2000. Type 2 diabetes in children and adolescents. *Pediatrics* 105(3):671–680.

American College of Epidemiology. 1995. Committee on Minority Affairs Statement of Principles on Epidemiology and Minority Populations. *Ann Epidemiol* 5:505–508.

Anderson LM, Scrimshaw SC, Fullilove MT, Fielding JE, Normand J. Task Force on Community Preventive Services. 2003a. Culturally competent healthcare systems. A systematic review. *Am J Prev Health* 24(3 Suppl):68–79.

Anderson LM, Scrimshaw SC, Fullilove MT, Fielding JE, Task Force on Community Preventive Services. 2003b. The community guide's model for linking the social environment to health. *Am J Prev Med* 24(3 Suppl):12–20.

Anderson LM, Brownson RC, Fullilove MT, Teutsch SM, Novick LF, Fielding J, Land GH. 2005. Evidence-based public health policy and practice: Promises and limits. *Am J Prev Med* 28(5 Suppl):226–230.

Andrulis DP. 2005. Moving beyond the status quo in reducing racial and ethnic disparities in children's health. *Public Health Rep* 120(4):370–377.

Annie E. Casey Foundation. 2006. *2006 Kids Count Data Book.* [Online]. Available: http://www.aecf.org/kidscount/sld/databook.jsp [accessed July 10, 2006].

Baruffi G, Hardy CJ, Waslien CI, Uyehara SJ, Krupitsky D. 2004. Ethnic differences in the prevalence of overweight among young children in Hawaii. *J Am Diet Assoc* 104(11):1701–1707.

Beech BM, Klesges RC, Kumanyika SK, Murray DM, Klesges L, McClanahan B, Slawson D, Nunnally C, Rochon J, McLain-Allen B, Pree-Cary J. 2003. Child- and parent-targeted interventions: The Memphis GEMS Pilot Study. *Ethnic Dis* 13(1 Suppl 1):S40–S53.

Boon CS, Clydesdale FM. 2005. A review of childhood and adolescent obesity interventions. *Crit Rev Food Sci Nutr* 45(7–8):511–525.

Brach C, Fraserirector I. 2000. Can cultural competency reduce racial and ethnic health disparities? A review and conceptual model. *Med Care Res Rev* 57(Suppl 1):181–217.

Burdette HL, Whitaker RC. 2005. A national study of neighborhood safety, outdoor play, television viewing, and obesity in preschool children. *Pediatrics* 116(3):657–662.

Burgeson CR, Wechsler H, Brener ND, Young JC, Spain CG. 2001. Physical education and activity: Results from the school health policy and program study 2000. *J School Health* 7(17):279–293.

Caballero B, Himes JH, Lohman T, Davis SM, Stevens J, Evans M, Going S, Pablo J. 2003. Body composition and overweight prevalence in 1704 schoolchildren from 7 American Indian communities. *Am J Clin Nutr* 78(2):308–312.

Cardon G, De Clercq D, De Bourdeaudhuij I, Breithecker D. 2004. Sitting habits in elementary schoolchildren: A traditional versus a "Moving School." *Patient Educ Couns* 54(2):133–142.

CDC (Centers for Disease Control and Prevention). 2004. REACH 2010 surveillance for health status in minority communities—United States, 2001–2002. *MMWR* 53(SS-6):1–36.

Chen E, Martin AD, Matthews KA. 2006. Understanding health disparities: The role of race and socioeconomic status in children's health. *Am J Public Health* 96(4):702–708.

Cohen DA, Finch BK, Bower A, Sastry N. 2006. Collective efficacy and obesity: The potential influence of social factors on health. *Soc Sci Med* 62(3):769–778.

Dabelea D, Hanson RL, Lindsay RS, Pettit DJ, Imperatore G, Gabir MM, Roumain J, Bennett PH, Knowler WC. 2000. Intrauterine exposure to diabetes conveys risks for type 2 diabetes and obesity: A study of discordant sibships. *Diabetes* 49(12):2208–2211.

Datar A, Sturm R. 2004. Physical education in elementary school and BMI: Evidence from the Early Childhood Longitudinal Study. *Am J Public Health* 94(9):1501–1506.

Day K. 2006. Active living and social justice: Planning for physical activity in low-income, black, and Latino communities. *J Am Planning Assoc* 72(1):88–99.

DeNavas-Walt C, Proctor BD, Lee CH. 2005. *Income, Poverty, and Health Insurance Coverage in the United States: 2004.* Current Population Reports, P60-229. U.S. Bureau of the Census. Washington, DC: U.S. Government Printing Office. [Online]. Available: http://www.census.gov/prod/2005pubs/p60-229.pdf [accessed July 12, 2006].

Dey AN, Lucas JW. 2006. Physical and mental health characteristics of U.S.- and foreign-born adults: United States, 1998–2003. *Advance Data from Vital and Health Statistics.* No. 369. Hyattsville, MD: National Center for Health Statistics.

DHHS (U.S. Department of Health and Human Services). 2001. *Mental Health: Culture, Race, and Ethnicity. A Supplement to Mental Health: A Report of the Surgeon General.* Rockville, MD: Office of the Surgeon General. Public Health Service.

DHHS. 2006a. *2006 Federal Poverty Guidelines.* [Online]. Available: http://www.dhhs. state.nh.us/DHHS/PIO/LIBRARY/Policy-Guideline/federal-poverty-guidelines.htm [accessed May 29, 2006].

DHHS. 2006b. *Best Practice Initiative: Latino Health Access Latino Childhood Obesity Prevention Initiative Demonstration Project.* [Online]. Available: http://phs.os.dhhs.gov/ ophs/BestPractice/LatinoObesity.htm [accessed May 29, 2006].

DHHS and AHRQ (Agency for Healthcare Research and Quality). 2005. *2005 National Healthcare Disparities Report.* [Online]. Available: http://www.ahrq.gov/qual/nhdr05/ nhdr05.pdf [accessed April 13, 2006].

Diez-Roux AV, Nieto FJ, Muntaner C, Tyroler HA, Comstock GW, Shahar E, Cooper LS, Watson RL, Szklo M. 1997. Neighborhood environments and coronary heart disease: A multilevel analysis. *Am J Epidemiol* 146(1):48–63.

Dirks LG, Ross-Tsilkowski A, Ballew C. 2006. *Rural Alaska Native Pediatric Height and Weight Survey 2005.* Alaska Native Tribal Health Consortium, Anchorage, AK. Indian Health Service 17th Annual Research Conference, April 24–26. Abstract.

Donnelly JE. 2005 (June 29). *Physical Activity Across the Curriculum/Take 10!* Presentation at the Institute of Medicine Symposium Progress in Preventing Childhood Obesity: Focus on Schools, Wichita, Kansas. Institute of Medicine Committee on Progress in Preventing Childhood Obesity.

Duncan GE. 2006. Prevalence of diabetes and impaired fasting glucose levels among U.S. adolescents. *Arch Pediatr Adolesc Med* 160(5):523–528.

Duran E, Duran B, Brave Heart MYH, Yellow-Horse-Davis S. 1998. Healing the American Indian soul wound. In: Danieli Y, ed. *International Handbook of Multigenerational Legacies of Trauma.* New York: Plenum Press.

Finkelstein EA, Khavjou OA, Mobley LR, Haney DM, Will JC. 2004. Racial/ethnic disparities in coronary heart disease risk factors among WISEWOMAN enrollees. *J Women's Health* 13(5):503–518.

Freedman DS, Khan LK, Serdula MK, Ogden CL, Dietz WH. 2006. Racial and ethnic differences in secular trends for childhood BMI, weight, and height. *Obesity* 14(2):301–308.

Gahagan S, Silverstein J. American Academy of Pediatrics Committee on Native American Child Health. American Academy of Pediatrics Section on Endocrinology. 2003. Prevention and treatment of type 2 diabetes mellitus in children, with special emphasis on American Indian and Alaska Native children. American Academy of Pediatrics Committee on Native American Child Health. *Pediatrics* 112(4):e328.

Garden Mosaics. 2006. *TRUCE Carrie McCracken Community Garden.* New York, NY: Garden Mosaics. [Online]. Available: http://www.gardenmosaics.cornell.edu/pgs/data/ inventoryread.aspx?garden=84 [accessed June 3, 2006].

Gil EF, Bob S. 1999. Culturally competent research: An ethical perspective. *Clin Psychol Rev* 19(1):45–55.

Gillman MW, Rifas-Shiman S, Berkey CS, Field AE, Colditz GA. 2003. Maternal gestational diabetes, birth weight, and adolescent obesity. *Pediatrics* 111(3):e221–e226.

Glanz K, Sallis JF, Saelens BE, Frank LD. 2005. Healthy nutrition environments: Concepts and measures. *Am J Health Promot* 19(5):330–333.

Goel MS, McCarthy EP, Phillips RS, Wee CC. 2004. Obesity among U.S. immigrant subgroups by duration of residence. *J Am Med Assoc* 292(23):2860–2867.

Goodman E. 1999. The role of socioeconomic status gradients in explaining differences in U.S. adolescents health. *Am J Public Health* 89(10):1522–1528.

Goodman E. 2003. Letting the "gini" out of the bottle: Social causation and the obesity epidemic. *J Pediatr* 142(3):228–230.

Goodman E, Whitaker RC. 2002. A prospective study of the role of depression in the development and persistence of adolescent obesity. *Pediatrics* 109(3):497–504.

Gordon-Larsen P, Harris KM, Ward DS, Popkin BM. 2003. Acculturation and overweight-related behaviors among Hispanic immigrants to the U.S.: The National Longitudinal Study of Adolescent Health. *Soc Sci Med* 57(11):2023–2034.

Gordon-Larsen P, Nelson MC, Page P, Popkin BM. 2006. Inequality in the built environment underlies key health disparities in physical activity and obesity. *Pediatrics* 117(2):417–424.

Gostin LO, Powers M. 2006. What does social justice require for the public's health? Public health ethics and policy imperatives. *Health Aff* 25(4):1053–1060.

Green LW, Mercer SL. 2001. Can public health researchers and agencies reconcile the push from funding bodies and the pull from communities? *Am J Public Health* 91(12):1926–1943.

Halfon N, Hochstein M. 2002. Life course health development: An integrated framework for developing health, policy, and research. *Milbank Q* 80(3):433–479.

Halfon N, Inkelas M. 2003. Optimizing the health and development of children. *J Am Med Assoc* 290(23):3136–3138.

Harris KM, Gordon-Larsen P, Chantala K, Udry JR. 2006. Longitudinal trends in race/ethnic disparities in leading health indicators from adolescence to young adulthood. *Arch Pediatr Adolesc Med* 160(1):74–81.

Hedley AA, Ogden CL, Johnson CL, Carroll MD, Curtin LR, Flegal KM. 2004. Prevalence of overweight and obesity among U.S. children, adolescents, and adults, 1999–2002. *J Am Med Assoc* 291(23):2847–2850.

Hobbs F, Stoops N. 2002. *Demographic Trends in the 20th Century. Census 200 Special Reports.* [Online]. Available: http://www.census.gov/prod/2002pubs/censr-4.pdf [accessed July 31, 2006].

Hofferth S, Curtin S. 2005. Poverty, food programs, and childhood obesity. *J Policy Anal Manage* 24(4):703–726.

Hopson R. 2003. *Overview of Multicultural and Culturally Competent Program Evaluation.* Oakland, CA: Social Policy Research Associates. [Online]. Available: http://www.calendow.org/reference/publications/pdf/evaluations/TCE0 509-2004_Overview_of_Mu.pdf [accessed April 18, 2006].

Huang ZJ, Yu SM, Ledsky R. 2006. Health status and health service access and use among children in U.S. immigrant families. *Am J Public Health* 96(4):634–640.

IHS (Indian Health Service). National Diabetes Program, Department of Health and Human Services. 2004. *Interim Report to Congress: Special Diabetes Program for Indians.* [Online]. Available: http://www.ihs.gov/MedicalPrograms/diabetes/resources/r_rtc2004 index.asp [accessed July 12, 2006].

ILSI (International Life Sciences Institute). 2006. *What Is Take 10!®?* [Online]. Available: http://www.take10.net/whatistake10.asp [accessed May 23, 2006].

ILSI Center for Health Promotion. 2005. *A General Overview of Physical Activity and Nutrition Intervention Programs.* [Online]. Available: http://chp.ilsi.org/NR/rdonlyres/ 1287022A-3300-426A-ACCF-C87D5CEA1348/0/SchoolHCCommtyProgramsList ILSICHP041206.pdf [accessed May 31, 2006].

IOM (Institute of Medicine). 1994. *Balancing the Scales of Opportunity: Ensuring Racial and Ethnic Diversity in the Health Professions.* Washington DC: National Academy Press.

IOM. 2001. *Health and Behavior: The Interplay of Biological, Behavioral, and Societal Influences*. Washington DC: National Academy Press.

IOM. 2003. *The Future of the Public's Health in the 21st Century*. Washington, DC: The National Academies Press.

IOM. 2005. *Preventing Childhood Obesity: Health in the Balance*. Washington DC: The National Academies Press.

IOM. 2006. *Examining the Health Disparities Research Plan of the National Institutes of Health: Unfinished Business*. Washington DC: The National Academies Press.

IOM. 2007. *Joint U.S.–Mexico Workshop on Preventing Obesity in Children and Youth of Mexican Origin*. Washington, DC: The National Academies Press.

Jackson MY. 1993. Height, weight, and body mass index of American Indian school children, 1990–1991. *J Am Diet Assoc* 93(10):1136–1140.

James SA, Fowler-Brown A, Raghunathan TE, Van Hoewyk J. 2006a. Life-course socioeconomic position and obesity in African American women: The Pitt County study. *Am J Public Health* 96(3):554–560.

James SA, Van Hoewyk J, Belli RF, Strogatz DS, Williams DR, Raghunathan TE. 2006b. Life-course socioeconomic position and hypertension in African American men: The Pitt County study. *Am J Public Health* 96(5):812–817.

Jargowsky PA. 1997. *Poverty and Place: Ghettos, Barrios and the American City*. New York, NY: Russell Sage Foundation.

Jenkins C, McNary S, Carlson BA, King MG, Hossler CL, Magwood G, Zheng D, Hendrix K, Beck LS, Linnen F, Thomas V, Powell S, Ma'at I. 2004. Reducing disparities for African Americans with diabetes: Progress made by the REACH 2010 Charleston and Georgetown Diabetes Coalition. *Public Health Rep* 119(3):322–330.

Jetter KM, Cassady DL. 2005. The availability and cost of healthier food alternatives. *Am J Prev Med* 30(1):38–44.

Kaiser LL, Melgar-Quinonez HR, Lamp CL, Johns MC, Sutherlin JM, Harwood JO. 2002. Food security and nutritional outcomes of preschool-age Mexican-American children. *J Am Diet Assoc* 102(7):924–929.

Kreuter MW, McClure SM. 2004. The role of culture in health communication. *Annu Rev Public Health* 25:439–455.

Krieger N. 1994. Epidemiology and the web of causation: Has anyone seen the spider? *Soc Sci Med* 39(7):887–903.

Krieger N. 2001. A glossary for social epidemiology. *J Epidemiol Community Health* 55(10): 693–700.

Krieger N, Davey Smith G. 2004. "Bodies count" and body counts: Social epidemiology and embodying inequality. *Epidemiol Rev* 26(1):92–103.

Kumanyika SK. 1994. Obesity in minority populations: An epidemiologic assessment. *Obes Res* 2(2):166–182.

Kumanyika SK. 2005. Obesity, health disparities, and prevention paradigms: Hard questions and hard choices. *Prev Chronic Dis* [Online]. Available: http://www.cdc.gov/Pcd/issues/2005/oct/05_0025.htm [accessed July 23, 2006].

Kumanyika SK, Golden PM. 1991. Cross-sectional differences in health status in U.S. racial/ethnic minority groups: Potential influence of temporal changes, disease, and lifestyle transitions. *Ethn Dis* 1(1):50–59.

Kumanyika SK, Grier S. 2006. Targeting interventions for ethnic minority and low-income populations. In: Paxon C, ed. *Future Child* 16(1):187–207.

Kumanyika SK, Gary TL, Lancaster KJ, Samuel-Hodge CD, Banks-Wallace J, Beech BM, Hughes-Halbert C, Karanja N, Odoms-Young AM, Prewitt TE, Whitt-Glover MC. 2005. Achieving healthy weight in African-American communities: Research perspectives and priorities. *Obes Res* 13(12):2037–2047.

Lavizzo-Mourey R, Richardson WC, Ross RK, Rowe JW. 2005. A tale of two cities. *Health Aff* 24(2):313–315.

Levy SR, Anderson EE, Issel LM, Willis MA, Dancy BL, Jacobson KM, Fleming SG, Copper ES, Berrios NM, Sciammarella E, Ochoa M, Hebert-Beirne J. 2004. Using multilevel, multisource needs assessment data for planning community interventions. *Health Promot Pract* 5(1):59–68.

Li X, Li S, Ulusoy E, Chen W, Srinivasan SR, Berenson GS. 2004. Childhood adiposity as a predictor of cardiac mass in adulthood: The Bogalusa Heart Study. *Circulation* 110(22): 3488–3492.

Liburd LC, Jack L Jr, Williams S, Tucker P. 2005. Intervening on the social determinants of cardiovascular disease and diabetes. *Am J Prev Med* 29(5 Suppl 1):18–24.

Lloyd LK, Cook CL, Kohl HW. 2005. A pilot study of teachers' acceptance of a classroom-based physical activity curriculum tool: Take 10!® *Texas Assoc Health Phys Educ Rec Dance J* 73(3):8–11.

Lumeng JC, Gannon K, Cabral HJ, Frank DA, Zuckerman B. 2003. Association between clinically meaningful behavior problems and overweight in children. *Pediatrics* 112(5): 1138–1145.

Lurie N, Jung M, Lavizzo-Mourey R. 2005. Disparities and quality improvement: Federal policy levers. *Health Aff* 24(2):354–364.

Lynch JW, Kaplan GA, Shema SJ. 1997. Cumulative impact of sustained economic hardship on physical, cognitive, psychological, and social functioning. *N Engl J Med* 337(26): 1889–1895.

Ma'at I, Owens M, Hughes M. 2002. Observations from the CDC. REACH 2010 coalitions: Reaching for ways to prevent cardiovascular disease and diabetes. *J Womens Health* 11(10):829–839.

Matheson DM, Varady J, Varady A, Killen JD. 2002. Household food security and nutritional status of Hispanic children in the fifth grade. *Am J Clin Nutr* 76(1):210–217.

MBDA (Minority Business Development Agency). U.S. Department of Commerce. 1999. *Minority Population Growth: 1995–2050*. [Online]. Available: http://www.mbda.gov/documents/mbdacolor.pdf [accessed June 16, 2006].

McAllister CL, Green BL, Terry MA, Herman V, Mulvey L. 2003. Parents, practitioners, and researchers: Community-based participatory research with early Head Start. *Am J Public Health* 93(10):1672–1679.

McEwen BS. 2001. From molecules to mind: Stress, individual differences, and the social environment. *Ann NY Acad Sci* 935:42–49.

Miech RA, Kumanyika SK, Stettler N, Link BG, Phelan JC, Chang VW. 2006. Trends in the association of poverty with overweight among U.S. adolescents, 1971–2004. *J Am Med Assoc* 295(20):2385–2393.

Narayan KM, Hoskin M, Kozak D, Kriska AM, Hanson RL, Pettitt DJ, Nagi DK, Bennett PH, Knowler WC. 1998. Randomized clinical trial of lifestyle interventions in Pima Indians: A pilot study. *Diabet Med* 15(1):66–72.

National Diabetes Information Clearinghouse. 2005. *National Diabetes Statistics*. [Online]. Available: http://diabetes.niddk.nih.gov/dm/pubs/statistics/index.htm [accessed July 12, 2006].

NCHS (National Center for Health Statistics). 2005. *Health United States, 2005 with Chartbook on Trends in the Health of Americans*. Hyattsville, MD: NCHS. [Online]. Available: http://www.cdc.gov/nchs/data/hus/hus05.pdf [accessed February 11, 2006].

New York City Department of Health and Mental Hygiene. 2006. *Obesity in Early Childhood: More Than 40% of Head Start Children in NYC Are Overweight or Obese.* [Online]. Available: http://www.nyc.gov/html/doh/downloads/pdf/survey/survey-2006childobesity.pdf [accessed April 9, 2006].

Nord M, Andrews M, Carlson S. 2005. *Household Food Security in the United States, 2004.* Economic Research Report Number 11. Washington, DC: Economic Research Service, U.S. Department of Agriculture.

North KE, MacCluer JW, Williams JT, Welty TK, Best LG, Lee ET, Fabsitz RR, Howard BV. 2003. Evidence for distinct genetic effects on obesity and lipid-related CVD risk factors in diabetic compared to nondiabetic American Indians: The Strong Heart Family Study. *Diabetes Metab Res Rev* 19(2):140–147.

NRC (National Research Council). 2001. *New Horizons in Health: An Integrative Approach.* Washington DC: National Academy Press.

NRC. 2006a. *Hispanics and the Future of America.* Washington DC: The National Academies Press.

NRC. 2006b. *Multiple Origins, Uncertain Destinies: Hispanics and the American Future.* Washington DC: The National Academies Press.

NRC and IOM. 2000. *From Neurons to Neighborhoods: The Science of Early Childhood Development.* Washington DC: National Academy Press.

NRC and IOM. 2004. *Children's Health, the Nation's Wealth.* Washington, DC: The National Academies Press.

Oeltmann JE, Liese AD, Heinze HJ, Addy CL, Mayer-Davis EJ. 2003. Prevalence of diagnosed diabetes among African-American and non-Hispanic white youth, 1999. *Diabetes Care* 26(9):2531–2535.

Ogden CL, Carroll MD, Flegal KM. 2003. Epidemiologic trends in overweight and obesity. *Endocrinol Metab Clin N Am* 32(4):741–760, vii.

Ogden CL, Carroll MD, Curtin LR, McDowell MA, Tabak CJ, Flegal KM. 2006. Prevalence of overweight and obesity in the United States, 1999–2004. *J Am Med Assoc* 295(13): 1549–1555.

Ogunwole SU. 2006. *We the People: American Indians and Alaska Natives in the United States.* Census 2000 Special Reports. U.S. Census Bureau. [Online]. Available: http://www.census.gov/prod/2006pubs/censr-28.pdf [accessed July 31, 2006].

Parsons TJ, Power C, Logan S, Summerbell CD. 1999. Childhood predictors of adult obesity: A systematic review. *Int J Obes Relat Metab Disord* 23(Suppl 8):S1–S107.

Pinhas-Hamiel O, Zeitler P. 2005. The global spread of type 2 diabetes mellitus in children and adolescents. *J Pediatr* 6(5):693–700.

Popkin BM, Udry JR. 1998. Adolescent obesity increases significantly in second and third generation U.S. immigrants: The National Longitudinal Study of Adolescent Health. *J Nutr* 128(4):701–706.

Powell LM, Slater S, Chaloupka FJ. 2004. The relationship between community physical activity settings and race, ethnicity and socioeconomic status. *Evidence-Based Prev Med* 1(2):135–144.

Pyramid Communications. 2003. *Communities Helping Children Be Healthy: A Guide to Reducing Childhood Obesity in Low-income African-American, Latino and Native American Communities.* [Online]. Available: http://www.rwjf.org/files/publications/HealthyChildren.pdf [accessed March 13, 2006].

Reilly JJ, Armstrong J, Dorosty AR, Emmett PM, Ness A, Rogers I, Steer C, Sherriff A. 2005. Early life risk factors for obesity in childhood: Cohort study. *Br Med J* 330(7504):1357–1364.

Robert SA, House JS. 2000. Socioeconomic inequalities in health: Integrating individual-, community-, and societal-level theory and research. In: Abrecht GL, ed. *Handbook of Social Studies in Health and Medicine.* New York: Sage Publications.

Robinson TN, Killen JD, Kraemer HC, Wilson DM, Matheson DM, Haskell WL, Pruitt LA, Powell TM, Owens AS, Thompson NS, Flint-Moore NM, Davis GJ, Emig KA, Brown RT, Rochon J, Green S, Varady A. 2003. Dance and reducing television viewing to prevent weight gain in African-American girls: The Stanford GEMS pilot study. *Ethnic Dis* 13(1 Suppl 1):S65–S77.

Rogers EM. 2003. *Diffusion of Innovations*, 5th ed. New York, NY: Free Press.

Rosenbloom AL. 2002. Fetal nutrition and insulin sensitivity: The genetic and environmental aspects of "thrift." *J Pediatr* 141(4):459–462.

Rosenbloom AL, Joe JR, Young RS, Winter WE. 1999. Emerging epidemic of type 2 diabetes in youth. *Diabetes Care* 22(2):345–354.

Ruiz-Beltran M, Kamau JK. 2001. The socio-economic and cultural impediments to well-being along the US-Mexico border. *J Community Health* 26(2):123–132.

Sallis JF, Glanz K. 2006. The role of built environments in physical activity, eating, and obesity in childhood. In: Paxon C, ed. *Future Child* 16(1):89–108.

Sallis JF, Cervero RB, Ascher W, Henderson KA, Kraft MK, Kerr J. 2006. An ecological approach to creating active living communities. *Annu Rev Public Health* 27:297–322.

Sherry B, Mei Z, Scanlon KS, Mokdad AH, Grummer-Strawn LM. 2004. Trends in state-specific prevalence of overweight and underweight in 2- through 4-year-old children from low-income families from 1989 through 2000. *Arch Pediatr Adolesc Med* 158(12):1116–1124.

Sloane D, Nascimento L, Yancey AK, Flynn G, Lewis LB, Guinyard JJ, Diamant A, Galloway-Gilliam L, Yancey AK. 2006. Assessing resource environments to target prevention interventions in community chronic disease control. *J Health Care Poor Underserved* 17(2):146–159.

Srinivasan SR, Myers L, Berenson GS. 2002. Predictability of childhood adiposity and insulin for developing insulin resistance syndrome (syndrome X) in young adulthood: The Bogalusa Heart Study. *Diabetes* 51(1):204–209.

Stewart JA, Dennison DA, Kohl HW, Doyle A. 2004. Exercise level and energy expenditure in the Take 10!® in-class physical activity program. *J School Health* 74(10):397–400.

Strauss RS, Knight J. 1999. Influence of the home environment on the development of obesity in children. *Pediatrics* 103(6):e85.

Strauss RS, Pollack HA. 2001. Epidemic increase in childhood overweight, 1986–1998. *J Am Med Assoc* 286(22):2845–2848.

TFAH (Trust for America's Health). 2005. *F as in Fat: How Obesity Policies are Failing in America 2005*. Washington, DC: The Trust for America's Health. [Online]. Available: http://healthyamericans.org/reports/obesity2005/Obesity2005Report.pdf [accessed May 9, 2006].

Thomson Medstat. 2006. *Childhood Obesity: Costs, Treatment Patterns, Disparities in Care, and Prevalent Medical Conditions*. Research brief. [Online]. Available: http://www.medstat.com/pdfs/childhood_obesity.pdf [accessed February 2, 2006].

Troiano RP, Flegal KM. 1998. Overweight children and adolescents: Description, epidemiology, and demographics. *Pediatrics* 101(3):497–504.

Tucker P, Liao Y, Giles WH, Liburd L. 2006. The REACH 2010 logic model: An illustration of expected performance. *Prev Chronic Dis* [Online]. Available: http://www.cdc.gov/Pcd/issues/2006/jan/05_0131.htm [accessed July 23, 2006].

Unger JB, Reynolds K, Shakib S, Spruijt-Metz D, Sun P, Johnson CA. 2004. Acculturation, physical activity, and fast-food consumption among Asian-American and Hispanic adolescents. *J Community Health* 29(6):467–481.

USDA (U.S. Department of Agriculture). 2006. *WIC Farmers' Market Nutrition Program*. [Online]. Available: http://www.fns.usda.gov/wic/FMNP/FMNPfaqs.htm [accessed June 13, 2006].

van der Kolk BA, Fisler RE. 1994. Childhood abuse and neglect and loss of self-regulation. *Bull Menninger Clin* 58(2):145–168.

Villa-Caballero L, Caballero-Solano V, Chavarria-Gamboa M, Linares-Lomeli P, Torres-Valencia E, Medina-Santillan R, Palinkas LA. 2006. Obesity and socioeconomic status in children of Tijuana. *Am J Prev Med* 30(3):197–203.

Whitaker RC, Orzol SM. 2006. Obesity among US urban preschool children: Relationships to race, ethnicity, and socioeconomic status. *Arch Pediatr Adolesc Med* 160(6):578–584.

Williams DR, Collins C. 1995. U.S. socioeconomic and racial differences in health: Patterns and explanations. *Annu Rev Sociol* 21(1):349–386.

Williams DE, Cadwell BL, Cheng YJ, Cowie CC, Gregg EW, Geiss LS, Engelgau MM, Narayan KM, Imperatore G. 2005. Prevalence of impaired fasting glucose and its relationship with cardiovascular disease risk factors in U.S. adolescents, 1999–2000. *Pediatrics* 116(5):1122–1126.

Williamson DF, Thompson TJ, Anda RF, Dietz WH, Felitti V. 2002. Body weight and obesity in adults and self-reported abuse in childhood. *Int J Obes Relat Metab Disord* 26(8): 1075–1082.

Wong MD, Shapiro MF, Boscardin WJ, Ettner SL. 2002. Contribution of major diseases to disparities in mortality. *N Engl J Med* 347(20):1585–1592.

Yancey AK, Lewis LB, Sloane DC, Guinyard JJ, Diamant AL, Nascimento LM, McCarthy WJ. 2004. Leading by example: A local health department-community collaboration to incorporate physical activity into organizational practice. *J Public Health Manage Pract* 10(2):116–123.

Yancey AK, Robinson RG, Ross RK, Washington R, Goodell HR, Goodwin NJ, Benjamin ER, Langie RG, Galloway JM, Carroll LN, Kong BW, Leggett CJ, Williams RA, Wong MJ, American Heart Association Advocacy Writing Group. 2005. Discovering the full spectrum of cardiovascular disease: Minority Health Summit 2003: Report of the Advocacy Writing Group. *Circulation* 111(10):e140–e149.

Yancey AK, Ortega AN, Kumanyika SK. 2006a. Effective recruitment and retention of minority research participants. *Annu Rev Pub Health* 27:1–28.

Yancey AK, Ory M, Davis SM. 2006b. Dissemination of physical activity promotion interventions in underserved populations. *Am J Prev Med*. 31(4S):82–91.

Yancey AK, Simon PA, McCarthy WJ, Lightstone AS, Fielding JE. 2006c. Ethnic and sex variations in overweight self-perception: Relationship to sedentariness. *Obesity* 14(5):1–9.

Yancy CW, Benjamin EJ, Fabunmi RP, Bonow RO. 2005. Discovering the full spectrum of cardiovascular disease: Minority Health Summit 2003: Executive summary. *Circulation* 111(10):1339–1349.

Yu S. 2006. The life-course approach to health. *Am J Public Health* 96(5):768.

Zephier E, Himes JH, Story M, Zhou X. 2006. Increasing prevalences of overweight and obesity in Northern Plains American Indian children. *Arch Pediatr Adolesc Med* 160(1): 34–39.

Zimring C, Joseph A, Nicoll GL, Tsepas S. 2005. Influences of building design and site design on physical activity: Research and intervention opportunities. *Am J Prev Med* 28(2 Suppl 2):186–193.

4

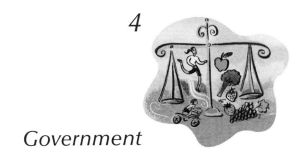

Government

G overnment serves several vital functions in a national public health crisis such as the childhood obesity epidemic. First and foremost the government provides leadership, which it demonstrates by making the response to the obesity epidemic an urgent public health priority and coordinating the public- and private-sector response. Galvanizing the response involves political commitment, policy development, prioritized funding, and coordination of programs. Other necessary elements of an adequate government response to the obesity epidemic are a strong governmental workforce, an enhanced organizational capacity, and a robust information-gathering system to monitor progress and guide programs and policies (Baker et al., 2005). Another key governmental function at the federal, state, and local levels is to improve the health status of the population and reduce inequities in health status among population groups (Health Canada, 2001; IOM, 2003).

In responding to the obesity epidemic, federal, state, and local government agencies across the nation share in the core public health responsibilities listed in Box 4-1 (IOM, 1988, 2003; NACCHO, 2005). Research and technical assistance for implementing, evaluating, and achieving national and regional objectives are primarily the responsibilities of the federal government, whereas program planning, implementation, and evaluation are state and local government responsibilities in partnership with other sectors (TFAH, 2006).

Two major recommendations in the *Health in the Balance* report were that "government at all levels should provide coordinated leadership for the

---

BOX 4-1
Public Health Mission and Government Responsibilities

Mission: The mission of public health is to fulfill society's interest in ensuring the existence of conditions in which people can be healthy.

Core Functions: All levels of government are responsible for conducting health assessments, health policy development, and the assurance of health. To accomplish its mission, public health agencies should establish operational linkages with other public sector agencies responsible for health-related functions. The execution of public health functions requires technical, political, management, program, and fiscal capacities at all levels. State government is the central force in public health and is the public-sector entity that bears primary responsibility for health.

Federal Government Responsibilities
- Support knowledge development and dissemination through data collection, research, and information exchange
- Establish national objectives and priorities on interstate and national health issues
- Provide technical assistance to support states and localities in determining objectives and carrying out actions on national and regional objectiveness
- Provide funds to states to strengthen their capacity for services to achieve adequate minimum health services and achieve national health objectives
- Ensure that its actions and services are in the interest of the entire nation, as in the case of epidemics, interstate environmental actions, and food and drug inspections

State Government Responsibilities
- Conduct health assessments based on statewide data
- Ensure an adequate statutory base for health activities in the state
- Establish health objectives, delegate responsibilities, and hold local governments accountable

---

prevention of obesity in children and youth" and an "increased level and sustained commitment of federal and state funds and resources are needed" to sufficiently address the childhood obesity epidemic. Additionally, the report recommended that state and local government should "provide co-ordinated leadership and support for childhood obesity efforts, particularly for populations at high risk of childhood obesity, by increasing resources and strengthening policies that promote opportunities for physical activity and healthful eating" (IOM, 2005a, p. 147–148).

Many of the efforts that have already been implemented by federal, state, and local governments play an essential role in the response to child-hood obesity in the United States. The number of existing governmental

- Ensure organized statewide efforts for personal, educational, and environmental health; provide access to health services; and solve health problems
- Guarantee the availability of a minimum set of health care services
- Support local health care service capacity, especially when disparities in local abilities exist with fiscal, administrative, technical capacity, and direct action

Local Government Responsibilities

- Assess, monitor, and provide surveillance for local health problems and resources with consideration of physical, behavioral, environmental, social, and economic conditions
- Prevent, investigate, minimize, and contain adverse health effects
- Ensure compliance with public health laws and ordinances
- Lead planning and response for public health emergencies
- Develop policy and leadership to engage the community, ensure the equitable distribution of public resources, and develop public-private partnerships to deliver activities commensurate with community needs
- Implement health promotion programs
- Coordinate public health system efforts in an intentional, noncompetitive, and nonduplicative manner
- Address health disparities.
- Ensure that high-quality services for the protection of public health, including personal health care, are accessible to all people; that the community receives proper consideration in the allocation of federal, state, and local resources for public health; and that the community and media are informed about how to obtain public health services
- Serve as a resource to local governing bodies, policy makers, community-based organizations, other governmental agencies, entities engaged in public health issues, and researchers

---

SOURCES: Adapted from IOM (1988, 2003); NACCHO (2005).

---

activities with the potential to reverse the childhood obesity epidemic is vast, dynamic, and difficult to track systematically over time. The prevention of childhood obesity will require contributions from all sectors of society. Government can play a special role by augmenting its own capacity in such a way that it stimulates and enhances the capacities and activities of other sectors of society. In order to continue to focus attention on the childhood obesity epidemic and encourage sustained efforts from all sectors of society, government will need to consistently acknowledge the importance of preventing childhood obesity.

In addition to implementing and sustaining new programs, governmental agencies at all levels need to reexamine their existing policies and initiatives that may hinder progress toward childhood obesity prevention. Examples include school siting policies that locate schools far outside of walking distance from the neighborhoods that those schools serve; U.S. agricultural policies including marketing practices, nutrition standards, agricultural subsidies, and procurement policies for agricultural commodity programs that affect the types and quantities of foods and beverages available in schools, communities, and through federal food assistance programs; land use policies that do not encourage mixed use of residential and business space and that subsequently discourage walking to neighborhood stores or businesses; and school policies that shorten the length of time in the school day devoted to healthy school meals and physical activity.

This chapter provides an overview of the role of government at all levels in the response to the childhood obesity epidemic. It provides examples of the policies, programs, and activities undertaken by federal, state, and local governmental agencies to reverse the current obesity epidemic and prevent a future rise in childhood obesity rates. The chapter examines the approaches needed to effectively evaluate policies and interventions and explores the factors that constitute success for the governmental sector. The chapter also recommends next steps in assessing progress with regard to leadership; implementing and evaluating policies and interventions and developing evaluation capacity; enhancing surveillance, monitoring, and research efforts; and using and disseminating the evidence from evaluation results.

SETTING THE CONTEXT

The severity of the obesity epidemic in the United States was first observed and publicized with data from the Behavioral Risk Factor Surveillance System (BRFSS). BRFSS is a system that uses telephone interviews for health surveillance and is jointly managed by the 50 state health departments and the Centers for Disease Control and Prevention's (CDC's) National Center for Chronic Disease Prevention and Health Promotion. In 1991, BRFSS data showed that four states had adult obesity prevalence rates of 15 to 19 percent and that no states had rates of 20 percent or greater. By 2004, BRFSS showed that 7 states had adult obesity prevalence rates of 15 to19 percent, 33 states had adult obesity rates of 20 to 24 percent, and 9 states had adult obesity rates of 25 percent or greater (CDC, 2005a).

The National Health and Nutrition Examination Survey (NHANES), a CDC surveillance system that is based on personal interviews and a physical examination and that was initiated in 1971, also revealed a rapidly evolving obesity epidemic in children, adolescents, and adults (Flegal et al., 2002; Ogden et al., 2002, 2006; Troiano et al., 1995). CDC presented the emerging data to the U.S. Congress at a House Appropriations Hearing in

2000 and warned of a growing obesity epidemic in children and adults. These data, coupled with evidence that obesity is not merely a cosmetic issue but leads to an array of serious health problems and comorbidities (Williams et al., 2005) as well as increasing health care costs (DHHS, 2001; Finkelstein et al., 2003, 2004; Wang and Dietz, 2002), were sufficient to raise national concern about the urgency of the epidemic and to stimulate congressional action. In 2001, the U.S. Surgeon General issued the *Surgeon General's Call to Action to Prevent and Decrease Overweight and Obesity* to stimulate the development of specific agendas and actions targeting this growing public health problem (DHHS, 2001).

In 2002, the Institute of Medicine (IOM) undertook a congressionally mandated study to develop a blueprint for a comprehensive action plan that is summarized in the report, *Preventing Childhood Obesity: Health in the Balance* (IOM, 2005a). The recommendations from that report focused on the actions needed by multiple stakeholders; the report called on government at all levels to take a leadership role and to bring resources to bear on this important health concern. The present IOM committee recommends increased efforts to address the government recommendations of the *Health in the Balance* report (Boxes 4-2 to 4-4) and to incorporate an evaluation component into all policies, programs, and initiatives.

To explore the breadth of childhood obesity prevention activities currently under way in the government sector—and whether and how they are being evaluated—the committee reviewed and drew information from a variety of sources, including those described in Chapter 1, as well as information and data from federal and state government surveillance and reporting systems, reports, and websites and from interviews conducted with selected state health officials; federal regulatory agencies; and federal representatives of the health, agriculture, and education sectors. A complete and systematic inventory of federal, state, and local government policies, programs, and activities relevant to childhood obesity prevention was beyond the charge of the committee and the scope of this progress report. However, a selected list of recent federal agency programs, initiatives, and surveillance systems relevant to childhood obesity prevention is compiled in Appendix D.

FEDERAL GOVERNMENT

The federal government has a responsibility to address public health crises including the childhood obesity epidemic through ensuring sufficient capacity to provide essential public health services; responding when a health threat is apparent across the entire country, region, or many states; providing assistance when the responses are beyond the jurisdictions of individual states; helping to formulate the public health goals of state and

BOX 4-2
Recommendations for Federal, State, and Local Government from the 2005 IOM report *Preventing Childhood Obesity: Health in the Balance*

Government at all levels should provide coordinated leadership for the prevention of obesity in children and youth. The president should request that the Secretary of the U.S. Department of Health and Human Services (DHHS) convene a high-level task force that includes the Secretaries or senior officials from DHHS, Agriculture, Education, Transportation, Housing and Urban Development, Interior, Defense, and other relevant agencies to ensure coordinated budgets, policies, and program requirements and to establish effective interdepartmental collaboration and priorities for action. An increased level and a sustained commitment of federal and state funds and resources are needed.

To implement this recommendation, the **federal government should:**
• Strengthen research and program efforts addressing obesity prevention, with a focus on experimental behavioral research and community-based intervention research and on the rigorous evaluation of the effectiveness, cost-effectiveness, sustainability, and scaling up of prevention interventions.
• Support extensive program and research efforts to prevent childhood obesity in high-risk populations with health disparities, with a focus on both behavioral and environmental approaches.
• Support nutrition and physical activity grant programs, particularly in states with the highest prevalence of childhood obesity.
• Strengthen support for relevant surveillance and monitoring efforts, particularly the National Health and Nutrition Examination Survey (NHANES).
• Undertake an independent assessment of federal nutrition assistance programs and agricultural policies to ensure that they promote healthful dietary intake and physical activity levels for all children and youth.
• Develop and evaluate pilot programs within the nutrition assistance programs that would promote healthful dietary intake and physical activity and scale up those found to be successful.

To implement this recommendation, **state and local governments should:**
• Provide coordinated leadership and support for childhood obesity prevention efforts, particularly those focused on high-risk populations, by increasing resources and strengthening policies that promote opportunities for physical activity and healthful eating in communities, neighborhoods, and schools.
• Support public health agencies and community coalitions in their collaborative efforts to promote and evaluate obesity prevention interventions.

Community Programs
Local governments, public health agencies, schools, and community organizations should collaboratively develop and promote programs that encourage healthful eating behaviors and regular physical activity, particularly for populations at high risk of childhood obesity. Community coalitions should be formed to facilitate and promote crosscutting programs and communitywide efforts.

SOURCE: IOM (2005a).

BOX 4-3
Recommendations for the U.S. Department of Health and Human Services from the 2005 IOM report *Preventing Childhood Obesity: Health in the Balance*

Advertising and Marketing
Industry should develop and strictly adhere to marketing and advertising guidelines That minimize the risk of obesity in children and youth.

To implement this recommendation:
- The Secretary of the U.S. Department of Health and Human Services should convene a national conference to develop guidelines for the advertising and marketing of foods, beverages, and sedentary entertainment directed at children and youth with attention to product placement, promotion, and content.

Multimedia and Public Relations Campaign
The U.S. Department of Health and Human Services should develop, implement, and evaluate a long-term national multimedia and public relations campaign focused on obesity prevention in children and youth.

To implement this recommendation:
- The campaign should be developed in coordination with other federal departments and agencies and with input from independent experts to focus on building support for policy changes, providing information to parents, and providing information to children and youth. Rigorous evaluation should be a critical component.
- Reinforcing messages should be provided in diverse media and effectively coordinated with other events and dissemination activities.
- The media should incorporate obesity issues into its content, including the promotion of positive role models.

Nutrition Labeling
Nutrition labeling should be clear and useful so that parents and youth can make informed product comparisons and decisions to achieve and maintain energy balance at a healthy weight.

To implement this recommendation:
- The Food and Drug Administration should revise the Nutrition Facts panel to prominently display the total calorie content for items typically consumed at one eating occasion in addition to the standardized calorie serving and the percent Daily Value.
- The Food and Drug Administration should examine ways to allow greater flexibility in the use of evidence-based nutrient and health claims regarding the link between the nutritional properties or biological effects of foods and a reduced risk of obesity and related chronic diseases.

Built Environment
The U.S. Department of Health and Human Services and the U.S. Department of Transportation should:
- Fund community-based research to examine the impact of changes to the built environment on the levels of physical activity in the relevant communities and populations.

SOURCE: IOM (2005a).

BOX 4-4
Recommendations for Other Relevant Federal Agencies
Recommendations from the 2005 IOM report
Preventing Childhood Obesity: Health in the Balance

U.S. Department of Education

Schools
Schools should provide a consistent environment that is conducive to healthful eating behaviors and regular physical activity.

To implement this recommendation:
Federal and state departments of education and health and professional organizations should
- Develop, implement, and evaluate pilot programs to explore innovative approaches to both staffing and teaching about wellness, healthful choices, nutrition, physical activity, and reducing sedentary behaviors. Innovative approaches to recruiting and training appropriate teachers are also needed.

U.S. Department of Transportation

Built Environment
The U.S. Department of Health and Human Services and the U.S. Department of Transportation should
- Fund community-based research to examine the impact of changes to the built environment on the levels of physical activity in the relevant communities and populations.

Federal Trade Commission

Advertising and Marketing
Industry should develop and strictly adhere to marketing and advertising guidelines that minimize the risk of obesity in children and youth.

To implement this recommendation:
- The Federal Trade Commission should have the authority and resources to monitor compliance with food and beverage and sedentary entertainment advertising practices.

U.S. Department of Agriculture

Schools
Schools should provide a consistent environment that is conducive to healthful eating behaviors and regular physical activity.

To implement this recommendation:
The U.S. Department of Agriculture, state and local authorities, and schools should
- Develop and implement nutritional standards for all competitive foods and beverages sold or served in schools.
- Ensure that all school meals meet the Dietary Guidelines for Americans.
- Develop, implement, and evaluate pilot programs to extend school meal funding in schools with a large percentage of children at high risk of obesity.

SOURCE: IOM (2005a).

local governments; and assisting states when they lack resources or expertise to adequately respond to a public health crisis (TFAH, 2006).

The U.S. Congress and several federal executive branch departments have become actively engaged in obesity prevention. The U.S. Department of Health and Human Services (DHHS) and the U.S. Department of Agriculture (USDA) are demonstrating leadership in these efforts, with growing involvement of the U.S. Department of Education and the U.S. Department of Transportation. However, a great deal more must be accomplished. Examples of the federal agency programs, initiatives, and surveillance systems that support and monitor the prevention of obesity in U.S. children and youth are discussed throughout this chapter, with additional information provided in Appendix D, including information on the extent and the nature of federal evaluation efforts based on the available data. It should be noted that this report is not a complete and systematic inventory of government programs and initiatives, as this was not the charge to the committee. Rather, the committee highlights some of the efforts that illustrate the key roles of government and that point to further work that can be done to increase the opportunities for children and youth to become more physically active and improve their eating patterns and diets.

Leadership

Leadership is an essential function of the federal government as it determines the priorities for funding and brings its considerable resources to bear on the problem. Government leadership influences the actions of those working within the federal government and across other sectors. Evidence of leadership includes the acknowledgement of and commitment to address a problem, followed by the development of a plan of action, the establishment of policies, and the commitment of financial and human resources to carry out a comprehensive and coordinated plan. The *Health in the Balance* report recommended federal leadership through the following actions (IOM, 2005a):

1. The president should appoint a high-level task force to coordinate federal agency responses.
2. DHHS and the Federal Trade Commission (FTC) should develop guidelines with broad stakeholder input for the advertising and marketing of foods, beverages, and sedentary entertainment directed at children and youth, with attention to product placement, promotion, and content.
3. The U.S. Food and Drug Administration (FDA) should revise the Nutrition Facts panel on packaged food and beverage products.
4. FDA should allow industry to have greater flexibility to use evidence-based nutrient and health claims regarding the link between

the nutritional properties or the biological effects of foods and a reduced risk of obesity and related chronic diseases.
5. USDA should develop nutritional standards for competitive foods and beverages available in schools.

An example of demonstrated federal leadership is an initial stakeholder workshop, jointly organized by FTC and DHHS, to develop guidelines for the advertising and marketing of foods, beverages, and sedentary entertainment to children and youth. In July 2005, FTC and DHHS held a joint workshop, *Marketing, Self-Regulation, and Childhood Obesity*, that provided a forum for industry, academic, public health advocacy, and government stakeholders, as well as consumers, to examine the role of the private sector in addressing the rising childhood obesity rates. A summary of the workshop (FTC and DHHS, 2006) contains recommendations and next steps for industry stakeholders, including a request that industry strengthen self-regulatory measures to advertise responsibly to children through the Children's Advertising Review Unit (CARU). FTC and DHHS indicated that both of these federal institutions plan to closely monitor the progress made on the recommendations in the joint FTC and DHHS summary report (FTC and DHHS, 2006). Moreover, Congress has requested that the FTC compile information on food and beverage marketing activities and expenditures targeted to children and adolescents. The FTC will be soliciting public comment on these issues, and the results will be submitted in a report to Congress as mandated in Public Law 109-108 (FTC, 2006) (Chapter 5).

Recent actions by FDA are providing steps toward improving consumer nutrition information. In April 2005, FDA released two advance notices of proposed rulemaking to elicit stakeholder and public input about two recommendations of the FDA Obesity Working Group: the first action was to make calorie information more prominent on the Nutrition Facts label and the second action provides more information about serving sizes on packaged foods (FDA, 2006). In September 2005, FDA issued a final rule on the nutrient content claims definition of sodium levels for the term *healthy* (FDA, 2006). The IOM committee awaits further progress that FDA can make toward finalizing the rulemaking and exploring the use of evidence-based nutrient and health claims regarding the link between the nutritional properties or biological effects of foods and a reduced risk of obesity and related chronic diseases.

Joint efforts by USDA and DHHS resulted in the release of the sixth edition of the Dietary Guidelines for Americans 2005, which provide specific recommendations on the consumption of foods in different food groups, fats, carbohydrates, sodium and potassium, and alcoholic beverages; food safety; and physical activity (DHHS and USDA, 2005). The Dietary Guidelines and their graphic representation, MyPyramid, are an important source of consumer nutrition information that should provide the basis for federal food and nutrition assistance programs, nutrition education, and nutrition policies.

The Child Nutrition and WIC Reauthorization Act (P.L. 108-265) provided another step forward for childhood obesity prevention efforts. In 2004, Congress initiated and passed the legislation, which requires school districts participating in the National School Lunch Program (NSLP) or School Breakfast Program (SBP) to establish a local school wellness policy by the beginning of the 2006–2007 school year (CNWICRA, 2004). As outlined in the legislation, the school wellness policies should include goals for nutrition education, physical activity, guidelines for foods and beverages served throughout school campuses, and other school-based activities that are designed to promote student wellness in a manner that the local educational agency determines is appropriate. The USDA secretary, in coordination with the secretary of education and in consultation with the DHHS secretary, acting through CDC, are charged with providing technical assistance to establish healthy school nutrition environments, reducing childhood obesity, and preventing diet-related chronic diseases. The act establishes a plan for measuring the implementation of the local school wellness policy, supported by $4 million in appropriated funds (CNWICRA, 2004) (Chapter 7). The committee encourages the systematic monitoring and evaluation of the implementation and the impacts and outcomes of these policies throughout the nation's school districts and local schools.

Progress is also under way to develop nutrition standards for competitive foods and beverages that are available in schools. In fiscal year (FY) 2005, Congress directed IOM to conduct a study to develop comprehensive recommendations for appropriate nutritional standards for competitive foods (Hartwig, 2004; IOM, 2006a). The study is in progress and when it is complete, the committee recommends that Congress, USDA, CDC, and other relevant agencies take expeditious action on developing national nutrition standards for competitive foods and beverages in schools.

The federal government has also demonstrated leadership in setting specific goals for childhood obesity prevention. DHHS incorporated into its *Strategic Plan FY 2004–2009* an objective for the Indian Health Service to decrease obesity rates among American Indian/Alaska Native (AI/AN) children by 10 percent during this 5-year period (DHHS, 2004).

However, the committee noted that federal leadership fell short of an important recommendation in the *Health in the Balance* report, in that no progress was made toward the establishment of a presidentially appointed high-level task force to make childhood obesity prevention a national priority and to coordinate activities and budgets for this goal across federal agencies. Because childhood obesity prevention is a national priority that requires the collective efforts of many federal departments and agencies, the establishment of a high-level task force to address this issue is essential for making progress.

Program Resources, Funding, and Evaluation

A public health program is a coordinated set of complementary activities designed to produce desirable health outcomes. Consistent with this consideration, substantial resources from a variety of federal government entities are designated for programs relevant to childhood obesity prevention. However, the level of funding and the resources invested in these efforts and their evaluation are not commensurate with the seriousness of this public health problem. Coordinated and sustained funding continues to be strengthened, however, as does the emphasis on program evaluation and the dissemination of evaluation results. For example, in 2005, the average per-capita federal investment in public health through CDC was $20.99. An estimated 80 percent of CDC funds are redistributed to states and private partners (TFAH, 2006). Throughout the country, the funding strategies that states and private partners use to support programs that promote healthy lifestyles and obesity prevention goals include making better use of existing resources, maximizing federal and state revenues, creating more flexibility in existing categorical funding, building public-private partnerships, and creating new dedicated revenue streams.

The amount of federal support that the states receive varies substantially. The following federal funding streams are especially relevant:

(1) *Formula and block grants*, in which states receive a fixed allocation of funds based on a formula prescribed by law to address particular issues of national priority (e.g., preventive health and health services block grants, maternal and child health block grants, and Safe Routes to School grants);

(2) *Entitlements*, which guarantee that individuals who meet the eligibility criteria for a specific program (e.g., low-income children and families participating in federal assistance programs such as the Food Stamps Program [FSP] and school meals) are served;

(3) *Discretionary or competitive project grants*, which target particular federal efforts such as obesity prevention, fund states on the basis of the merits of their grant applications, and are awarded for a specific time frame (e.g., CDC's Nutrition and Physical Activity Program to Prevent Obesity and Other Chronic Diseases; USDA's Special Supplemental Nutrition Program for Women, Infants, and Children [WIC] and Fresh Fruit and Vegetable Program [FFVP]);

(4) *Cooperative agreements*, which have prescriptive project agreements (e.g., CDC's Steps to a HealthierUS Initiative); and

(5) *Need-based formula grants*, which are often based on the prevalence of a condition and that match the states' costs on a formula basis (e.g., Medicaid, and USDA's Food Stamp Nutrition Education [FSNE] program) (Finance Project, 2004; TFAH, 2006).

In assessing the overall progress in funding support for obesity prevention programs, however, it is important to ensure that double counting does not take place or that an increase in funding from one source (e.g., federal funding) is not accompanied by a reduction in funding from existing sources (e.g., state funding). Of the numerous federally funded programs relevant to childhood obesity prevention, only a few are highlighted below or in subsequent chapters and Appendix D.

The *Health in the Balance* report (IOM, 2005a) recommended that the federal government undertake an independent assessment of federal nutrition assistance programs and agricultural policies to ensure that they promote healthful dietary intake and increase physical activity levels for all children and youth. To date, there have been limited analyses examining the relationships among U.S. food supply-related agricultural, industrial, and economic policies (or the environment resulting from these policies) and consumer demand-driven nutrition policies (e.g., dietary guidance) (Tillotson, 2004). Future efforts to improve the U.S. food and agricultural system will need to create connections among health, food, and farm policies that support the Dietary Guidelines for Americans 2005. The 2007 U.S. Farm Bill, which contains a multitude of programs and provisions that will impact the U.S. food and agricultural system, is an opportunity to foster changes that support both healthier diets and strengthen agricultural economies (Schoonover and Muller, 2006).

USDA has many programs designed to directly influence dietary behaviors. In FY 2005, expenditures for USDA's 15 federal food assistance programs totaled $50.7 billion. An estimated 55 percent of USDA's budget supported programs that provide low-income families and children with access to food for a healthful diet and nutrition education (USDA, 2006b) (Table 4-1). USDA has indicated that it is committed to aligning its programs with the Dietary Guidelines for Americans 2005 (Food, Nutrition, and Consumer Services, 2006). The contents of the WIC food packages are currently undergoing review, with a focus on implementing the recommendations of the IOM report, *WIC Food Packages: Time for a Change* (IOM, 2005b). The USDA Food and Nutrition Service (FNS) is presently seeking public comments on proposed revisions to the regulations governing the contents of the WIC food packages to align them with the Dietary Guide-

TABLE 4-1 Expenditures for and Rates of Participation in Major Federal Food and Nutrition Assistance Programs, FY 2005

Federal Food and Nutrition Assistance Programs	Average Monthly Participation or Nutrition Provided	Annual Expenditures ($ billion)
Food Stamp Program	25.7 million participants	31.0
Special Supplemental Nutrition Program for Women, Infants, and Children	8.0 million participants	5.0
National School Lunch Program	29.6 million participants	8.0
School Breakfast Program	9.3 million participants	1.9
Child and Adult Care Food Program	1,099.0 million meals served in child-care centers; 72.1 million meals served in family child-care centers; 57.3 million meals served in adult day-care centers	2.1

SOURCE: USDA (2006b).

lines for Americans 2005 and current infant feeding practice guidelines of the American Academy of Pediatrics (USDA, 2006d). The committee recommends that Congress and USDA expeditiously complete the revision of the contents of the WIC food packages and thoroughly examine other relevant food and nutrition assistance programs so that they can be strengthened to fully address childhood obesity prevention goals and to monitor and evaluate relevant outcomes.

In 1999, USDA funded a childhood obesity prevention initiative called Fit WIC to support and evaluate social and environmental approaches to prevent and reduce obesity in preschool-aged children. Four state WIC programs (California, Kentucky, Vermont, and Virginia) and the Inter-Tribal Council of Arizona received funds for a 3-year period to identify ways in which the WIC program could respond to the childhood obesity epidemic for program participants. The main finding from the five pilot projects was that many parents of obese preschool-aged children neither saw their children as being obese nor were they concerned about their children's weight. However, the pilot program also found that parents demonstrated interest in receiving information on ways to promote healthy behaviors in their families, WIC program staff requested information on effective methods to reach parents, and community groups expressed interest in working on the issue of childhood obesity prevention (USDA, 2005b) (Chapters 6 and 8).

USDA's Food and Nutrition Service and Agricultural Marketing Service have collaborated with the Department of Defense (DoD) since 1995 through the DoD Fresh Program to supply fresh fruit and vegetable produce directly to school food services to improve school meals (USDA, 2006a). The DoD uses its high volume and effective purchasing and delivery mechanisms to deliver fresh produce to schools, along with military installations and other sites. The DoD Fresh Program, which began in 1995 with 8 states, is now a permanent program that provided fresh produce to schools in 46 states and the District of Columbia in the 2005–2006 school year and which was funded at $50 million in FY 2005; produce is also supplied to over 100 Indian tribal organizations (David Leggett, USDA, personal communication, July 13, 2006; USDA, 2006a).

Another federal effort focused on increasing student consumption of fruits and vegetables in schools is the USDA Fresh Fruit and Vegetable Program (FFVP). In the 2002 Farm Bill, Congress initiated the FFVP that provides schools with the funding to offer fresh and dried fruits and fresh vegetables as snacks to students outside of the regular school meal periods. Initiated in the 2002–2003 school year as a pilot program funded at $6 million in 100 schools in four states (Indiana, Iowa, Michigan, and Ohio) and seven schools in New Mexico's Zuni Indian Tribal Organization, the program has since expanded to 14 states and three tribal organizations and legislation has been drafted to expand the program nationwide (Branaman, 2003; Buzby et al., 2003; ERS, 2002; UFFVA, 2006) (Chapter 7). Quantitative outcomes data were not collected in the pilot program, but a qualitative process evaluation suggested satisfaction with the program in many schools and by food service staff (Buzby et al., 2003). An evaluation of 25 schools in Mississippi that participated in the FFVP suggests that the distribution of free fruit to middle school students might be effective as a component of a more comprehensive approach to improve dietary behaviors (Schneider et al., 2006). The committee encourages more extensive evaluations of the FFVP and DoD Fresh Program that examine a variety of relevant outcomes to preventing childhood obesity.

The *Health in the Balance* report (IOM, 2005a) recommended that DHHS develop, implement, and evaluate a long-term national multimedia and public relations campaign focused on obesity prevention in children and youth. Inherent in this recommendation was the need to develop a campaign, in coordination with other federal departments and agencies, and with input from independent experts to focus on building support for obesity prevention policy changes and providing information to parents as well as children and youth. The report emphasized the need for a rigorous evaluation to be a critical component of the campaign; that reinforcing messages be provided in diverse media and effectively coordinated with other events and dissemination activities; and that the media incorporate obesity issues into its content, including the promotion of positive role models.

The committee acknowledges that as a component of the DHHS Steps to a HealthierUS Cooperative Agreement Program (Steps Program), DHHS partnered with the Ad Council to create SmallStep and SmallStep Kids!, which target parents, teens, and children and which includes public service advertisements (PSAs), a public relations campaign, a health care provider's tool kit, and consumer information materials. The component targeted to children includes games and activities, television advertisements, and links to other materials. In addition to the advertising components, the Ad Council plans to implement a curriculum-based program with a major educational partner to educate children about the importance of healthy lifestyles and anticipates expanding the program through additional partnerships.

BOX 4-5
Case Study of the VERB™ Campaign

Background

The VERB™ campaign, coordinated by CDC from FY 2001 through 2006, was a 5-year, national, multicultural, social marketing initiative designed to increase and maintain physical activity among 21 million U.S. tweens (children ages 9–13 years) (Huhman et al., 2004; Wong et al., 2004). The national program initially included augmented media in selected markets where local coalitions coordinated community activities to complement the media campaign. Beginning in the second year, national marketing promotions were initiated that invited schools and communities to participate in the campaign. Parents and other intermediaries that influence tweens (e.g., teachers and youth program leaders) were secondary target audiences of the campaign. The VERB campaign is an example of behavioral branding, which raises the awareness of a brand that encourages a behavior or lifestyle such as increased physical activity. The primary goal during the first year of the campaign was to build brand awareness among tweens followed by messaging that encouraged them to find "their verb" and become physically active. All forms of media (e.g., television, print, the Internet) were used to reach tweens of various racial/ethnic groups. The campaign combined paid advertising, modern media marketing strategies, and partnerships to reach the distinct audiences of young people and their adult influencers.

Formative Evaluation

Before CDC launched the 5-year youth media campaign, VERB—It's what you do.—it used exploratory research techniques to gain insights into a variety of factors relevant to understanding how to increase and maintain physical activity levels in the multiethnic U.S. tweens. Formative research was conducted with the target group to inform the design of the social marketing campaign. The research showed that tweens would respond positively to messages that promoted physical activities that are fun, occur in a socially inclusive environment and that emphasize self-

The campaign has received approximately $210 million in donated media support. An evaluation of SmallStep has shown that respondents who had seen at least one of the PSAs were more likely than those who had not seen the campaign to report that they had already changed their diet and physical activity habits (27 percent compared with 14 percent) (Ad Council, 2006). Ongoing support and evaluation of this program are recommended given the potential reach and influence of the media in socializing the public, especially young people. Further, DHHS and its partners should work to further coordinate this campaign and related dissemination activities with other federal agencies. Print, broadcast, and electronic media should include the promotion of positive role models and healthy lifestyles.

However, the CDC's VERB™—It's what you do., described in Box 4-5, is an example of a federal program initially funded at scale that even

efficacy, self-esteem, and belonging to their peer group (Aeffect, Inc., 2005; CDC, 2006a).

Process Evaluation
Evaluations have examined process measures to ensure that the campaign was being implemented as planned. A quarterly tracking survey was conducted to assess that the brand and messages continued to appeal to tweens and that the high awareness of the campaign was maintained over time (CDC, 2006d).

Outcome Evaluation
The cognitive and behavioral outcomes of the VERB campaign have been tracked annually through the Youth Media Campaign Longitudinal Survey (YMCLS). During the first years of the campaign, the level of awareness of the VERB campaign among the target audience was high, and was associated with higher levels of physical activity in tweens who were exposed to and aware of VERB (Huhman et al., 2005, 2007). Evaluation of VERB through FY 2006, monitored through the YMCLS, will allow continued comparison of physical activity levels in tweens who were exposed to the campaign and those who were not exposed (Huhman, 2006). Additionally, surveillance data collected through the YMCLS will be publicly available in 2008 (Faye Wong, CDC, personal communication, August 8, 2006).

Lessons Learned
Despite evidence of success and widespread knowledge of the importance of physical activity in preventing childhood obesity, there was inadequate support in the administration and Congress for continuing VERB, and insufficient external support to encourage sustained funding. A major challenge for the VERB campaign was to sustain children's awareness and motivation to be physically active despite the progressive reduction in federal support over its 5-year authorization. Federal funding for the campaign was $125 million in FY 2001, reduced to $68 million in FY 2002, $51 million in FY 2003, $36 million in FY 2004, and increased to $59 million in FY 2005. Over the 5-year period, the average cost of the VERB campaign was $68 million/year.

with positive evaluation results has not received sustained funding. Multiyear evaluations of VERB were appropriately built into the campaign from its inception. Evaluation of the campaign's first 2 years demonstrated the program's effectiveness in raising awareness of the VERB brand and achieving increased free-time physical activity in tweens (Huhman et al., 2005, 2007). However, it was not included in the president's FY 2006 budget and received no congressional support for continuation beyond FY 2006 because of competing policy priorities. The campaign will be phased out by September 2006 (Huhman, 2006). Evaluation activities will be completed in early 2007 with plans to publish the summative evaluation results of the campaign (Faye Wong, CDC, personal communication, August 8, 2006). The termination of an adequately funded, well-designed, and effective program to increase physical activity and combat childhood obesity calls into question the commitment to obesity prevention within government and by multiple stakeholders who could have supported the continuity of the VERB campaign.

Capacity Development

Capacity building is a multidimensional process that improves the ability of individuals, groups, communities, organizations, and governments to meet their objectives or enhance performance to address population health. In public health, capacity building or capacity development involves the performance of essential functions, such as developing and sustaining partnerships, leveraging resources, surveillance and monitoring, providing training and technical assistance, and conducting evaluations. It is a function of the size, training, and experience of the workforce and the resources available to the workforce to accomplish the task (IOM, 2003).

The *Health in the Balance* report recommended that the federal government support nutrition and physical activity grant programs, particularly in states with the highest prevalence of childhood obesity (IOM, 2005a). Although specific definitions and measures of the capacities of federal, state, and local governments to adequately carry out the activities necessary to halt and reverse the childhood obesity epidemic are not readily available, the committee concluded that existing evidence suggests serious shortfalls. Recent surveys conducted by the Council of State and Territorial Epidemiologists noted that the epidemiologic capacity for terrorism preparedness and emergency response had increased between 2001 and 2004, whereas capacities in six other areas, including the capacity for epidemiologic analysis of chronic diseases, had decreased, with less than half of the states reporting that they had a substantial capacity for the epidemiologic analysis of chronic diseases (CDC, 2005b; CSTE, 2004). The *Health in the Balance* report recommended that the federal government should support nutrition and physical activity grant programs, particularly in states with the highest prevalence of childhood obesity (IOM, 2005a).

Nutrition and Physical Activity Program to Prevent Obesity and Other Chronic Diseases

CDC's Nutrition and Physical Activity Program to Prevent Obesity and Other Chronic Diseases is an example of a federal initiative designed to build the capacity of states to prevent obesity in adults, children, and youth. In 2005 and 2006, a total of 28 states received funding under this program: 21 states received funding of $400,000 to $450,000 for capacity development and seven states (Colorado, Massachusetts, North Carolina, New York, Oregon, Pennsylvania, and Washington) received funding of $750,000 to $1.3 million for basic implementation (CDC, 2006b). CDC has provided technical assistance and tools to help all states develop and evaluate their obesity prevention strategic plans (Yee et al., 2006). The states have hired approximately 130 individuals to work on the strategic plans, and CDC has hired staff to provide program oversight and technical assistance to the states (CDC and RTI, 2006). This initiative was first funded in FY 2000, and appropriations grew from $1.6 million in FY 2000 to $16.2 million in FY 2005 and declined slightly to $16.0 in FY 2006 (Table 4-2). Despite applications from nearly every state, the relatively stable level of funding since FY 2004 has limited the expansion of this program to other states. An assessment is needed to identify the appropriate level of funding required to support all states and territories in capacity building and program implementation to prevent obesity.

TABLE 4-2 CDC's Nutrition and Physical Activity Program to Prevent Obesity and Other Chronic Diseases

Fiscal Year	Number of States Funded	Funding ($ million)
2000	6	$ 1.6
2001	12	$ 4.0
2002	12	$ 5.6
2003	20	$ 9.7
2004	28	$14.6
2005	28	$16.2
2006	28	$16.0

SOURCE: Robin Hamre, NCCDPHP/CDC, personal communication, July 27, 2006.

A process evaluation of the efforts in 28 of the CDC-funded states has been conducted. The evaluation focuses on policies, legislation, and environmental changes affecting nutrition and physical activity, implementation and coordination, and the inclusion of relevant partners. The evaluation found that the funded states had successfully involved partner organizations in planning and implementing interventions and cosponsored events aimed at improving body mass index (BMI) in children and adults; however, the evaluation also revealed potential service gaps, overlap with other programs aimed at preventing and controlling obesity, opportunities for additional services, and potential barriers to delivering services (CDC and RTI, 2006).

Steps to a HealthierUS Program

The Steps to a HealthierUS Program, initiated in 2003 by DHHS and administered by CDC, is another federal program intended to increase the capacity of local public health systems to address chronic health concerns. The Steps Program enables communities to develop an action plan, a community consortium, and an evaluation strategy that supports chronic disease prevention and health promotion to lower the prevalence of obesity, type 2 diabetes, and asthma through healthful eating, physical activity, and tobacco avoidance in disproportionately affected, at-risk and low-income populations including African Americans, Hispanics/Latinos, American Indians/Alaska Natives, Asian Americans, and Pacific Islanders (DHHS, 2005b,c). The Steps Program funds communities in three categories: large cities or urban areas, state-coordinated small cities or rural areas, and tribes or tribal entities. Initially funded at $13.6 million in FY 2003, during FY 2004 to FY 2006 the Steps Program received $35.8 million per year to support 40 communities nationwide. Aside from financial resources, CDC provides capacity through technical assistance to support evidence-based program planning and implementation, disease and risk factor surveillance, and program evaluation with the 40 funded communities participating in the annual BRFSS and biennial Youth Risk Behavior Surveillance System (YRBSS). The allocation of resources to support both surveillance and evaluation comprises 10 percent of the total program funding in the majority of the funded communities (Mac-Donald et al., 2006).

The Steps Program uses indicators developed by CDC that provide a comprehensive set of measures for assessing programs in chronic disease prevention and health promotion. The most relevant indicators related to nutrition and physical activity among youth include fruit and vegetable consumption, vigorous physical activity, television viewing, and monitoring of obesity prevalence (CDC, 2004). The Steps Program uses data from the BRFSS and YRBSS to monitor the progress that has been made in achieving behavioral and health outcomes at national and community levels (MacDonald et al., 2006). An evaluation of the 40 Steps Program communities funded nationwide is in progress.

Food Stamp Nutrition Education Program

USDA's Food Stamp Nutrition Education (FSNE) program is an example of a federal innovation that encourages collaboration and that leverages resources. FSNE allows states to create social marketing networks, mobilize other organizations, and join efforts to conduct interventions with low-income participants to achieve healthier eating patterns and increased physical activity levels (Gregson et al., 2001; Hersey and Daugherty, 1999). Some states also encourage policy, systems, and environmental changes that increase access to foods and beverages that contribute to healthful diets and physical activity in low-income communities. Schools with limited resources are a common setting used by FSNE. In 2005, nearly all state Food Stamp Programs (FSP) submitted annual FSNE plans that qualified for federal financial participation funds, whereas only a decade earlier only seven states had done so. A review of state FSNE is near completion.

HealthierUS School Challenge

USDA's HealthierUS School Challenge is a more recent USDA initiative aimed at encouraging positive changes by recognizing schools that are creating a healthy environment. To qualify, elementary schools must enroll in Team Nutrition, conduct school assessments, provide lunches that meet specific nutrient requirements, offer physical activity, and achieve 70 percent participation in NSLP. Recognition programs such as these could help in disseminating promising practices; however, it is important that the efforts be disseminated broadly to media, parent-teacher associations, and others to provide incentive for schools to participate.

Further Efforts

It has been recommended that USDA improve coordination and strengthen linkages among its nutrition education efforts (GAO, 2004a), and state nutrition action plans are now required for USDA food and nutrition assistance programs. The committee encourages further efforts to develop policies that foster opportunities for collaboration among USDA programs relevant to childhood obesity prevention.

National Surveillance, Monitoring, and Research

Surveillance and Monitoring

Public health surveillance is the ongoing systematic process of collecting, analyzing, interpreting, and using data from generalizable samples that pertain to the public's health. Surveillance systems provide ongoing assessments of changes and trends related to public health concerns and provide evidence of the combined effect of all actions taken to address the concern. They can be viewed as an evaluation of the overall system, but surveillance systems rarely provide sufficient information about the factors that cause the changes to serve as the primary tools of evaluation.

The *Health in the Balance* report included the following recommendations related to surveillance (IOM, 2005a):

1. Support for relevant surveillance and monitoring systems, especially NHANES, should be strengthened;
2. FTC should monitor industry compliance with food and beverage and sedentary entertainment advertisement practices; and
3. All school meals programs should meet the Dietary Guidelines for Americans 2005 (DHHS and USDA, 2005).

Examples of federal surveillance activities that are conducted by CDC and that are used to monitor selected indicators and behavioral outcomes relevant to obesity in children and youth at national or state levels include (1) NHANES, which assesses the health and nutritional status of a nationally representative sample of U.S. adults, youth, and children through interviews and a direct physical examination; (2) the National Health Interview Survey (NHIS), which is conducted annually and which assesses physical activity, health care access, and health care coverage for household members; (3) the Pediatric Nutrition Surveillance System (PedNSS), which collects data on health care and health status of low-income children, especially participants in the WIC program; (4) the Youth Media Campaign Longitudinal Survey (YMCLS), which is used to track older children's physical activity levels and media use, and to evaluate the VERB campaign; and (5) the Youth Risk Behavior Surveillance System (YRBSS), which was initiated in 1991 as a system of national, state, and local school-based surveys conducted biennially. YRBSS obtains self-reported information about six categories of health-related behaviors, including dietary and physical activity behaviors for students in grades 9 to 12. Since 1999, the Youth Risk Behavior Survey (YRBS) has included self-reported height and weight, from which the BMI is calculated. Although NHANES uses directly measured height and weight, it provides only national estimates, whereas YRBS provides national, state, and city data only for those participating and only those organizations that have the capacity to administer the survey. A national YRBS is not conducted with students in grades 6 to 8. The most current YRBSS summarizes the results from the national survey, 40 state surveys, and 21 local surveys conducted with students in grades 9 to 12 from 2004 to 2006 (Eaton et al., 2006).

Other national surveillance systems include the U.S. Department of Labor's (DoL's) National Longitudinal Survey of Youth (NLSY), which has provided data on income and BMI for two youth cohorts since 1979 and 1997 (DoL, 2006); the American Community Survey, which is conducted by the U.S. Census Bureau (U.S. Census Bureau, 2006); and the National Household Travel Survey (NHTS), which is conducted by the Bureau of Transportation Statistics and the Federal Highway Administration to assess motorized and nonmotorized travel (BTS, 2006). Federally funded surveillance and monitoring systems also examine changes in policies and programs. Examples include the School Health Policies and Programs Study (SHPPS) and the School Health Profiles (SHP) survey. A more detailed description of these surveys is found in Chapter 7 and Appendixes C and D. Given the urgency of the childhood obesity epidemic, it is important to conduct frequent assessments of changes in the school environment. For example, USDA's School Nutrition Dietary Assessment Study (SNDA), which provides information about the nutritional quality of meals served in public schools that participate in the school meals programs (USDA, 2001), was conducted in the 1991–1992 and 1998–1999 school years, and a report on the most recent SNDA is anticipated in fall 2006. Adequate funding and expansion of this survey is needed to ensure ongoing and regularly scheduled assessments. Additionally, the committee recommends that USDA explore other approaches for tracking and monitoring the nutritional quality, monetary sales, and levels of consumption of foods and beverages sold in schools.

An assessment has been conducted to identify national data systems that could track the outcomes of USDA food assistance and nutrition programs (Biing-Hwan et al., 2006). At present, however, no reporting systems are in place to identify how the precursors of childhood obesity are being addressed in the populations, organizations, and communities served by the WIC program, FSP, or the school meals programs. Examples of outcome measures that could be monitored include the degree to which individual hunger and household food insecurity are reduced by FSP and whether the recommended performance-based school meals reimbursement system provides incentives for the NSLP meals to meet the Dietary Guidelines for Americans 2005 (OMB, 2005).

USDA, in collaboration with other stakeholders, has opportunities to assist states and localities by improving surveillance and monitoring capacity to fill essential data gaps. Some larger state WIC programs have developed reporting systems that could help identify effective approaches to address obesity in young children (National WIC Association, 2003). For example, new state registries for school wellness policies could be used to track progress toward achieving important obesity-related national goals. FSNE state systems that monitor the outcomes of programs at the state and local levels might be tapped for adoption nationwide. Such actions would require administrative decisions but not statutory changes. For example, USDA could allow the WIC program to invest in computers or permit FSNE to fund surveys of individuals with incomes above 130 percent of the federal poverty level. For the WIC program, many large states already have made the investment in computers, so automation in smaller states could be offered at a modest incremental cost. These opportunities could improve the monitoring of the effectiveness of USDA interventions and programs (USDA, 2006c).

As noted earlier, both BRFSS and NHANES were the first surveillance systems to document the growing obesity epidemic in U.S. adults and children (Flegal et al., 2002; Hedley et al., 2004; Mokdad et al., 1999; Ogden et al., 2002, 2006; Troiano et al., 1995). The NHANES and NHIS are administered through CDC's National Center for Health Statistics (NCHS); and BRFSS, YRBSS, SHP, and SHPPS are administered through CDC's National Center for Chronic Disease Prevention and Health Promotion (NCCDPHP). The funding for these surveillance systems in FY 2001 and FY 2005 is provided in Table 4-3.

Comparison of the FY 2001 and FY 2005 budgets for NHIS and NHANES reveals a relatively flat funding structure to support these two important national surveillance systems[1] (Edward Hunter, NCHS/CDC, personal communication, June 28, 2006). Similarly, federal funding levels have been static for other surveillance systems, including YRBSS, SHP, PedNSS, and Pregnancy Nutrition Surveillance System (PNSS). The only survey that showed a marked increase in funding during this time frame was BRFSS, which was due to a congressional appropriation of $5 million in FY 2003 and small incremental increases until FY 2005. These increases occurred so that Congress could rectify the funding gap between BRFSS expenses and the congressional funding line. Even with these increases, BRFSS has never been fully funded; thus, funds from other categorical

---

[1]Both surveys, particularly NHANES, rely on funding from many different sources including other federal agencies. The funding sources differ from fiscal year to fiscal year. The funds appropriated to CDC's NCHS to support these surveys may fluctuate considerably across fiscal years, without representing substantial program changes.

TABLE 4-3 CDC Surveillance Systems Funding

	FY 2001 ($ million)	FY 2005 ($ million)
NHANES	21.0	20.5
NHIS	12.9	15.4
BRFSS	1.92	7.64
YRBSS	1.96	2.5
SHP	0.712	0.767
SHPPS	data unavailable	1.74
PedNSS and PNSS	0.248	0.274

SOURCES: Edward Hunter, NCHS/CDC, personal communication, June 28, 2006; NCCDPHP/CDC Financial Management Office, personal communication, July 17, 2006.

awards and from state budgets are used to fully fund this surveillance system (NCCDPHP/CDC, Financial Management Office, personal communication, July 17, 2006).

A sufficient investment in health statistics and surveillance systems is essential to track a national public health crisis such as the obesity epidemic. Although these funds have been used to increase sample sizes necessary for these surveys and to provide information on population subgroups, including children and youth (DHHS, 2006), the committee concluded that substantial funding increases are needed not only to ensure the continuation of these important surveillance systems but also to enhance and expand data collection for the range of outcomes relevant to the childhood obesity epidemic.

Research

Conducting and supporting obesity-related research are important governmental functions (IOM, 2003). Research helps provide an understanding of the fundamental and intermediate causes of childhood obesity and the determinants of and the relationships between eating and physical activity behaviors. Research also helps to refine theories about behavioral change that are necessary for the development of effective programs and promising practices. Ongoing research is examining the developmental changes of children and youth and the risk and protective factors that affect vulnerable periods during the life course relevant to childhood obesity. Given the complex interplay among environmental, social, economic, and behavioral factors that influence childhood obesity, considerably more research is necessary to inform an adequate and comprehensive response to the obesity epidemic.

In 2005, the Federal Interagency Working Group on Overweight and Obesity Research was formed to strengthen federal leadership in the area of obesity research. The working group is cochaired by the U.S. Office of Science and Technology Policy, DHHS, and USDA (Appendix D). Its purpose is threefold: to facilitate constructive, coordinated research across diverse federal agencies and departments; identify areas in which interagency collaboration can extend progress in obesity prevention; and advise OSTP's Committee on Science about the research needs and opportunities related to overweight and obesity and associated adverse health effects (NSTC, 2006). The intent of the working group is not to duplicate the research initiatives of other federal agencies, such as the NIH Obesity Research Task Force (see below); rather, it is intended to enhance and strengthen the total federal research effort by interdepartmental collaboration (Yanovski, 2006). The working group is in its initial phases, and its efforts have not yet been evaluated. The working group could serve as a component of the broader federal coordinating task force described earlier in this chapter.

The NIH Obesity Research Task Force was established in FY 2003 to accelerate progress in obesity research across the NIH institutes, centers, and offices and is another example of federal leadership in research. An important charge to the task force was the development and implementation of a Strategic Plan for NIH Obesity Research (Spiegel and Alving, 2005), the coordination of obesity-related research activities across NIH, and the development of new research efforts (NIH, 2004; Spiegel and Alving, 2005). The Strategic Plan for NIH Obesity Research focuses on goals for basic, clinical, and population-based obesity research and has the following strategies for achieving the goals:

- Identify modifiable behavioral and environmental factors that contribute to the development of obesity in children and adults through research for the prevention and treatment of obesity through lifestyle modification;
- Identify genetic factors and biologic targets related to obesity and identify pharmacologic, medical, and surgical approaches for preventing and treating obesity; and
- Identify the connections between obesity and type 2 diabetes, cardiovascular diseases, cancer, and other diseases and approaches for addressing these chronic conditions.

The strategic plan focuses on enhancing crosscutting research by encouraging interdisciplinary research teams; focusing on specific populations such as children and racial/ethnic minorities; conducting translational research that progresses from basic science to clinical studies, trials, and community interventions; and disseminating research results to the public (NIH, 2005).

It is unclear what proportion of the NIH research effort is dedicated to obesity prevention research and what proportion is dedicated to clinical research on treatment methods or basic research on the endocrine or metabolic mechanisms of obesity. To achieve the strategic plan's goals, activities must be coordinated among the NIH institutes, offices, and centers. Effective coordination has been identified as a formidable challenge for the implementation of other NIH strategic plans, including the Health Disparities Research Program, because of the research's scope and complexity and NIH's organizational and functional setting (IOM, 2006b). The committee's perspective is that similar challenges exist for effectively coordinating the Strategic Plan for NIH Obesity Research.

CDC's Prevention Research Center (PRC) programs also play an important role in obesity prevention research. The 33 currently funded PRC programs have established academic and community-based partnerships that collaboratively conduct research addressing the immediate health needs of communities. The community and university research partners identify the successful aspects of projects that can be disseminated to other communities (CDC, 2006c). Seven PRCs have projects that focus on obesity prevention such as Preventing Obesity in the United States. Other projects are Guidelines for Obesity Prevention and Control (Yale University), Adapting the Coordinated Approach To Child Health (CATCH) for Obesity Prevention and Control (University of Texas at Houston), Planet Health—A Health Education Program for School Children (Harvard University), Dietary Contributions to Obesity and Adolescents (Harvard University), and Impact of Neighborhood Design and Availability of Public Transportation on Physical Activity and Obesity Among Chicago Youths (Harvard University) (CDC, 2006c). A network of PRCs, referred to as the Physical Activity Policy Research Network, is collaborating to study policies and policy development pertaining to physical activity. Additionally, 7 PRCs and 12 state health departments are collaborating with the Center for Weight and Health at the University of California at Berkeley to review the dietary and developmental influences on obesity (Woodward-Lopez et al., 2006).

STATE AND LOCAL GOVERNMENTS

The *Health in the Balance* report called for state and local governments to implement the report's recommendations through the provision of coordinated leadership and support for childhood obesity efforts, particularly those focused on high-risk populations, by increasing resources and strengthening policies that promote opportunities for healthful eating and physical activity in communities, neighborhoods, and schools (IOM, 2005a). It encouraged the provision of support for public health agencies and local coalitions in their collaborative efforts to promote and evaluate obesity prevention interventions. State and local government agencies have traditionally and constitutionally been the primary overseers and implementers of public health activities. The important functions of state and local governments mirror those of the federal government and include leadership; the provision of program resources, funding, and evaluation; the conduct of statewide and local surveillance, monitoring, and research; and the dissemination and use of the evidence resulting from evaluations.

Leadership

Many states and communities throughout the nation are providing leadership through focused efforts to increase opportunities for physical activity and improve the dietary intake of children and youth. The National Governors Association made obesity prevention a priority as early as 2002 and has established a bipartisan task force of governors to provide further direction on this issue (NGA, 2003, 2006). As administrators of state programs, governors are in a central position to promote the societal norms and a culture that supports physical activity, healthful eating, and obesity prevention in their states (NGA, 2006). The Council of State Governments has developed a tool kit for policy options to promote healthy lifestyles and prevent obesity in youth (CSG, 2006).

Obesity prevention was also identified as a priority for local governments in a resolution at the 72nd Annual Meeting of the U.S. Conference of Mayors, which encouraged and supported local leadership through the implementation of policies, public health programs, and partnerships, including a focus on under-represented, low-income, and socially disadvantaged populations (USCM, 2004).

Several states have developed action plans focused on reducing obesity in children, youth, and adults. Many of these plans were developed through the collaborative efforts of voluntary health organizations, state agencies, nonprofit organizations, and health plans and other business partners (e.g., Georgia Department of Human Resources and Division of Public Health, 2005; North Carolina Department of Health and Human Services, 2005; West Virginia Healthy Lifestyle Coalition, 2005). Some plans originated with the action of a state agency to convene stakeholders, whereas other plans coalesced under the leadership of a nonprofit organization and then became an integral part of the state effort. In Texas, for example, the state strategic plan includes measurable objectives and sector-specific strategies for families, schools and child-care centers, communities, worksites, the health care sector, local businesses and private industry, and state government (Texas Statewide Obesity Taskforce, 2003).

As states and local governments work to develop and implement action plans, it is important that they sustain an active task force or standing committee to coordinate and oversee the efforts related to preventing childhood obesity. Task forces or committees function in ways that are appropriate for state and local conditions and practices, in general, and are expected to coordinate and leverage resources, ensure the capacity of government agencies to conduct surveillance and monitoring of programs, and ensure that childhood obesity prevention activities are appropriately evaluated at all levels.

In September 2005, the California Governor's Summit for a Healthy California brought together a diverse group of stakeholders to discuss the next steps for obesity prevention and health promotion in the state as outlined in a 10-point vision for healthy living (Box 4-6). Strategic planning efforts are under way to follow through on the actions discussed at the summit (Strategic Alliance, 2005) (Appendix F).

A number of states and communities have introduced or adopted bills and resolutions that represent legislative and policy actions related to childhood obesity prevention (Boehmer et al., 2006; TFAH, 2005) (Table 4-4).

BOX 4-6
A Vision for California—10 Steps Toward Healthy Living

1. Californians will understand the importance of physical activity and healthy eating, and they will make healthier choices based on that understanding.
2. Every child will participate in physical activities every day.
3. California's adults will be physically active every day.
4. Schools will offer only healthful foods and beverages to students.
5. Only healthful foods and beverages will be marketed to children ages 12 years and younger.
6. Produce and other fresh, healthful food items will be affordable and available in all neighborhoods.
7. Neighborhoods, communities and buildings will support physical activity, including safe walking, stair climbing, and bicycling.
8. Healthful foods and beverages will be accessible, affordable, and promoted in grocery stores, restaurants, and entertainment venues.
9. Health insurers and health care providers will promote physical activity and healthful eating.
10. Employees will have access to physical activity and healthful food and beverage options.

SOURCE: California Health & Human Services Agency and The California Endowment (2005).

TABLE 4-4 State Legislation Relevant to Childhood Obesity, 2003–2005

Topic	Description	Bills[a] # adopted/ # introduced (% adopted)	Resolutions[b] # adopted/ # introduced (% adopted)
School Environment			
Nutrition Standards, Vending Machines	Provide students with nutritious food and beverage items. Restrict access to vending machines and competitive foods. Regulate marketing of foods and beverages with minimal nutritional value. Report nutritional information and vending machine revenue.	27/213 (13%)	9/25 (36%)
Physical Education, Physical Activity	Ensure that schools have a physical education (PE) program. Set time and frequency for PE classes. Restrict substitutions and waivers for PE. Promote physical activity in other classes.	26/165 (16%)	14/26 (54%)
Health Education	Ensure that schools include nutrition, physical activity, and obesity prevention in health education curriculum.	12/68 (18%)	3/5 (60%)
Curriculum for Health and Physical Education Classes	Govern changes to the state's curriculum related to health, nutrition, and physical education. Require set hours of PE per week. Establish graduation requirements.	9/61 (15%)	2/7 (29%)
Local Authority	Provide local districts with the ability to set policies and create committees that focus on reducing the prevalence of obesity among school-age children through the regulation of low-nutrient food and beverages and physical activity requirements.	12/58 (21%)	1/4 (25%)
Safe Routes to School	Provide bicycle facilities, sidewalks, crossing guards, and traffic-calming measures to enable children to bicycle or walk safely to school.	12/43 (28%)	3/4 (75%)
Body Mass Index (BMI)	Require or allow schools to measure, monitor, and report student's BMI in conjunction with intervention strategies to help reduce childhood obesity.	8/37 (50%)	1/2 (22%)
Model School Policies	Require state agencies or state education officials to develop model school policies relating to nutrition and physical education.	4/14 (29%)	1/1 (100%)

TABLE 4-4 continued

Topic	Description	Bills[a] # adopted/ # introduced (% adopted)	Resolutions[b] # adopted/ # introduced (% adopted)
Community Environment			
Study/Council/ Task Force	Establish a commission, committee, council, task force, or study to address obesity within schools or communities.	11/68 (16%)	15/42 (36%)
Farmers' Markets	Support and make appropriations for farmers' market initiatives. Promote the implementation of locally grown nutritious foods in school systems.	31/87 (36%)	3/3 (100%)
Statewide Initiative	Establish initiatives, often though the state's department of health, to reduce the prevalence of obesity among residents statewide.	11/37 (30%)	28/35 (80%)
Walking/ Biking Paths	Support (through appropriations and regulations) physical activity through the creation or maintenance of bicycle trails, walking paths, and sidewalks. Promote bicycle and pedestrian safety.	17/46 (37%)	2/2 (100%)
Soda and Snack Tax	Increase or establish a tax on snacks and soft drinks. May use revenue to promote nutrition and health in schools.	0/49 (0%)	0/0 (0%)
Restaurant Menu and Product Labeling	Regulates the labeling of nutrition content on food items. Requires restaurants to post nutritional information on menus.	0/25 (0%)	0/0 (0%)
Total[c]		123/717 (17%)	71/134 (53%)

[a]A *bill* is a proposed law or amendment to an existing law that is presented to a state legislature for consideration. A bill requires approval by both chambers of the legislature and action by the governor in order to become law.

[b]A *resolution* is a formal expression of the will, opinion, or direction of one or both houses of the state legislature on a matter of public interest. Joint and concurrent resolutions are voted on by both houses but require no action on the part of the governor. Typically, resolutions are temporary in nature and do not have the power of law.

[c]Numbers and percents do not add up to the total because some bills and resolutions were listed in more than one topic area.

SOURCE: Adapted from Boehmer et al. (2006).

Many of these efforts are primarily focused on changing the school environment. However, there are some proposals relevant to childhood obesity prevention through its influence on communities (e.g., establishing farmers' markets, creating walking or bike paths, supporting smart growth, preserving green spaces, and addressing urban sprawl issues and industry (e.g., restaurant menu and product labeling, proposing taxes on soda or snack foods) (Boehmer et al., 2006; TFAH, 2005).

State legislation specific to schools has largely been focused on establishing nutritional standards for school foods, with growing attention being paid to mandating physical activity standards (Chapter 7). For example, legislation and regulations in Texas have mandated a minimum number of minutes of physical education for students in elementary, middle, and junior high schools; created local school health advisory councils; and established nutritional requirements for foods, beverages, and meals served in schools (TAHPERD, 2006; Texas Department of Agriculture, 2003). Arkansas Act 1220 was enacted in 2003 and included several school-related mandates, such as eliminating access to vending machines in public elementary schools, disclosing contracts for competitive foods and beverages, conducting annual BMI assessments for all students, and establishing nutrition and physical activity advisory committees to develop local policies (Ryan et al., 2006). The committee encourages the states to develop accountability mechanisms that provide the general public with information on the extent to which schools are meeting obesity prevention standards and evaluation results of innovative obesity prevention programs. Additionally, the committee supports increased legislative and other state and local government actions that will facilitate childhood obesity prevention efforts at the community, regional, and state levels.

Program Resources and Evaluation

Many state and local agencies have essential roles to play in designing, funding, implementing, and evaluating effective programs to support childhood obesity prevention goals. The obesity prevention efforts of local governments are complementary to those of the state and federal governments. In particular, local public health departments are involved in providing leadership for the horizontal integration of interventions, communications, and funding requirements, as well as developing an adequate infrastructure in which policies and programs can be implemented and evaluated at the local level.

Horizontal integration is a useful public health approach that encourages partners at the same level of operation—the neighborhood, city, county, regional, or state level—to work across organizational lines to deliver consistent, comprehensive, and multicomponent interventions. Examples of horizontal integration are the coordination of obesity prevention interventions through a local WIC program, a community youth agency, and a local business or a corporate-sponsored community-based program. Vertical integration is also used when partners work at different levels—the national, regional, state, county, and community levels—to deliver interventions planned at a higher level and delivered at a lower level in a coordinated way. The use of both the vertical and the horizontal integration approaches allow maximum synergy to facilitate effective collaboration.

The USDA's State Nutrition Action Plans have promoted horizontally and vertically integrated efforts across agency lines by local health departments, school districts, county extension agencies, and social service departments (USDA, 2006c). For example, the members of the Florida Interagency Food and Nutrition Agency include the Florida Department of Children and Families, the Department of Health, the Department of Education, the Department of Agriculture, and Consumer Services, among others, that coordinate nutrition campaigns and activities (FIFNC, 2006). Utah's Blueprint to Promote Healthy Weight for Children, Youth, and Adults addresses actions by families, schools, communities, worksites, health care, media, and government that are needed including forming a team of leaders to assume active roles in addressing issues of overweight and obesity (Bureau of Health Promotion, 2006).

At times, however, the division of authority among governments at the federal, state, and local levels has led to inconsistencies, ineffective resource allocation, and uncertainty about the respective roles and responsibilities of the units at each level that is challenging for the task of effective coordination (Baker et al., 2005; TFAH, 2006). A sustained effort that includes adequate planning and cooperation among governmental agencies and departments and other stakeholder groups is needed so that the units at each of these levels can effectively work together.

In addition, the overall capacity to address childhood obesity is not enhanced when increases in federal funding are responded to by decreases at the state level. Current funding for obesity prevention is also often tied to funding for other public health issues; thus, decision makers at the state and local levels are challenged by coordinating funds from a variety of funding strategies and sources (Finance Project, 2004).

Similar to other states, California has only recently begun to recognize the need to develop policies related to nutrition, physical activity, and food security and an infrastructure to enhance those provided by the federal government or to fill gaps where the federal government does not meet the state's needs in these areas. Like the federal government, California is starting to integrate the efforts of its categorical programs and establish crosscutting approaches to address obesity prevention. Some federal requirements, however, do not allow programs to address crosscutting problems, such as issues related to physical activity and the built environment. Methods such as consumer empowerment and community development to create more livable communities are not yet fully employed in nutrition and physical activity promotion programs.

Many states are exploring or implementing innovative programs related to childhood obesity prevention, and evaluation of these initiatives is the critical next step. For example, in Pennsylvania, the state department of health established Pennsylvania Advocates for Nutrition and Activity (PANA), a coalition-based organization supported by state and federal funds that provides technical assistance and resources for obesity prevention efforts and that serves as a communication clearinghouse. In 2005, PANA began the Keystone Healthy Zone Schools campaign, which recognizes schools that are working toward a healthier school environment (PANA, 2006). In West Virginia, the program WV Walks is a joint effort of the Monongalia County Health Department and West Virginia University that promotes walking through the use of the media, the Internet, and community-based campaigns (WV Walks, 2006). In Arkansas, efforts are under way to examine the link between receiving FSP benefits and childhood obesity.

The committee encourages the implementation and evaluation of innovative approaches and pilot programs that create incentives for the purchase of fruits and vegetables and other foods and beverages that contribute to healthful diets by participants in the FSP and other federal food assistance programs.

State- and Local-Level Surveillance and Monitoring

Existing surveillance systems have provided sufficient information to justify the implementation of actions that can address the obesity epidemic at the federal and state levels, but these systems often do not provide sufficient data that allow careful monitoring of long-term trends or the assessment of progress at the state and local levels.

Federally funded surveys may be designed to collect data at the national, state, and local levels; they may also collect only national data but provide technical assistance to state and local areas that collect state or local data. For example, CDC had conducted SHPPS every 6 years (e.g., 1994, 2000, and 2006) to assess school health-related policies and programs at the state, district, and local levels. In contrast, states and selected municipal health departments have conducted the SHP survey every 2 years since 1994, with technical assistance provided by CDC. In 2004, 27 states and 11 municipalities successfully completed the SHP survey. YRBSS has been conducted every 2 years since 1991. CDC provides technical assistance to states and municipalities that conduct YRBS at the state or local levels concurrent with CDC's performance of YRBS at the national level. In 2005, weighted results (which required a 60 percent or higher response rate) were collected for 40 states and 21 school districts (Eaton et al., 2006).

For younger children, state-based WIC programs measure height, weight, and dietary intake for participating infants and young children up to age 5 years. The WIC program provides information on the prevalence of obesity in high-risk groups from low-income families (IOM, 2005b).

Several states and localities also fund surveillance systems that can provide obesity-related data at state, county, and local levels. For example, the California Health Interview Survey (CHIS) is a biennial telephone survey of adults, adolescents, and children that provides extensive data on demographics, health outcomes, and health-related behaviors (CHIS, 2006). CHIS is funded by the joint efforts of the California Department of Health Services, other state agencies, several county health departments, federal agencies, foundations, and nonprofit organizations. CHIS provides data that allow the prevalence of obesity to be tracked at the county level, which is important in engaging local decision makers in this issue. In Los Angeles County (which, with approximately 10 million residents, has a population larger than that of 42 states), local surveillance sampling strategies and survey content have been coordinated, where feasible, with CHIS to permit corroboration of local findings and better comparisons with statewide findings. The Los Angeles County Health Survey is a random-digit-dial telephone survey of a representative sample of more than 8,000 adults with similar domains to those of CHIS conducted every 2 to 3 years (1997, 1999, 2002, and 2005). Hennepin County in Minnesota conducted its Survey of the Health of All the Population and the Environment (SHAPE) in 1998, 2002, and 2006 (SHAPE, 2006). This partnership of the Hennepin County Human Services and Public Health Departments and the University of Minnesota's School of Public Health collects data on lifestyle, environmental, and health-related indicators (e.g., height and weight).

Specifically focused datasets may also be available on a state-by-state basis. For example, the Arkansas Center for Health Improvement collects and analyzes data provided by the Arkansas school height and weight assessments. Prevalence of obesity can be analyzed by grade level and demographics (Thompson et al., 2006) (Chapter 7).

Although there are a limited number of surveillance systems that provide local and regional data, few provide the depth of information needed by local decision makers. Surveillance of funding and resources, the implementation of programs and policies, the availability of foods and beverages that contribute to healthful diets, the availability of places for physical activity, and the mapping of advocacy activities and grassroots efforts are a few of the other actions and outcomes that need to be monitored. One area in which evidence of progress has been noted is the monitoring of state legislation. Currently, several organizations track this information and provide online reports including CDC's Nutrition and Physical Activity Legislative Database (CDC, 2006e), the National Conference of State Legislatures summary of childhood obesity policy options (NCSL, 2006), the Trust for America's Health annual report of federal and state policies and legislation (TFAH, 2004, 2005), and NetScan's Health Policy Tracking Services for state legislation related to school nutrition and physical activity (NetScan, 2005). Enhanced coordination of these state legislative tracking efforts is needed.

A second area of general surveillance deficiency is in the surveillance of certain age or population groups, for which gaps certain gaps exist. This is particularly problematic for heterogeneous ethnic groups, for example, Asian Americans/Pacific Islanders. Pacific Islanders' obesity rates more closely mirror those of Latinos than those of Asian Americans, and in many Asian subgroups, obesity-related comorbidities are associated with BMIs lower than those for other populations (even BMIs considered nonoverweight or obese). As another example, state-specific information about elementary school-aged children and children ages 1 to 5 years who do not participate in the WIC program are not available.

Finally, few local surveillance systems have been established. Although community-level agencies and other sources are sampled and these data comprise the data used to make national and state estimates, the information from any given local area is generally insufficient in size or frequency to be used for surveillance for the local area itself. With the exception of data systems that collect data on every event (e.g., death and hospitalization data), the sample size limitations of any given surveillance system preclude the collection of sufficient data to monitor all localities. As a result, communities and local agencies should consider developing systems of their own, such as the Los Angeles County Health Survey or the SHAPE in Hennepin County, Minnesota (SHAPE, 2006). Local surveillance can often be jointly funded to leverage state and federal funds and to build on shared interests. Such an effort could consist of a collaboration between the local department of public works and the local health department to collect data on bicycling and walking.

APPLYING THE EVALUATION FRAMEWORK TO GOVERNMENT

What Constitutes Progress for Government?

The success of government efforts to prevent childhood obesity—and for all other sectors—will be determined by the reversal of the rise in the obesity and at-risk obesity prevalence for children and youth and a reduction in their obesity-related morbidities. Although the desire is to reverse this trend as quickly as possible, the achievement of long-term success to prevent childhood obesity may take several years or decades (as it did for tobacco-control efforts) and will require the sustained and coordinated implementation of a comprehensive and integrated spectrum of strategies and actions to produce the necessary changes in a variety of outcomes including structural, institutional, systemic, environmental, behavioral, and health outcomes. For the government sector, the achievement of short- and intermediate-term success will require evidence of leadership, strategic planning, political commitment, adequate funding, and capacity development, and a wide range of new, revised, or expanded policies, programs, surveillance and monitoring systems, partnerships and collaborations, and communications activities.

For the federal government, leadership and political commitment are essential and are made tangible by the provision of increased resources to support surveillance and monitoring, innovative interventions, and program evaluation. Support for goal setting, research, and surveillance by the federal government is particularly important. Federal research efforts should emphasize intervention research, that is, scientific assessments of the values of policies, environments, programs, and other activities that are implemented to improve dietary and physical activity behaviors. Surveillance systems need to be expanded not only to include behavioral and health outcomes, but also to monitor levels of funding, research, public health capacity, programmatic activities, policy development and implementation, and structural, institutional, and systemic outcomes.

Current Approaches to Assess Government Progress in Childhood Obesity Prevention

Evaluation is a priority for many federally and state-funded programs, which are generally required to conduct an evaluation and report on its results. Evaluation of government policies is more difficult.

Federal agencies and departments are held accountable and are evaluated in several ways, although the level of specificity often does not allow a specific set of initiatives, such as childhood obesity prevention programs, to be the focus of the evaluation. Each agency or department submits an annual report summarizing how budgets are spent and the status of programs; these reports usually need to cover a broad array of information and provide an overview of the entire agency, with few specifics on individual issues provided (CDC, 2005c; DHHS, 2005a; FTC, 2005; USDA, 2005a). Additionally, the U.S. Government Accountability Office (GAO) frequently conducts evaluations of federal programs at the request of Congress, some of which are relevant to childhood obesity prevention (GAO, 2004c, 2005a).

For example, GAO has examined the availability of competitive foods in relation to the USDA-administered school meals programs, USDA's nutrition education activities, and other related topics, such as commercial activities in schools and the use of schools as community centers (GAO, 2000a,b, 2003, 2004b, 2005b).

A 2005 congressionally requested GAO study focused on the collection of information on childhood obesity prevention program strategies and elements identified by experts as being "likely to contribute to success." For that assessment, GAO surveyed 233 experts in academia, the private sector, and government at all levels and interviewed program officials. The GAO assessment, which has had limited application, found that no comprehensive national inventory of childhood obesity programs exists at present and that there is no general consensus about the outcome measures that should be used to determine the success of programs for childhood obesity prevention (GAO, 2005a) (Chapter 2).

Another mechanism for assessing federal agency accountability is the Office of Management and Budget's (OMB's) Program Assessment Rating Tool (PART), which is used to evaluate federal agency programs for each fiscal year. Many of these federal agencies either currently support or have the potential to initiate or support childhood obesity prevention efforts. PART involves a review of evidence pertaining to the program purpose and design, strategic planning, program management, and results. The results are weighted for each component of the assessment; and the final results are issued in the form of a report card, in which a grade is assigned using five rating categories: fully effective, moderately effective, adequate, results not demonstrated, and ineffective (OMB, 2006). OMB evaluated 234 programs in FY 2005 and FY 2006 and found that over half (50.5 percent) had not demonstrated results, mostly because of a "lack of performance measures and/or performance data." OMB also noted that a majority of programs have measures that emphasize inputs rather than outcomes. Moreover, obesity prevention was absent from the evaluations of many programs in several federal agencies that have obesity prevention programs and that could be integrating evaluation activities into the existing programs, including USDA, and the U.S. Departments of Education, Interior, and Transportation (OMB, 2006).

A general lack of consensus and clarity exists about the types of outcome measures that should be used to determine the effectiveness of childhood obesity prevention policies or programs. Additionally, no evaluative component exists that can be used to examine the leadership activities, political commitment, funding, and capacity development efforts adopted by federal government agencies to address childhood obesity in the United States. There is a need for objective public health expertise to provide this evaluative component.

At the state level, several organizations use report card approaches that

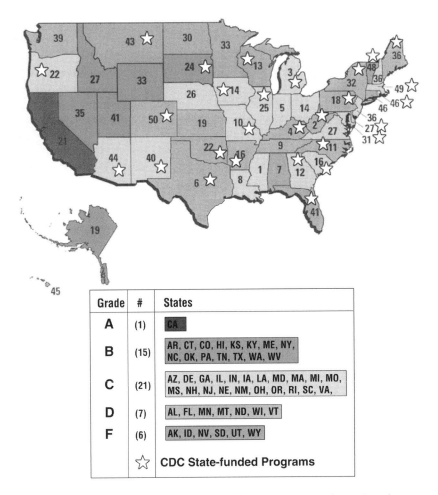

Grade	#	States
A	(1)	CA
B	(15)	AR, CT, CO, HI, KS, KY, ME, NY, NC, OK, PA, TN, TX, WA, WV
C	(21)	AZ, DE, GA, IL, IN, IA, LA, MD, MA, MI, MO, MS, NH, NJ, NE, NM, OH, OR, RI, SC, VA,
D	(7)	AL, FL, MN, MT, ND, WI, VT
F	(6)	AK, ID, NV, SD, UT, WY
	☆	**CDC State-funded Programs**

FIGURE 4-1 The University of Baltimore's Obesity Report Card™ ratings for state efforts to control childhood obesity.
NOTE: The number within each state represents its rank from the highest prevalence (1) to the lowest prevalence (50) of obesity in adults. The states receiving CDC grants for capacity building or implementation are identified by a star.
SOURCES: Adapted from the University of Baltimore (2005a); CDC (2006a).

rate states on the extent of legislative and policy activity. For example, the University of Baltimore (UB) issued the UB Obesity Report Card™ in 2004 and 2005 as an assessment of state efforts to pass obesity control policies (Figure 4-1). The evaluation is based on eight different types of legislation that have been introduced or passed in each of the 50 states (e.g., nutrition standards; recess and physical education standards; vending machine usage; BMI measurement in schools; and obesity-related programs and education, research, treatment, or task forces) (University of Baltimore, 2004, 2005b). UB also developed a report card specifically for state efforts to control childhood obesity (University of Baltimore, 2005a). The grade for each state is a composite of the score for each of the eight types of legislation, and the successful passage of a law in one of each area is necessary to obtain a grade of "A." Because the introduction of legislation may be an indicator of an increased awareness of the problem and the presence of a state's political will to prevent or control obesity, points are awarded even if the proposed legislation is not currently active. On the basis of the 2005 UB Obesity Report Card™, California was the only state to receive an "A" for its legislative efforts to control childhood obesity, whereas five states received an "F" for taking no legislative actions at all. No state received an "A" for its overall efforts to address the obesity epidemic. Although it is valuable to have this type of evaluation, it is important to recognize that this approach examines only one aspect of state prevention efforts, that is, those efforts that require legislative action, and does not take into account other policies, programs, and interventions. Figure 4-1 indicates the state ratings and delineates the grade for the 28 states currently receiving CDC grants for capacity building or implementation (CDC, 2006a).

Applying the Evaluation Framework

The evaluation framework introduced in Chapter 2 can be used to assess progress for government actions at all levels. Figure 4-2 highlights some of the strategies and actions to be considered when the extent to which government is demonstrating leadership and commitment in making childhood obesity prevention a national priority is evaluated. As discussed earlier in this chapter, federal and state high-level task forces could serve to coordinate and prioritize budgets, policies, and programs and serve as a basis for new initiatives.

Selected outcomes that assess the adequacy of government leadership are shown in Figure 4-2 and include assessments of the following:

1. *Policies and Programs:* assessments of whether a federal task force and 50 state-level task forces have been established, have developed and implemented strategic plans, and have produced annual progress reports showing that activities have been evaluated;
2. *Research:* assessments of whether childhood obesity prevention is incorporated into strategic research plans and activities across many federal agencies, such as CDC, NIH, and USDA;
3. *Coordination:* assessments of whether federal, state, and local gov-

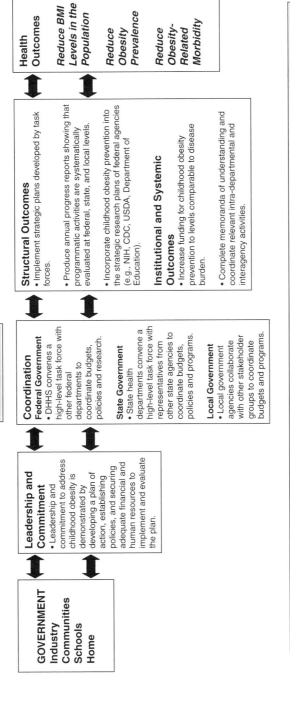

FIGURE 4-2 Evaluating government leadership to prevent childhood obesity.

ernment funding levels for childhood obesity prevention are comparable to funding for efforts on health outcomes of similar disease burden and whether relevant activities and budgets are coordinated across agencies and categorical programs; and

4. *Collaboration:* assessments of the implementation of memorandums of understanding and of intradepartmental and interagency activities.

Finally, the desirable health outcome that these changes could be linked to is an overall reduction in the prevalence of obesity in children and youth.

Figure 4-3 provides a framework for evaluating government efforts to support capacity development for preventing childhood obesity. A number of strategies and actions can be undertaken to support capacity development for programs, coordination, training, surveillance, and research. Programmatic activities for the prevention of childhood obesity will need to be expanded; and interventions will need to be implemented, monitored, and evaluated. The activities conducted by governmental and nongovernmental agencies will need to be coordinated for maximum efficiency. Training materials and methods for delivering the training will need to be developed. Surveillance systems will need to be improved, and new systems will need to be developed to enable monitoring of the full range of intervention activities displayed in the evaluation framework (Figure 4-3). Evaluation research needs to be conducted to confirm that promising interventions or best practices are being replicated. Selected outcomes for capacity development are shown in Figure 4-3 and include assessments of the following:

1. *Policies and programs:* assessments of whether federal programs have sufficient resources to provide adequate technical assistance to state agencies;
2. *Training:* assessments of whether state health departments have sufficient numbers of adequately trained staff to provide leadership and statewide training and whether all states meet the minimum staffing requirements recommended by CDC's State-Based Nutrition and Physical Activity Program to Prevent Obesity and Other Chronic Diseases;
3. *Surveillance and monitoring:* assessments of whether state and local health departments have adequate or improved surveillance systems to monitor trends in obesity, dietary patterns, and physical activity behaviors; and
4. *Research:* assessments of whether federally funded research that examines the causal relationships between exposure to specific physical and social environments and obesity is actively underway to reduce the prevalence of childhood obesity.

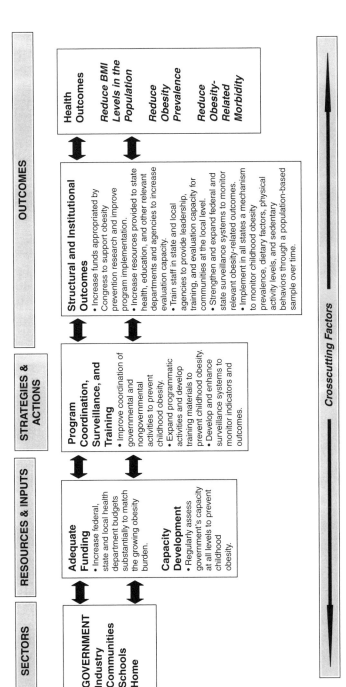

FIGURE 4-3 Evaluating government efforts to support capacity development for preventing childhood obesity.

Improved capacity will increase the knowledge base through the development, implementation, and evaluation of programs, policies, and interventions relevant to achieving and maintaining behavioral changes and improved health outcomes (Figure 4-3).

Needs and Next Steps in Assessing Progress

Leadership and Collaboration

Evidence of federal leadership and sustained political commitment is vital. The large number of federal programs related to preventing childhood obesity (Appendix D) and the examples described earlier in the chapter suggest that some progress in addressing the childhood obesity epidemic has been made. However, no progress on several important leadership actions has been made. The recommendation from the *Health in the Balance* report (IOM, 2005a) that "The President should request that the Secretary of DHHS convene a high-level task force to ensure coordinated budgets, policies, and program requirements and to establish interdepartmental collaboration and priorities for action" remains unfulfilled and should be a top priority.

Although leading administrative officials refer to the importance of the childhood obesity epidemic, the rhetoric has often not been matched with adequate resources to address it effectively. In addition to the activities identified above, the task force should also monitor federal obesity prevention activities and provide a biennial summary of relevant efforts across agencies, with particular attention given to the extent of federal resources appropriated for these efforts and evaluation results. The coordination of activities will improve efficiency but will not be sufficient without an infusion of resources to expand research and surveillance capabilities, increase agency capacity, facilitate the expansion of governmental and nongovernmental programs, and assure the evaluation of governmental policies, programs, and initiatives. Emphasis should be placed on intervention research, capacity improvement, and surveillance of strategies and actions. The committee recommends that the federal government, particularly DHHS, USDA, and the U.S. Department of Education, strengthen its leadership role by making childhood obesity prevention an urgent priority and reflecting this priority in the public statements, programs, research priorities, and budgets of federal departments and agencies.

Furthermore, state and local governments should provide coordinated leadership and support for childhood obesity prevention efforts by increasing resources and strengthening policies that promote opportunities for physical activity and healthful eating in communities, neighborhoods, and schools. This should include support for public health agencies and community coalitions so that they may promote and evaluate obesity prevention interventions. Local governments have the primary responsibility for shaping the built environment through general plans, land use ordinances, and capital improvement programs. Although changes to the built environment in communities can be part of obesity prevention efforts, many of the current efforts at the state and local levels have focused on improving nutrition and physical activity opportunities in schools. It is incumbent on state and local governments to also focus attention and funding on community-based programs and evaluations of those efforts (Chapter 6).

Develop, Sustain, and Support Evaluation and Evaluation Capacity

Evaluation should be a key component of all interventions funded by federal, state, and local government. The capacities of federal, state, and local agencies to conduct activities and interventions to prevent childhood obesity need to be strengthened.

The resources needed for capacity building of evaluation come from diverse funding streams, including a variety of federal and state agencies and departments, foundations, voluntary health organizations, and other sources. It is important that these resources be managed effectively and that funding for evaluation be increased to address the numerous childhood obesity prevention efforts that are planned and under way. The federal government is not expected to provide sole support for that capacity, but it is the responsibility of the federal government to monitor the capacity and to stimulate its development where necessary. Although CDC's Nutrition and Physical Activity Program to Prevent Obesity and Other Chronic Diseases and the Steps to a HealthierUS initiative are examples of capacity development programs, federal funding has not increased over the past 3 years. There are few, if any, other examples of federal activities designed to enhance the capacity to implement and evaluate childhood obesity prevention activities.

A concerted effort should be undertaken to take advantage of the existing strengths, competencies, and resources to provide technical program evaluation support to states and local communities. CDC, through its Office on Smoking and Health, has published *Key Outcome Indicators for Evaluating Comprehensive Tobacco Control Programs* (CDC, 2005d) as a practical, well-documented resource to help state and local health agencies and departments in their ongoing efforts to evaluate tobacco control programs. Such tools should be developed for the evaluation of childhood obesity prevention interventions. One component of this effort may build on the Communities of Excellence in Nutrition, Physical Activity, and Obesity Prevention (CX^3) database that is under development by the California Department of Health Services (2006) (Chapter 6; Appendix D).

The committee recommends additional support for existing and new programs to increase the capacities of federal, state, and local agencies to conduct and evaluate activities for the prevention of childhood obesity. The committee recommends that CDC, USDA, and state agencies develop similar resources to guide childhood obesity prevention policies and interventions. Specifically, a *Key Outcome Indicators for Evaluating Childhood Obesity Prevention Programs* resource, which could be modeled after CDC's guide for evaluating tobacco control efforts (CDC, 2005d), should be developed. Furthermore, supported by the evidence generated by the findings from childhood obesity prevention evaluations and research, a technical support and training component should be developed for program managers implementing and evaluating childhood obesity prevention activities and programs at the local level.

Enhance Surveillance, Monitoring, and Research

Surveillance is essential to maximizing the probability of success and the efficiency of childhood obesity prevention efforts. Federal surveillance systems are to be credited for alerting the nation to the national epidemic of obesity. However, surveillance systems need to be expanded beyond the monitoring of behavioral and health outcomes to include surveillance of the full spectrum of intervention activities depicted in the evaluation framework (Figure 4-3). A routine compilation and summary of the programs and activities of federal agencies would be valuable evidence of leadership as well as an important augmentation of surveillance activities.

Surveillance of environmental and institutional changes that are being implemented to promote healthful eating and regular physical activity is particularly lacking. Furthermore, surveillance of state and local policies, regulations, and practices that pertain to the prevention of childhood obesity provide an inadequate assessment of status or progress. Data with which to make those assessments are often not available at the local level (Chapter 6). The development of such systems has been hampered by insufficient resources and a lack of consensus about the factors that require surveillance. As a first step, CDC, USDA, and relevant state agencies should develop guidelines for the surveillance of policies and environmental outcomes pertaining to the prevention of childhood obesity. The creation of linkages should be explored between existing surveillance systems (e.g., YRBS and SHHPS) that could potentially increase the utility of the data (Chapter 7).

The committee also recommends support for applied behavioral research to identify programs that improve relevant short-, intermediate-, and long-term outcomes depicted in the evaluation framework and to identify interventions that are cost-effective and sustainable and that can be scaled-up. Community-based intervention research should receive increased federal attention and funding. Intervention research identifies programs that improve the short-, intermediate-, and long-term outcomes that will lead to favorable health outcomes. Intervention research is a special form of evaluation that is scientifically sophisticated and expensive. Intervention research identifies not only effective programs but also assesses cost-effectiveness, sustainability, and the potential for expansion. Federal support for intervention research is essential and could be channeled through CDC's PRCs to enable more intervention research and the development of a thematic network for the prevention of childhood obesity.

One largely untapped research opportunity is found in natural experiments[2] (TRB and IOM, 2005) involving political, environmental, or social changes implemented for reasons that may or may not pertain to childhood obesity but that might be expected to affect dietary or physical activity behavior and childhood obesity. An example of a natural experiment currently underway is the NIH research on the effects of recent changes in the use of vending machines in schools. The Federal Interagency Working Group on Overweight and Obesity Research should make the documentation of its progress publicly transparent, specify the areas of research that need to be emphasized, and prioritize obesity prevention and evaluation as areas for interagency collaboration.

SUMMARY AND RECOMMENDATIONS

Government is an integral part of the response to the childhood obesity epidemic. At the federal, state, and local levels, government has the authority and the resources to make childhood obesity prevention a public health priority and to act on that priority by authorizing and appropriating adequate funding, training personnel, and supporting technical capabilities directed to efforts that will increase opportunities for physical activity and improved diets for the population to engage in healthy lifestyles.

Efforts at all levels of government are evident and the committee could highlight here only selected policies, programs, and activities. However, opportunities abound for improving coordination between government agencies; increasing or sustaining funding for programs proven to be effective; and enhancing surveillance, technical assistance, and evaluation capacity. An increased emphasis on evaluation and increased funding for evalua-

---

[2]Natural experiments are naturally occurring circumstances in which different populations are exposed or not exposed to a potential causal factor or intervention such that it resembles a true experiment in which study participants are assigned to exposed and unexposed groups.

tion are urgently needed so that effective interventions can be scaled up, adapted to different contexts, and widely disseminated.

Each of the report's four recommendations presented in Chapter 2 is directly relevant to promoting leadership and collaboration and improving the evaluation efforts of government policies and interventions. The following text provides the report's recommendations and summarizes the specific implementation actions for government that are needed.

Recommendation 1: **Government, industry, communities, schools, and families should demonstrate leadership and commitment by mobilizing the resources required to identify, implement, evaluate, and disseminate effective policies and interventions that support childhood obesity prevention goals.**

Implementation Actions for Government
Federal, state, and local government should each establish a high-level task force to identify priorities for action, coordinate public-sector efforts, and establish effective interdepartmental collaborations.

To accomplish this,
- The president of the United States should request that the secretary of the DHHS convene a high-level task force involving the secretaries or senior officials from all relevant federal government departments and agencies (e.g., the U.S. Departments of Agriculture, Education, Defense, Interior, and Transportation; the Federal Communications Commission; and the Federal Trade Commission) to coordinate departmental budgets, policies, and research efforts and establish effective interdepartmental collaboration and priorities for action.
- State governments should convene high-level task forces involving the state departments of health, education, agriculture; the land-grant cooperative extension services, and other relevant agencies. Childhood obesity prevention should be a priority that is reflected in each state government's public statements, policies and programs, budgets, research efforts, and interagency collaboration.
- Local government agencies should convene community- or regional-level task forces to provide coordinated leadership in preventing childhood obesity by increasing resources, collaborating with community stakeholders, and developing or strengthening policies and programs that promote opportunities for physical activity and healthful eating in communities and neighborhoods.

Recommendation 2: Policy makers, program planners, program implementers, and other interested stakeholders—within and across relevant sectors—should evaluate all childhood obesity prevention efforts, strengthen the evaluation capacity, and develop quality interventions that take into account diverse perspectives, that use culturally relevant approaches, and that meet the needs of diverse populations and contexts.

Implementation Actions for Government

Federal and state government departments and agencies should consistently evaluate the effects of all actions taken to prevent childhood obesity and strengthen the evaluation capacity, paying particular attention to culturally relevant evaluation approaches.

To accomplish this,

- The actions of federal agencies, including policies that have been implemented, should be consistently evaluated to determine whether these actions and policies provide evidence of leadership and to identify the promising actions that are likely to be the most effective in preventing childhood obesity.
- The U.S. Congress should increase federal support for capacity-building activities such as the CDC's State-Based Nutrition and Physical Activity Program to Prevent Obesity and Other Chronic Diseases and Steps to a HealthierUS Program.
- Federal and state agencies should assess and strengthen the capacities of state and territorial health departments to provide leadership and technical assistance, enhance surveillance efforts, and implement and evaluate programs to prevent childhood obesity.
- DHHS, other federal agencies, and private-sector partners should work toward evaluating existing media efforts (including Small Step and Small Step Kids!) with the goal of developing, coordinating, and evaluating a more comprehensive, long-term, national multimedia and public relations campaign focused on obesity prevention in children and youth.

Recommendation 3: Government, industry, communities, and schools should expand or develop relevant surveillance and monitoring systems and, as applicable, should engage in research to examine the impact of childhood obesity prevention policies, interventions, and actions on relevant outcomes, paying particular attention to the unique needs of diverse groups and high-risk populations. Additionally, parents and caregivers should monitor changes in their family's food, beverage, and physical activity choices and their progress toward healthier lifestyles.

Implementation Actions for Government
Government at all levels should develop new surveillance systems or enhance existing surveillance systems to monitor relevant outcomes and trends and should increase funding for obesity prevention research.

> *To accomplish this,*
> - Federal and state government surveillance systems should monitor the full range of outcomes in the evaluation framework. Surveillance systems—such as NHANES, SHPPS, YMCLS, YRBSS, and NHTS—should be expanded to include relevant obesity-related outcomes. Surveillance systems that monitor the precursors of dietary and physical activity behaviors, including policies that have been implemented and structural, institutional, and environmental outcomes should be expanded or developed.
> - All states should have a mechanism in place to monitor childhood obesity prevalence, dietary factors, physical activity levels, and sedentary behaviors through population-based sampling over time.
> - The U.S. Congress should appropriate sufficient funds to support research on obesity prevention research (e.g., efficacy, effectiveness, quasiexperimental, cost-effectiveness, sustainability, and scaling up research) to improve program implementation and outcomes for children and youth.

Recommendation 4: Government, industry, communities, schools, and families should foster information-sharing activities and disseminate evaluation and research findings through diverse communication channels and media to actively promote the use and scaling up of effective childhood obesity prevention policies and interventions.

Implementation Actions for Government
Government at all levels should commit to the long-term support and dissemination of childhood obesity prevention policies and interventions that have been proven to be effective.

> *To accomplish this,*
> - Federal, state, and local governments should publicly disseminate and promote the results of evaluations of childhood obesity prevention policies and interventions.
> - The federal government should provide a sustained commitment and long-term investment to adequately support and disseminate childhood obesity prevention interventions that are proven to be effective—such as the VERB campaign. Further,

the federal government should provide sustained support for surveillance systems that are vital to the monitoring of trends and progress in response to the childhood obesity epidemic.

- Incentives and rewards should be developed for state and local government agencies to coordinate efforts that improve obesity-related outcomes for children and youth.

REFERENCES

Ad Council. 2006. *Obesity Prevention: Campaign Results Summary*. Washington DC.

Aeffect, Inc. 2005. Excerpts from research to support development of the Youth Media Campaign: Revealing target audience receptiveness to potential message concepts. *Soc Market Q* 11(1):47–56.

Baker EL, Potter MA, Jones DL, Mercer SL, Cioffi JP, Green LW, Halverson PK, Lichtveld MY, Fleming DW. 2005. The public health infrastructure and our nation's health. *Annu Rev Public Health* 26:303–318.

Biing-Hwan L, Logan C, Fox MK, Smallwood D. 2006. Data for assessing outcomes of food assistance and nutrition programs. *Nutr Today* 41(1):32–37.

Boehmer TK, Brownson RC, Haire-Joshu D, Dreisinger ML. 2006. *Patterns of Childhood Obesity Prevention: Legislation in the United States*. Working Paper. St. Louis University School of Public Health, St. Louis, Mo.

Branaman B. 2003. *Fruits and Vegetables: Issues for Congress*. Congressional Research Service, The Library of Congress. [Online]. Available: http://ncseonline.org/NLE/CRS reports/03Feb/IB10098.pdf [accessed May 10, 2006].

BTS (Bureau of Transportation Statistics). 2006. *National Household Travel Survey*. [Online]. Available: http://www.bts.gov/programs/national_ household_travel_survey/ [accessed May 16, 2006].

Bureau of Health Promotion. 2006. *Tipping the Scales Toward a Healthier Population: The Utah Blueprint to Promote Healthy Weight for Children, Youth, and Adults*. Salt Lake City, UT: Utah Department of Health. [Online]. Available: http://health.utah.gov/obesity/ [accessed July 19, 2006].

Buzby JC, Guthrie JF, Kantor LS. 2003. *Evaluation of the USDA Fruit and Vegetable Pilot Program: Report to Congress*. E-FAN-03-006. Washington, DC: USDA. [Online]. Available: http://www.fns.usda.gov/cnd/Research/FV030063.pdf [accessed May 8, 2006].

California Department of Health Services. 2006. *Communities of Excellence in Nutrition, Physical Activity, and Obesity Prevention (CX³)*. [Online]. Available: http://www.ca5aday.org/CX3 [accessed July 14, 2006].

California Health & Human Services Agency and The California Endowment. 2005. *Governor's Vision for a Healthy California*. [Online]. Available: http://www.mrmib.ca.gov/MRMIB/Gov_vision.pdf [accessed July 12, 2006].

CDC (Centers for Disease Control and Prevention). 2004. Indicators for chronic disease surveillance. *MMWR* 3(RR-11):1–120.

CDC. 2005a. *Obesity Trends: U.S. Obesity Trends 1985–2004*. [Online]. Available: http://www.cdc.gov/nccdphp/dnpa/obesity/trend/maps/index.htm [accessed March 6, 2006].

CDC. 2005b. Assessment of epidemiologic capacity in states and territorial health departments—United States, 2004. *MMWR* 54(18):457–459.

CDC. 2005c. *CDC Now: Protecting Health for Life. The State of the CDC, Fiscal Year 2005*. [Online]. Available: http://www.cdc.gov/about/stateofcdc/fy05/cd/SOCDC/SOCDC2005.pdf [accessed June 15, 2006].

CDC. 2005d. *Key Outcome Indicators for Evaluating Comprehensive Tobacco Control Programs*. [Online]. Available: http://www.cdc.gov/tobacco/Indicators/Key_Indicators.pdf [accessed June 12, 2006].

CDC. 2006a. *Formative Research*. [Online]. Available: http://www.cdc.gov/youthcampaign/research/formative.htm [accessed August 8, 2006].

CDC. 2006b. *Overweight and Obesity: State-Based Programs*. [Online]. Available: http://www.cdc.gov/NCCDPHP/DNPA/obesity/state_programs/index.htm [accessed June 26, 2006].

CDC. 2006c. *Prevention Research Centers Profiles*. [Online]. Available: http://www.cdc.gov/prc/centers/index.htm [accessed March 9, 2006].

CDC. 2006d. *Process Evaluation*. [Online]. Available: http://www.cdc.gov/youthcampaign/research/process.htm [accessed August 8, 2006].

CDC. 2006e. *State Legislative Information: Search for Bills*. [Online]. Available: http://apps.nccd.cdc.gov/DNPALeg/ [accessed July 19, 2006].

CDC and RTI International. 2006. *Improving Nutrition, Physical Activity, and Obesity Prevention: Performance Report of the Nutrition and Physical Activity Program to Prevent Obesity and Other Chronic Diseases: July 1 Through December 31, 2005*. CDC Contract No. 200-2001-00123, Task 29, RTI Project No. 08235.029.

CHIS (California Health Interview Survey). 2006. *California Health Interview Survey*. [Online]. Available: http://www.chis.ucla.edu [accessed June 13, 2006].

CNWICRA (Child Nutrition and WIC Reauthorization Act). 2004. *Child Nutrition and WIC Reauthorization Act of 2004*. P. L. 108-265, 108th Congress, June 30, 2004. [Online]. Available: http://www.fns.usda.gov/cnd/Governance/Legislation/PL_108-265.pdf [accessed March 22, 2006].

CSG (Council of State Governments). 2006. *Tool Kit on Trends and Policy Solutions for Youth Obesity*. [Online]. Available: http://www.healthystates.csg.org/Public+Health+Issues/Obesity/Obesity+Resources.htm [accessed June 19, 2006].

CSTE (Council of State and Territorial Epidemiologists). 2004. *National Assessment of Epidemiologic Capacity: Findings and Recommendations*. Atlanta, GA: Council of State and Territorial Epidemiologists.

DHHS (U.S. Department of Health and Human Services). 2001. *The Surgeon General's Call to Action to Prevent and Decrease Overweight and Obesity*. Rockville, MD: Public Health Service, Office of the Surgeon General, U.S. Public Health Service.

DHHS. 2004. *Strategic Plan FY 2004–2009*. Washington, DC: U.S. Department of Health and Human Services. [Online]. Available: http://aspe.hhs.gov/hhsplan/2004/hhsplan 2004.pdf [accessed May 17, 2006].

DHHS. 2005a. *FY2005 Performance and Accountability Report*. Office of Finance, DHHS. [Online]. Available: http://www.hhs.gov/of/library/par05/pdfmenu/ [accessed June 15, 2006].

DHHS. 2005b. *Steps to a HealthierUS*. [Online]. Available: http://www.cdc.gov/steps/about_us/index.htm [accessed July 3, 2006].

DHHS. 2005c. *Funding Communities to Prevent Obesity, Diabetes, and Asthma FY2004*. [Online]. Available: http://www.healthierus.gov/steps/grantees/2004/StepsCoopAgrmn.pdf [accessed July 20, 2006].

DHHS. 2006. *FY 2006 Budget in Brief*. [Online]. Available: http://www.hhs.gov/budget/06budget/cdc.html [accessed May 13, 2006].

DHHS and USDA (U.S. Department of Agriculture). 2005. *Dietary Guidelines for Americans 2005*. [Online]. Available: http://www.healthierus.gov/dietaryguidelines [accessed December 29, 2005].

DoL (U.S. Department of Labor). 2006. *National Longitudinal Surveys*. [Online]. Available: http://www.bls.gov/nls/ [accessed May 16, 2006].

Eaton DK, Kann L, Kinchen S, Ross J, Hawkins J, Harris WA, Lowry R, McManus T, Chyen D, Shanklin S, Lim C, Grunbaum JA, Wechsler H. 2006. Youth risk behavior surveillance—United States, 2005. *MMWR* 55(5):1–108.

ERS (Economic Research Service). 2002. *Farm Policy. Title IV Nutrition Programs.* [Online]. Available: http://www.ers.usda.gov/Features/farmbill/titles/titleIVnutritionprograms.htm [accessed May 8, 2006].

FDA (U.S. Food and Drug Administration). 2006. *Food Labeling and Nutrition.* [Online]. Available: http://www.cfsan.fda.gov/~dms/lab-ind.html [accessed May 16, 2006].

FIFNC (Florida Interagency Food and Nutrition Committee). 2006. *Florida Interagency Food and Nutrition Committee: SNAP, the Florida Way.* [Online]. Available: http://www. fns.usda.gov/oane/menu/NNEC/Files/Presentations/FloridaSNAP.pdf [accessed June 15, 2006].

Finance Project. 2004. *Financing Childhood Obesity Prevention Programs: Federal Funding Sources and Other Strategies.* [Online]. Available: http://www.financeproject.org/ Publications/obesityprevention.pdf [accessed May 16, 2006].

Finkelstein EA, Fiebelkorn IC, Wang G. 2003. National medical spending attributable to overweight and obesity: How much, and who's paying? *Health Aff* W3:219–226.

Finkelstein EA, Fiebelkorn IC, Wang G. 2004. State-level estimates of annual medical expenditures attributable to obesity. *Obes Res* 12(1):18–24.

Flegal KM, Carroll MD, Ogden CL, Johnson CL. 2002. Prevalence and trends in obesity among US adults, 1999–2000. *J Am Med Assoc* 288(14):1723–1727.

Food, Nutrition, and Consumer Services. 2006. *Statement of Eric Bost, Under Secretary, Food, Nutrition, and Consumer Services Before the Subcommittee on Agriculture, Rural Development, Food and Drug Administration and Related Agencies, U.S. House of Representatives.* [Online]. Available: http://appropriations.house.gov/_files/EricBost Testimony.pdf [accessed June 12, 2006].

FTC (Federal Trade Commission). 2005. *Performance and Accountability Report 2005.* [Online]. Available: http://www.ftc.gov/opp/gpra/index.htm [accessed June 15, 2006].

FTC. 2006. Request for information and comment: Food industry marketing practices to children and adolescents. *Fed Regist* 71(4):10535–10536. [Online]. Available: http:// a257.g.akamaitech.net/7/257/2422/01jan20061800/edocket.access.gpo.gov/2006/06- 1931.htm [accessed March 6, 2006].

FTC and DHHS. 2006. *Perspectives on Marketing, Self-regulation & Childhood Obesity: A Report on a Joint Workshop of the Federal Trade Commission & the Department of Health and Human Services.* [Online]. Available: http://www.ftc.gov/os/2006/05/ PerspectivesOnMarketingSelfRegulation&ChildhoodObesityFTCandHHSReporton JointWorkshop.pdf [accessed May 8, 2006].

GAO (U.S. General Accounting Office). 2000a. *Commercial Activities in Schools.* Report HEHS-00-156. Washington, DC: GAO. [Online]. Available: http://www.gao.gov/archive/ 2000/he00156.pdf [accessed June 12, 2006].

GAO. 2000b. *School Facilities: Construction Expenditures Have Grown Significantly in Recent Years.* Report HEHS-00-41. Washington, DC: GAO. [Online]. Available: http:// www.gao.gov/archive/2000/he00041.pdf [accessed June 12, 2006].

GAO. 2003. *School Lunch Program: Efforts Needed to Improve Nutrition and Encourage Healthy Eating.* Report GAO-03-506. Washington, DC: GAO. [Online]. Available: http:// www.gao.gov/new.items/d03506.pdf [accessed [accessed June 12, 2006].

GAO. 2004a. *Nutrition Education: USDA Provides Services Through Multiple Programs, but Stronger Linkages Among Efforts Are Needed.* Report No. GAO-04-528. Washington, DC: GAO. [Online]. Available: http://www.gao.gov/new.items/d04528.pdf [accessed June 13, 2006].

GAO. 2004b. *School Meal Programs: Competitive Foods Are Available in Many Schools: Actions Taken to Restrict Them Differ by State and Locality.* Report GAO-04-673. Washington, DC: GAO. [Online]. Available: http://www.gao.gov/new.items/d04673.pdf [accessed June 12, 2006].

GAO. 2004c. *Strategic Plan 2004–2009.* [Online]. Available: http://www.gao.gov/sp/d04534sp. pdf [accessed April 22, 2006].

GAO (U.S. Government Accountability Office). 2005a. *Childhood Obesity: Most Experts Identified Physical Activity and the Use of Best Practices as Key to Successful Programs.* Report GAO-06-127R. Washington, DC: GAO. [Online]. Available: http://www.gao. gov/new.items/d06127r.pdf [accessed June 12, 2006].

GAO. 2005b. *School Meal Programs: Competitive Foods are Widely Available and Generate Substantial Revenues for Schools.* Report GAO-05-563. Washington, DC: GAO. [Online]. Available: http://www.gao.gov/new.items/d05563.pdf [accessed June 12, 2006].

Georgia Department of Human Resources and Division of Public Health. 2005. *Georgia's Nutrition and Physical Activity Plan: 2005–2015.* [Online]. Available: http://health. state.ga.us/pdfs/familyhealth/nutrition/Nutritionand PhysicalActivityPlanFINAL.pdf [accessed June 13, 2006].

Gregson J, Foerster SB, Orr R, Jones L, Benedict J, Clark B, Hersey J, Lewis J, Zotz K. 2001. System, environmental, and policy changes: Using the social-ecological model as a framework for evaluating nutrition education and social marketing programs with low-income audiences. *J Nutr Educ* 33(Suppl 1): S4–S15.

Hartwig M. 2004. *Harkin Enlists Institute of Medicine to Study Foods in Schools.* U.S. Senator Tom Harkin of Iowa. November 24. [Online]. Available: http://harkin.senate. gov/press/print-release.cfm?id=228717 [accessed May 16, 2005].

Health Canada. 2001. *The Population Health Template: Key Elements and Actions that Define a Population Health Approach.* [Online]. Available: http://www.phac-aspc.gc.ca/ ph-sp/phdd/pdf/discussion_paper.pdf [accessed April 17, 2006].

Hedley AA, Ogden CL, Johnson CL, Carroll MD, Curtin LR, Flegal KM. 2004. Prevalence of overweight and obesity among US children, adolescents, and adults, 1999–2002. *J Am Med Assoc* 291(23):2847–2850.

Hersey J, Daugherty S. 1999. *Evaluating Social Marketing in Nutrition: A Resource Manual.* Report prepared by Research Triangle Institute and Health Systems Research, Inc. Alexandria, VA: Food and Nutrition Service, U.S. Department of Agriculture.

Huhman M. 2006 (April 27). *Promoting Physical Activity Among Tweens: Evaluation Results of CDC's VERB™ Campaign.* Presentation at the Kaiser Family Foundation Forum on Assessing the Effectiveness of Public Education Campaigns, Washington, DC. [Online]. Available: http://www.kff.org/entmedia/upload/-Promoting-Physical-Activity-Among-Tweens-Evaluation-Results-of-CDC-s-VERB-Campaign-Marian-Huhman.pdf [accessed April 30, 2006].

Huhman M, Heitzler CD, Wong FL. 2004. The VERB™ campaign logic model: A tool for planning and evaluation. *Prev Chron Dis* 1(3):1–6. [Online]. Available: http:// www.cdc.gov/Pcd/issues/2004/jul/04_0033.htm [accessed July 23, 2006].

Huhman M, Potter LD, Wong FL, Banspach SW, Duke JC, Heitzler CD. 2005. Effects of a mass media campaign to increase physical activity among children: Year-1 results of the VERB™ campaign. *Pediatrics* 116(2):e277–e284.

Huhman ME, Potter LD, Duke JC, Judkins MA, Heitzler CD, Wong FL. 2007. Evaluation of a national physical activity intervention for children: VERB campaign, 2002–2004. *Am J Prev Med* 32(1):38–43.

IOM (Institute of Medicine). 1988. *The Future of Public Health.* Washington, DC: National Academy Press.

IOM. 2003. *The Future of the Public's Health in the 21st Century.* Washington, DC: The National Academies Press.

IOM. 2005a. *Preventing Childhood Obesity: Health in the Balance.* Washington, DC: The National Academies Press.

IOM. 2005b. *WIC Food Packages: Time for a Change.* Washington, DC: The National Academies Press.

IOM. 2006a. *Nutrition Standards for Foods in Schools.* [Online]. Available: http://www. iom.edu/project.asp?id=30181 [accessed May 15, 2006].

IOM. 2006b. *Examining the Health Disparities Research Plan of the National Institutes of Health: Unfinished Business.* Washington DC: The National Academies Press.

MacDonald G, Garcia D, Zaza S, Schooley M, Compton D, Bryant T, Bagnol L, Edgerly C, Haverkate R. 2006. Steps to a HealthierUS Cooperative Agreement Program: Foundational elements for program evaluation planning, implementation, and use of findings. *Prev Chronic Dis* [Online] Available: http://www.cdc.gov/pcd/issues/2006/jan/pdf/05_0136.pdf [accessed March 22, 2006].

Mokdad AH, Serdula MK, Dietz WH, Bowman BA, Marks JS, Koplan JP. 1999. The spread of the obesity epidemic in the United States, 1991–1998. *J Am Med Assoc* 282(16):1519–1522.

NACCHO (National Association of County and City Health Officials). 2005. *Operational Definition of a Functional Local Health Department.* [Online]. Available: http:// www. naccho.org/topics/infrastructure/documents/Operation-alDefinitionBrochure.pdf [accessed February 9, 2006].

National WIC Association. 2003. *National WIC Association.* [Online]. Available: http:// www.nwica.org/ [accessed June 28, 2006].

NCSL (National Conference of State Legislatures). 2006. *Childhood Obesity—2005 Update and Overview of Policy Options.* [Online]. Available: http://www.ncsl.org/programs/ health/ChildhoodObesity-2005.htm [accessed April 24, 2006].

NetScan. 2005. *School Nutrition & Physical Education Legislation: An Overview of 2005 State Activity.* [Online]. Available: http://www.rwjf.org/files/research/NCSL%20-%20 April%202005%20Quarterly%20Report.pdf [accessed April 24, 2006.

NGA (National Governors Association) Center for Best Practices. 2003. *Preventing Obesity in Youth Through School-Based Efforts.* [Online]. Available: http://www.nga.org/cda/ files/022603PREVENTING.pdf [accessed January 6, 2006].

NGA. 2006. *Healthy America: Wellness Where We Live, Work and Learn. Call to Action: An Agenda for America's Governors.* [Online]. Available: http://www.nga.org/Files/pdf/ 0602HEALTHYAMCALL.PDF [accessed March 2, 2006].

NIH (National Institutes of Health). 2004. *Strategic Plan for NIH Obesity Research.* [Online]. Available: http://obesityresearch.nih.gov/About/ObesityEntireDocument.pdf [accessed December 30, 2005].

NIH. 2005. *NIH Obesity Research.* [Online]. Available: http://obesityresearch.nih.gov/News/ background.htm [accessed June 7, 2006].

North Carolina Department of Health and Human Services. 2005. *Eat Smart, Move More. . . North Carolina.* [Online]. Available: http://www.eatsmart movemorenc.com/aboutus. htm [accessed June 14, 2006].

NSTC (National Science and Technology Council). 2006. *National Science and Technology Council.* Draft. [Online]. Available: http://www.ostp.gov/nstc/html/NSTCOrgChart.pdf [accessed July 30, 2006].

Ogden CL, Flegal KM, Carroll MD, Johnson CL. 2002. Prevalence and trends in overweight among US children and adolescents, 1999–2000. *J Am Med Assoc* 288(14):1728–1732.

Ogden CL, Carroll MD, Curtin LR, McDowell MA, Tabek CJ, Flegal KM. 2006. Prevalence of overweight and obesity in the United States, 1999–2004. *J Am Med Assoc* 295(13): 1549–1555.

OMB (Office of Management and Budget). 2005. *National School Lunch Program, Key Performance Measures, FY2004.* [Online]. Available: http://www.whitehouse.gov/omb/budget/fy2004/pma/nationalschool.pdf [accessed August 9, 2006].

OMB. 2006. *Program Assessment Rating Tool.* [Online]. Available: http://www.whitehouse.gov/omb/budget/fy2006/part.html [accessed April 22, 2006].

PANA (Pennsylvania Advocates for Nutrition and Activity). 2006. *Joining Forces to Create an Active and Healthy State.* [Online]. Available: http://www.panaonline.org/ [accessed June 7, 2006].

Ryan KW, Card-Higginson P, McCarthy SG, Justus MB, Thompson JW. 2006. Arkansas fights fat: Translating research into policy to combat childhood and adolescent obesity. *Health Aff* 25(4):992–1004.

Schneider DJ, Carithers T, Coyle K, Endahl J, Robin L, McKenna M, Debrot K, Seymour J. 2006. Evaluation of a fruit and vegetable distribution program—Mississippi, 2004–05 school year. *MMWR* (35):957–961.

Schoonover H, Muller M. 2006. *Food Without Thought. How U.S. Farm Policy Contributes to Obesity.* Minneapolis, MN: Institute for Agriculture and Trade Policy. [Online]. Available: http://www.iatp.org/iatp/publications.cfm?accounID=421&refID=80627#search=%22Food%20Without%20Thought%20IATP%22 [accessed August 24, 2006].

SHAPE (Survey on the Health of All the Population, and the Environment). 2006. *Survey on the Health of All the Population, and the Environment.* [Online]. Available: http://www.co.hennepin.mn.us/vgn/images/portal/cit_100003616/39/0/163356092Generic Handout.pdf [accessed July 19, 2006].

Spiegel AM, Alving BM. 2005. Executive summary of the Strategic Plan for National Institutes of Health Obesity Research. *Am J Clin Nutr* 82(1):211S–214S.

Strategic Alliance. 2005. *Governor's Summit Follow-up: Moving Forward on a Statewide and Local Level.* Oakland, CA. [Online]. Available: http://www.preventioninstitute.org/sa/documents/GovernorSummitReportPDF_000.pdf [accessed May 15, 2006].

TAHPERD (Texas Association for Health, Physical Education, Recreation, and Dance). 2006. *Physical Activity.* [Online]. Available: http://www.tahperd.org/LINKS/links_physical_ed.html [accessed July 18, 2006].

Texas Department of Agriculture. 2003. *Square Meals: Policy Implications.* [Online]. Available: http://www.squaremeals.org/fn/render/channel/items/0,1249,2348_2351_0_0,00.html [accessed March 1, 2006].

Texas Statewide Obesity Taskforce. 2003. *Strategic Plan for the Prevention of Obesity in Texas.* http://www.dshs.state.tx.us/phn/pdf/obesity-plan.pdf [accessed June 14, 2006].

TFAH (Trust for America's Health). 2004. *F as in Fat: How Obesity Policies Are Failing America.* Washington DC: The Trust for America's Health. [Online]. Available: http://healthyamericans.org/reports/obesity/Obesity Report.pdf [accessed June 27, 2006].

TFAH. 2005. *F as in Fat: How Obesity Policies Are Failing America 2005.* Washington DC: The Trust for America's Health. [Online]. Available: http://healthyamericans.org/reports/obesity2005/Obesity2005Report.pdf [accessed December 22, 2005].

TFAH. 2006. *Shortchanging America's Health 2006. A State-by-State Look At How Federal Public Health Dollars Are Spent.* Washington DC: The Trust for America's Health. [Online]. Available: http://healthyamericans.org/reports/shortchanging06/ [accessed June 27, 2006].

Thompson J, Shaw J, Card-Higginson P, Kahn R. 2006. Overweight among students in grades K–12: Arkansas, 2003–04 and 2004–05 school years. *MMWR* 55(1):5–8.

Tillotson JE. 2004. America's obesity: Conflicting public policies, industrial economic development, and unintended human consequences. *Annu Rev Nutr* 24:617–643.

TRB (Transportation Research Board) and IOM (Institute of Medicine). 2005. *Does the Built Environment Influence Physical Activity? Examining the Evidence.* TRB Special Report 282. Washington, DC: The National Academies Press. [Online]. Available: http://books.nap.edu/html/SR282/SR282.pdf [accessed December 29, 2005].

Troiano RP, Flegal KM, Kuczmarski RJ, Campbell SM, Johnson CL. 1995. Overweight prevalence and trends for children and adolescents. *Arch Pediatr Adolesc Med* 149(10):1085–1091.

UFFVA (United Fresh Fruit and Vegetable Association). 2006. *Fruit and Vegetable Snack Program Resource Center.* [Online]. Available: http://www.uffva.org/fvpilotprogram.htm [accessed May 10, 2006].

University of Baltimore. 2004. *UB Obesity Report Card.* [Online]. Available: http://www.ubalt.edu/experts/obesity/states.html [accessed June 30, 2006].

University of Baltimore. 2005a. *State Efforts to Control Childhood Obesity.* [Online]. Available: http://www.ubalt.edu/experts/obesity/large_state_childhood.jpg [accessed June 30, 2006].

University of Baltimore. 2005b. *The UB Obesity Report Card: An Overview.* [Online]. Available: http://www.ubalt.edu/experts/obesity/ [accessed June 30, 2006].

U.S. Census Bureau. 2006. *American Community Survey.* [Online]. Available: http://www.census.gov/acs [accessed August 7, 2006].

USCM (U.S. Conference of Mayors). 2004. *Supporting Efforts in the Prevention and Treatment of Obesity and Overweight.* [Online]. Available: http://www.usmayors.org/uscm/resolutions/72nd_conference/apes_05.asp [accessed July 5, 2006].

USDA (U.S. Department of Agriculture). 2001. *School Nutrition Dietary Assessment Study.* [Online]. Available: http://www.fns.usda.gov/OANE/MENU/Published/CNP/FILES/SNDAIIfindsum.htm [accessed May 16, 2006].

USDA. 2005a. *Performance and Accountability Report 2005.* Part I. [Online]. Available: http://www.usda.gov/ocfo/usdarpt/pdf/par04.pdf [accessed February 23, 2006].

USDA. 2005b. *Fit WIC: Programs to Prevent Childhood Overweight in Your Community.* Special Nutrition Program Report Series, No. WIC-05-FW. USDA Food and Nutrition Service. Alexandria, VA: Office of Analysis, Nutrition, and Evaluation. [Online]. Available: http://www.fns.usda.gov/oane/MENU/Published/WIC/FILES/fitwic.pdf [accessed February 28, 2006].

USDA. 2006a. *Department of Defense Fresh Fruit and Vegetable Program.* [Online]. Available: http://www.fns.usda.gov/fdd/programs/dod/DoD_Fresh FruitandVegetableProgram.pdf [accessed May 16, 2006].

USDA. 2006b. *The Food Assistance Landscape.* Economic Information Bulletin 6-2. USDA Economic Research Service. [Online]. Available: http://www.ers.usda.gov/publications/eib6-2/eib6-2.pdf [accessed February 21, 2006].

USDA. 2006c. *State Nutrition Action Plans.* [Online]. Available: http://www.fns.usda.gov/oane/SNAP/SNAP.htm [accessed February 28, 2006].

USDA. 2006d. Special Supplemental Nutrition Program for Women, Infants and Children (WIC): Revisions in the WIC food packages; Proposed Rule. *Fed Regist* 71(151):44784–44924. [Online]. Available: http://www.fns.usda.gov/wic/regspublished/foodpackages revisions-proposedrulepdf.pdf [accessed August 9, 2006].

Wang G, Dietz WH. 2002. Economic burden of obesity in youths aged 6–17 years: 1979–1999. *Pediatrics* 109(5): E81–E86. [Online]. Available: http//www.pediatrics.org/chi/content/full/109(5)e81 [accessed February 9, 2006].

West Virginia Healthy Lifestyle Coalition. 2005. *Taking Action to Address Obesity in West Virginia: Recommendations of the West Virginia Healthy Lifestyle Coalition.* [Online]. Available: http://www.healthywv.com/shared/content/page_objects/content_objects/action_plan_2005.pdf [accessed June 28, 2006].

Williams J, Wake M, Hesketh K, Maher E, Waters E. 2005. Health-related quality of life of overweight and obese children. *J Am Med Assoc* 293(1):70–76.

Woodward-Lopez G, Ritchie LD, Crawford PB. 2006. *Obesity: Dietary and Developmental Influences*. Taylor & Francis Group, LLC. Boca Raton, FL: CRC Press.

Wong F, Huhman M, Heitzler C, Ashbury L, Bretthauer-Mueller R, McCarthy S, Londe P. 2004. VERB™—A social marketing campaign to increase physical activity among youth. *Prev Chron Dis* [Online]. Available: http://www.cdc.gov/Pcd/issues/2004/jul/04_0043. htm [accessed July 23, 2006].

WVWalks. 2006. *WV Walks 30+ Minutes Daily*. [Online]. Available: http://www.wvwalks. org/ [accessed June 15, 2006].

Yanovski S. 2006 (January 11). *Prevention Research in Pediatric Obesity: An NIH Perspective*. Presentation at the Institute of Medicine Committee on Progress in Preventing Childhood Obesity meeting, Washington, DC. Institute of Medicine Committee on Progress in Preventing Childhood Obesity.

Yee SL, Williams-Piehota P, Sorensen A, Roussel A, Hersey J, Hamre R. 2006. The Nutrition and Physical Activity Program to Prevent Obesity and Other Chronic Diseases: Monitoring progress in funded states. *Prev Chron Dis* [Online]. Available: http://www.cdc.gov/ Pcd/issues/2006/jan/05_0077.htm [accessed July 23, 2006].

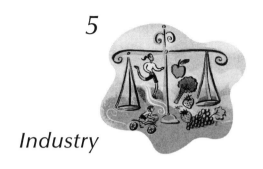

5

Industry

The Institute of Medicine's (IOM's) *Health in the Balance* report presented a set of comprehensive recommendations to guide industry's collective actions to support childhood obesity prevention goals (IOM, 2005). The report recommended that industry prioritize obesity prevention in children and youth by "developing and promoting products, opportunities, and information that will encourage healthful eating behaviors and regular physical activity." The report also recommended that "industry should develop and strictly adhere to marketing and advertising guidelines that minimize the risk of obesity in children and youth" (IOM, 2005, p. 166). The development of clear and useful nutrition labeling was a third area in which the report offered guidance to industry and the U.S. Food and Drug Administration (FDA) so that they may help parents and youth make informed purchases in the marketplace and select foods, beverages, and meal options that contribute to healthful diets (Box 5-1) (IOM, 2005).

After the release of the *Health in the Balance* report, another IOM committee released a related report, *Food Marketing to Children and Youth: Threat or Opportunity?*, which provides findings on the influence of marketing on children's and adolescents' food and beverage preferences, choices, purchase requests, dietary practices, and health-related outcomes (IOM, 2006). It also offers expanded recommendations for numerous industry stakeholders including food retailers, trade associations, entertainment companies, food and beverage companies, restaurants, and the media (Box 5-2).

This chapter explores the current and potential strategies that industry stakeholders use or could use to make progress toward meeting the recommendations made in those reports. The chapter provides examples of

BOX 5-1
Recommendations for Industry from the 2005 IOM report
Preventing Childhood Obesity: Health in the Balance

Industry should make obesity prevention in children and youth a priority by developing and promoting products, opportunities, and information that will encourage healthful eating behaviors and regular physical activity.

To implement this recommendation:
- Food and beverage industries should develop product and packaging innovations that consider energy density, nutrient density, and standard serving sizes to help consumers make healthful choices.
- Leisure, entertainment, and recreation industries should develop products and opportunities that promote regular physical activity and reduce sedentary behaviors.
- Full serve and fast food restaurants should expand healthier food options and provide calorie content and general nutrition information at point of purchase.

Industry should develop and strictly adhere to marketing and advertising guidelines that minimize the risk of obesity in children and youth.

To implement this recommendation:
- The Secretary of the Department of Health and Human Services should convene a national conference to develop guidelines for the advertising and marketing of foods, beverages, and sedentary entertainment directed at children and youth with attention to product placement, promotion, and content.
- Industry should implement the advertising and marketing guidelines.
- The Federal Trade Commission should have the authority and resources to monitor compliance with the food and beverage and sedentary entertainment advertising practices.

Nutrition labeling should be clear and useful so that parents and youth can make informed product comparisons and decisions to achieve and maintain energy balance at a healthy weight.

To implement this recommendation:
- The Food and Drug Administration should revise the Nutrition Facts panel to prominently display the total calorie content for items typically consumed at one eating occasion in addition to the standardized calorie serving and the percent Daily Value.
- The Food and Drug Administration should examine ways to allow greater flexibility in the use of evidence-based nutrient and health claims regarding the link between the nutritional properties or biological effects of foods and a reduced risk of obesity and related chronic diseases.
- Consumer research should be conducted to maximize use of the nutrition label and other food guidance systems.

SOURCE: IOM (2005).

BOX 5-2
Recommendations from the 2006 IOM Report
Food Marketing to Children and Youth: Threat or Opportunity?

Food and beverage companies should use their creativity, resources, and full range of marketing practices to promote and support more healthful diets for children and youth.

To implement this recommendation, companies should:
- Shift their product portfolios in a direction that promotes new and reformulated child- and youth-oriented foods and beverages that are substantially lower in total calories, lower in fats, salt, and added sugars, and higher in nutrient content.
- Shift their advertising and marketing emphasis to child- and youth-oriented foods and beverages that are substantially lower in total calories, lower in fats, salt, and added sugars, and higher in nutrient content (see later recommendations on public policy and monitoring).
- Work with government, scientific, public health, and consumer groups to develop and implement labels and advertising for an empirically validated industry-wide rating system and graphic representation that is appealing to children and youth to convey the nutritional quality of foods and beverages marketed to them and their families.
- Engage the full range of their marketing vehicles and venues to develop and promote healthier appealing and affordable foods and beverages for children and youth.

Full serve restaurant chains, family restaurants, and quick serve restaurants should use their creativity, resources, and full range of marketing practices to promote healthful meals for children and youth.

To implement this recommendation, restaurants should:
- Expand and actively promote healthier food, beverage and meal options for children and youth.
- Provide calorie content and other key nutrition information, as possible, on menus and packaging that is prominently visible at the point of choice and use.

Food, beverage, restaurant, retail, and marketing industry trade associations should assume transforming leadership roles in harnessing industry creativity, resources, and marketing on behalf of healthful diets for children and youth.

To implement this recommendation, trade associations should:
- Encourage member initiatives and compliance to develop, apply, and enforce industry-wide food and beverage marketing practice standards that support healthful diets for children and youth.
- Provide technical assistance, encouragement, and support for members' efforts to emphasize the development and marketing of healthier foods, beverages, and meals for children and youth.

continued

BOX 5-2 continued

- Exercise leadership in working with their members to improve the availability and selection of healthful foods and beverages accessible at eye level and reach for children, youth, and their parents in grocery stores and other food retail environments.
- Work to foster collaboration and support with public sector initiatives promoting healthful diets for children and youth.

The food, beverage, restaurant, and marketing industries should work with government, scientific, public health, and consumer groups to establish and enforce the highest standards for the marketing of foods, beverages, and meals to children and youth.

To implement this recommendation, the cooperative efforts should:
- Work through the Children's Advertising Review Unit (CARU) to revise, expand, apply, enforce, and evaluate explicit industry self-regulatory guidelines beyond traditional advertising to include evolving vehicles and venues for marketing communication (e.g., the Internet, advergames, branded product placement across multiple media).
- Assure that licensed characters are used only for the promotion of foods and beverages that support healthful diets for children and youth.
- Foster cooperation between CARU and the Federal Trade Commission in evaluating and enforcing the effectiveness of the expanded self-regulatory guidelines.

The media and entertainment industry should direct its extensive power to promote healthful foods and beverages for children and youth.

To implement this recommendation, media and the entertainment industry should:
- Incorporate into multiple media platforms (e.g., print, broadcast, cable, Internet, and wireless-based programming) foods, beverages, and storylines that promote healthful diets.
- Strengthen their capacity to serve as accurate interpreters and reporters to the public on findings, claims, and practices related to the diets of children and youth.

SOURCE: IOM (2006).

current private-sector efforts that support obesity prevention, including the efforts of food and beverage manufacturers; full serve restaurants and quick serve restaurants (QSR);[1] food retailers; trade associations; the media; corpo-

---

[1]A *QSR* is a category of restaurants characterized by foods, beverages, and meals that are supplied quickly after ordering, with minimal service, and may be consumed at the restaurant or served as takeout.

rate and private foundations; and the leisure, recreation, and sedentary entertainment industries. The strategies that industry uses to address childhood obesity prevention include product development and reformulation, product packaging, enhancing physical activity opportunities, advertising and marketing communications, public-private partnerships, employee wellness initiatives, and corporate social responsibility and public relations.[2] The chapter discusses the challenges in assessing the progress made by the private sector and recommends next steps for strengthening evaluation efforts.

A substantial amount of the discussion in this chapter focuses on the food, beverage, and restaurant industries, with fewer examples from the physical activity, leisure, recreation, and sedentary entertainment industries. This imbalance in coverage is due in part to the attention that has been placed on the responses to the obesity epidemic by the food, beverage, and restaurant industries. It is also possible that the segments of industry whose efforts are directly or indirectly related to changing physical activity behaviors may not perceive themselves to be part of the obesity prevention discourse or they may not want to be a focus of attention for this issue. Although a number of corporations are actively engaged in increasing opportunities for physical activity, there is need for further involvement. The committee also benefited from the work of the prior IOM committee on food marketing but did not have a similar compendium of recent efforts related to physical activity. A comprehensive review of the efforts by the physical activity, leisure, recreation, and sedentary entertainment industries[3] is needed, as there are many opportunities to increase and coordinate actions within and across this sector to promote physical activity among children and youth.

OPPORTUNITIES AND CHALLENGES

In December 2005, the committee held a symposium in Irvine, California that focused on the efforts by industry to engage in and contribute to childhood obesity prevention (Appendix H). This IOM symposium explored the challenges and opportunities that exist in forging alliances between the public health community and industry. Acknowledging the po-

---

[2]A list of acronyms and a glossary of definitions are provided in Appendixes A and B. Box 5-3 provides the definitions of common marketing terms.

[3]Examples of active leisure and recreation industries include companies that promote sporting goods, fitness, gyms, and dance. Sedentary entertainment requires minimal physical activity. Examples of sedentary entertainment industries include companies that promote spectator sports, broadcast and cable television, videogames, DVDs, and movies (IOM, 2006; Sturm, 2004).

tential tension among stakeholder groups, it is important to nurture and strengthen partnerships supporting obesity prevention efforts by

- Conveying consistent, appealing, and specific messages to children, adolescents, and adults;
- Ensuring transparency through the sharing of data between the public health community and industry;
- Making long-term commitments to obesity prevention;
- Ensuring company-wide commitments (large corporations in particular need to ensure that the entire organization and not just isolated sectors of the business is engaged in obesity prevention efforts);
- Balancing the free market system with protecting children's health. While public health advocates acknowledge the values and realities of the competitive marketplace and recognize that many companies are making positive changes, companies should accept responsibility for engaging in marketing practices that promote healthy lifestyles for children and youth;
- Understanding the interactions between companies, marketing practices, and consumer demand;
- Exploring potential avenues of impact. One area that has not been fully examined is the potential impact that business leaders can have in advocating for policy changes and initiatives that promote improvements in diet and increased levels of physical activity; and
- Making a commitment to monitor and evaluate efforts.

UNDERSTANDING THE MARKETPLACE

Companies use a variety of integrated marketing strategies to influence consumer preferences, stimulate consumer demand for specific products, increase sales, and expand their market share. Integrated marketing is a planning process designed to ensure that all promotional activities of a company—including media advertising, direct mail, sales promotion, and public relations—produce a unified, customer-focused promotion message that is relevant to a customer and that is consistent over time. The allocation of companies' marketing budgets differs on the basis of the nature and the size of the company. Food companies usually spend approximately 20 percent of their total marketing budgets for advertising, 25 percent for consumer promotion, and 55 percent for trade promotion (GMA Forum, 2005; IOM, 2006) (Box 5-3). The committee had no data with which it could assess how the leisure, recreation, and entertainment industries allocate their marketing budgets.

The U.S. Department of Agriculture (USDA), which tracks trends in

BOX 5-3
Industry Definitions

Marketing
A set of processes for creating, communicating, and delivering value to customers and for managing customer relationships in ways that benefit an organization and its stakeholders. Marketing encompasses a wide range of activities including conducting market research; analyzing the competition; positioning a new product; pricing products and services; and promoting products and services through advertising, consumer promotion, trade promotion, public relations, and sales. All of these activities are integral tools used by companies in the marketplace that can be potentially directed toward healthier products, diets, and lifestyles.

Advertising
Advertising represents the paid public presentation and promotion of ideas, goods, or services by a company or sponsor and is intended to bring a product to the attention of consumers through various media channels. It is often the most recognizable form of marketing.

Consumer Promotion
Consumer promotion is a marketing activity distinct from advertising. It is also referred to as "sales promotion" and represents companies' promotional efforts that have an immediate impact on sales. Examples of consumer or sales promotion include coupons, discounts and sales, contests, point-of-purchase displays, rebates, gifts, incentives, and product placement.

Trade Promotion
Trade promotion is a type of marketing that targets intermediary industry stakeholders such as supermarkets, grocery stores, convenience stores, and other food retail outlets. Examples of trade promotion strategies include in-store displays, agreements with retailers to provide specific shelf space and product positioning, free merchandise, and sales contests to encourage food wholesalers or retailers to sell more of a specific company's branded products or product lines.

Public Relations
Public relations are a company's communications and relationships with various groups including customers, employees, suppliers, stockholders, government, and the public.

Proprietary Data
Proprietary data consist of information obtained from private companies or firms that hold the exclusive rights to distribute those data, which are often collected for specific commercial purposes intended for a targeted audience. They may be available to customers who can purchase the data, and are usually not widely available to the public due to the expense.

SOURCES: AMA (2005); Boone and Kurtz (1998); IOM (2006).

food and beverage marketplace expenditures, estimated that in 2005, total food and beverage sales in the United States were $1.023 trillion. The growth in food expenditures has been steady since 1967, with a growth of nearly 6.4 percent per year (ERS/USDA, 2006).[4] Between 1987 and 2001 there was also considerable growth in the industries associated with leisure and recreation (e.g., sporting goods, spectator sports, and entertainment) (Sturm, 2004), but the committee was unable to find recent data that accurately quantified the total expenditures made by these industries.

In 2004, marketing expenditures for all products—including food, beverages, and other manufactured items—totaled $264 billion, which included $141 billion for advertising in measured media[5] (Brown et al., 2005). The IOM Committee on Food Marketing and the Diets of Children and Youth found that corporations spent more than $10 billion in 2004 to advertise foods, beverages, and meals to children and youth, of which $5 billion of the total was for television advertising (IOM, 2006). The total advertising spending by companies in measured media for selected categories of products was used to approximate the amount spent by the food, beverage, and restaurant industries in 2004. An estimated $6.84 billion was spent on advertising in the food, beverage, and candy category and $4.42 billion was spent on advertising for restaurants and fast food, for a total of $11.26 billion. An additional $10.89 billion was spent on advertising for toys and games; sporting goods; media; and sedentary entertainment, including movies, DVDs, and music (Brown et al., 2005). Company data on how marketing budgets are allocated are often proprietary, however, and are thus not available to the public. Therefore, industry data that can be used to assess recent investments in healthful products are not widely available. As discussed later in the chapter, despite the high level of product innovation toward healthier choices that has been forecasted by industry analysts, most companies do not provide publicly accessible information on the investments that they make in research and development on healthier products (Lang et al., 2006). Furthermore, there is currently limited evidence that companies with product portfolios comprised largely of less healthful products are merging with or acquiring companies with healthier products (Insight Investment, 2006).

---

[4]The USDA differentiates food sales from food expenditures. The latter includes noncash sales in the Economic Research Service food expenditure series. The Bureau of Labor Statistics Consumer Price Index for Food grew at a rate of 4.6 percent from 1967 to 2005 so more than half of the growth in food sales was due to higher retail prices (ERS/USDA, 2006).

[5]*Measured media* represent the categories of media tracked by media research companies, including television (e.g., major networks; national spots; and cable, syndicated, and Spanish-language networks), radio (e.g., network, national spot, and local radio), magazines (e.g., local and Sunday magazines), business publications, newspapers (e.g., local and national newspapers), outdoor advertising, direct mail, telephone directory advertising, and the Internet.

Branding is a goal of most companies and involves providing a name or symbol that legally identifies a company, a specific product, or a product line and that distinguishes it from other companies or similar products in the marketplace (Roberts, 2004). Branding has become a normalized part of life for American children and adolescents (Schor, 2004). The rate of brand loyalty is highest among adolescents, especially for carbonated soft drinks and QSRs. Brand loyalty may be related to the increased trend over the past 20–30 years in sweetened beverage consumption and the proportion of calories that children and youth receive from away-from-home foods, beverages, and meals, especially those purchased and consumed at full serve restaurants and QSRs. These products often contain higher amounts of fat and total calories than those products consumed at home (IOM, 2006).

After reviewing the available literature on branding and young consumers, the IOM Committee on Food Marketing to Children and Youth concluded that children are aware of particular food brands when they are as young as 2 to 3 years of age and that preschoolers demonstrate the ability to recognize particular brands when they are cued by spokescharacters and colorful packages. The committee also found that a majority of children's food requests are for branded products.

Although the use of child-oriented licensed cartoon and other fictional or real-life spokescharacters to promote the consumption of low-nutrient and high-calorie food and beverage products has been a prevalent practice over the past several decades, the use of licensed characters to promote foods and beverages that contribute to healthful diets, particularly for preschoolers, is relatively recent (IOM, 2006). Preliminary evaluation and research results from the Sesame Workshop suggests that preschoolers may view fruits, vegetables, and other foods that contribute to a healthful diet more favorably if they are endorsed by familiar and appealing spokescharacters or mascots (Appendix H).

More recently, businesses, institutions, and communities are using branding to promote behavioral changes, often called *lifestyle branding* or *behavioral branding*. Such branding encourages individuals to associate a brand or a product line with a specific behavior, lifestyle, or social cause (Holt, 2004; IOM, 2006; Roberts, 2004; Tillotson, 2006a). Examples of initiatives that promote this type of branding are Active Living by Design (RWJF, 2006), Balanced Active Lifestyles (McDonald's Corporation, 2006), Healthy Eating, Active Living (Kaiser Permanente, 2006), Health is Power! (PepsiCo, 2006a), Fruits and Veggies—More Matters!™ (PBH, 2006), the VERB™ campaign (Wong et al., 2004) (Chapter 4), and the American Legacy Foundation's truth® campaign (Evans et al., 2005).

Given the growing concerns linking corporate marketing practices and the obesity epidemic among children, youth, and adults in the United States

(Dorfman et al., 2005; Freudenberg, 2005; Kreuter, 2005) and internationally (Lang et al., 2006; WHO, 2003, 2004; Yach et al., 2005), industry and individual companies should be involved in changing how they conduct business to address social and economic pressures and consumer demands. This is what marketers refer to as the "strategic inflection point" (Parks, 2002).

The *Health in the Balance* report emphasized that market forces may be influential in changing both consumer and industry behaviors. To lead healthier and more active lifestyles, young consumers and their parents will need to make positive changes in their own lives, including developing preferences for and selecting foods and beverages that contribute to healthful diets and regularly engaging in more active pursuits. All industries—the food, beverage, restaurant, recreation, entertainment, and leisure industries—should share responsibility for supporting consumer changes and childhood obesity prevention goals. These industries can be instrumental in changing social norms throughout the nation and internationally so that obesity will be acknowledged as an important and preventable health outcome and healthful eating and regular physical activity will be the accepted and encouraged standard (IOM, 2005). The childhood obesity epidemic needs to reach a "tipping point" (Gladwell, 2000), which is the point at which the collective changes made by industry, in concert with efforts in other sectors and by other stakeholders, will produce a large effect to make healthy behaviors and lifestyles the social norm.

It is important to recognize that corporations as employers have an interest in a healthy workforce with healthy families, and many employers are placing an increasing emphasis on obesity prevention and improved employee well-being. Corporate responsibility, health care costs, and lost productivity are key drivers in the development and promotion of employee wellness opportunities. Such employee benefits may include the provision of discounts for health club memberships or gyms at the workplace; offering foods and beverages that contribute to healthful diets in cafeterias, vending machines, and at meetings; and the promotion of walking breaks or physical activity during the work day.

Although this chapter primarily focuses on corporations as the producers and the deliverers of goods and services, corporations are also major consumers of health care and have an increasing interest in the outcomes and impact of obesity on their current and future workforces and their families.

EXAMPLES OF PROGRESS

Building consumer demand for regular physical activity and for foods and beverages that contribute to a healthful diet is an ongoing process that is moving forward through the efforts of corporations that are willing to make changes to engage consumers in achieving healthy lifestyles. This will require the broad involvement of many sectors and stakeholders, including food, beverage, and restaurant companies; food retailers; trade associations; the leisure, recreation, and fitness industries; the entertainment industry; and the media (IOM, 2005, 2006).

Wansink and Huckabee (2005) have proposed three phases for the food and restaurant industries' and trade associations' response to the obesity epidemic. The first phase is to deny that they have a contributing role in the obesity epidemic by associating increasing obesity rates with the rising levels of physical inactivity and sedentary lifestyles. The second phase is to appeal to consumer sovereignty by emphasizing moderation and consumer choice in their food and beverage intake, promoting physical activity, and asserting the rights of customers to decide on the appropriate selections for their own or their families' lifestyles. The third phase is to develop win-win strategies that are profitable and that therefore satisfy company shareholder needs while concurrently meeting consumers' needs for healthful products, portion control, and other steps that can lead them toward healthy lifestyles. Wansink and Huckabee (2005) have suggested several different types of changes that food, beverage, and restaurant companies can consider making and pilot testing to offer products that are both healthful to consumers and profitable (Table 5-1).

Several groups have offered suggestions and guidelines to the food industry and restaurant sector to help them provide healthier food, beverage, and meal options. The American Heart Association's 2006 Diet and Lifestyle Recommendations provide several tailored recommendations specifically for these industry sectors (Lichtenstein et al., 2006; Box 5-4). The Keystone Forum on Away-From-Home Foods, supported by the FDA, also provides detailed recommendations on how consumers can make more healthful choices and what restaurants and food retailers can do to cater to consumer choices (Keystone Center, 2006). The following sections highlight some examples of changes that are in progress, many of which need to be evaluated. The committee highlights promising practices and raises issues relevant to increasing corporate involvement in this issue.

Product and Meal Development and Reformulation

Many industry leaders are testing a variety of new product development strategies, such as incorporating more nutritious ingredients into products (e.g., whole grains) and expanding healthier meal options at full serve restaurants and QSRs (e.g., fruit, salads, and low-fat yogurt). Making small changes to existing products to improve their healthfulness and continuing

TABLE 5-1 Influences on Consumption to Promote Healthier Diets

Consumption Driver	Implications for Marketers
Convenience *Increase convenience by modifying the package and portion size.*	• Recognize that a proportion of consumers may be willing to pay a premium for package modifications that help them control how much they consume. • Consider smaller-serving multipackages. • Place smaller volume inside packages—"implied servings" (e.g., five cookies instead of ten cookies) or calorie-controlled servings (e.g., 100-calorie snack packages). • Design packages that require slightly more effort to open, access, and consume. • Angle the bottoms of boxes for high-calorie snacks to limit consumption of the contents.
Cost *Change the product but not the price.*	• Reduce selected sizes but not the price. • Reduce portions for individual packages using a "just noticeable difference" principle (e.g., "just a taste" size). • Consider premium-priced smaller packaging.
Taste *Change the recipe but retain good taste.*	• Reformulate foods to make them less energy dense but sized similarly. • Reduce energy density by adding fewer or no calorie-containing ingredients (e.g., vegetables, fruits, water, air) and reducing calorie-containing and flavoring ingredients (e.g., sugar, fat, salt).
Knowledge *Provide understandable labels and nutrition information but be realistic.*	• Place markers on the side of a package to show how much a serving size is and to help consumers see a natural stopping point. • Put indicator lines inside packages to assist consumers to monitor how much they have eaten in a single serving. • Place messages with links on packaging to educate and remind consumers. • Use the package to promote healthy options, recipes, or complementary products.

SOURCE: Adapted from Wansink and Huckabee (2005).
Copyright ©2005 by the Regents of the University of California. Reprints from the *California Management Review*, Vol. 47, No. 4. By permission of The Regents.

to change these products over time by making incremental and systematic changes may help consumers develop preferences for more healthful choices.

There is evidence, however, of a greater segmentation of demand both within and between consumers. Thus, the health trend is not uniform across the entire population. Many consumers seeking healthful diets will exchange certain foods for healthier choices; at the same time, however, they may seek indulgent and high-calorie treats (IRI, 2006) that may offset the

---

BOX 5-4
Suggestions for Restaurants and the Food Industry
to Adopt the AHA 2006 Diet and Lifestyle Recommendations

Restaurants
- Display the calorie content on menus, and make nutrition information easily accessible to consumers at the point of decision and the point of purchase.
- Reduce portion sizes and provide options for selecting smaller portions.
- Reformulate products to reduce calories, sodium, saturated fats, and *trans* fats.
- Use *trans* fat-free and low-saturated fat oils in food preparation.
- Provide vegetable options prepared with minimal added calories and salt.
- Provide fruit options served without added sugar.
- Develop innovative approaches to market fruits and vegetables to make them more appealing to consumers.
- Allow substitution of nonfried and low-fat vegetables for side dishes such as french fries and potato salad.
- Make whole-grain options available for bread, crackers, pasta, and rice.

Food Industry
- Decrease the salt and sugar contents of processed foods.
- Replace the saturated fat and *trans* fat in prepared foods with low-saturated fat liquid vegetable oils.
- Increase the proportion of whole-grain foods available.
- Redesign food packaging in smaller individual portion sizes.
- Develop packaging that allows greater preservation and palatability of fresh fruits and vegetables without added salt.

SOURCE: Adapted with permission from Lichtenstein et al. (2006).

---

benefits of the healthier choices. The restaurant industry reports that two out of three consumers surveyed indicate that their favorite restaurant foods provide flavor and taste sensations that they cannot easily replicate at home (Cohn, 2006; NRA, 2006). Additionally, more consumer segments seek different types of benefits from products (e.g., their purchases are for natural, organic, low-fat, low-calorie, or calorie-free products) (Sloan, 2006; Tillotson, 2006b).

New product development, product reformulation, and packaging are all important components of the marketing process. Companies are continuously developing new products or meal options or reformulating existing products and brands to keep pace with changing consumer preferences, technological developments, and the activities of their competitors. In 2000, a typical large supermarket offered approximately 40,000 products from more than 16,000 food manufacturers (Harris, 2002). Many of these products were developed for children and youth, as reflected by the annual sales of food and beverages to children and youth, which were more than $27 billion in 2002 (Packaged Facts, 2003).

An analysis conducted by the IOM Committee on Food Marketing and the Diets of Children and Youth assessed the trends in introduction of new products targeted to children and youth. The analysis used ProductScan®, an online global database that has tracked new consumer products and packaged goods introductions into the U.S. marketplace since 1980 (Marketing Intelligence Service, 2005), and examined 50 product categories and 16 beverage categories contained in the ProductScan® database (IOM, 2006; Williams, 2005). The analysis showed that for both food and beverage products, the overall trend lines increased upward from 1994 to 2004, indicating that the growth rate of introduction of both new food and new beverage products targeted to children and youth was greater than the growth rate for food and beverage products targeted to the general market. Overall, from 1994 to 2004, products high in total calories, sugar, or fat and low in nutrients dominated among the new foods and beverages targeted to children and youth (IOM, 2006). A decline in the numbers of both food and beverage products targeted to children and youth relative to those targeted to the general market occurred between 2003 and 2004. The decline may be attributed to recent scrutiny directed to the introduction of new products targeted to children and youth. It is uncertain whether the recent decline in new products targeted to children and youth is attributed to an overall decrease in the numbers of all new products introduced or whether it represents a selective reduction in the introduction of products in certain categories, such as those products deemed to be less healthful for children and youth (Williams, 2005).

Industry analysts recognize that there are many new product growth opportunities in the child- and youth-specific food and beverage market, especially for the categories of fresh produce, ready-to-eat meals, sauces and condiments, and fortified products (Business Insights, 2006; Sloan, 2006). Companies have begun to explore the development of new convenience foods and beverages (Blake, 2006; JPMorgan, 2006). The products that contribute to healthful diets of children and youth have been projected to be among the most active and profitable new product categories for industry from 2005 to 2009 (Business Insights, 2005). A recent industry analysis report suggests that 18 of the 24 fastest growing food categories globally are perceived to be healthier by consumers (Insight Investment, 2006).

There has also been a trend toward a decline in sales of high-calorie beverages and snacks. Analyses conducted for the beverage industry suggest that there has been a recent decrease in the volume of sales in the carbonated soft drink category (Beverage Digest, 2006). Morgan Stanley's consumer marketing research forecasts that there will be an annual 1.5 percent decline in carbonated soft drink sales volume in the United States over the next 5 years. The reasons for the projected decline are attributed to an increased concern about health and rising obesity rates that are influencing parents to monitor their own and their children's carbonated soft drink intake (Wilbert, 2006). Marketing research also suggests that in 2005 the sales of high-calorie packaged snack foods, such as cookies and bakery items, decreased, whereas the sales of more nutrient-dense snacks, such as yogurt and food bars, increased (Packaged Facts, 2006). It is important to track these trends because the prevalence of snacking and the number of snacking occasions by children and youth have increased steadily over the past 25 years (IOM, 2006).

As emphasized in the *Health in the Balance* report, high energy-dense foods, such as potato chips and sweets, tend to be palatable but may not be satiating for consumers, calorie for calorie, thereby encouraging greater food consumption (IOM, 2005). The Dietary Guidelines for Americans 2005 encourages Americans to consume adequate nutrients within their calorie needs. More specifically, the Dietary Guidelines recommend that individuals consume a variety of nutrient-dense foods and beverages within and among the basic food groups while selecting foods and beverages that limit their intake of saturated fat, *trans* fat, cholesterol, added sugars, salt, and alcohol. There is presently no consensus or guidelines that define a healthful food or beverage. However, an analysis of cross-sectional, nationally representative dietary intake data have found that low energy-dense diets, which include a relatively large proportion of foods high in micronutrients and water and low in fat, such as fruits and vegetables, are associated with better dietary quality and lower total calorie intake when compared to high energy-dense diets (Ledikwe et al., 2006). Longitudinal data are needed to support this relationship.

Both diversity and quality are important components of children's and adolescents' intakes, and energy balance may be more difficult to achieve when diets are high in total calories and fat (Kennedy, 2004). The Dietary Guidelines for Americans 2005 introduced the concept of "discretionary calories," which represents the amount of calories that remain in a person's energy allowance after he or she has consumed sufficient nutrient-dense foods to meet his or her nutrient requirements each day. An individual's energy allowance is the amount of calories needed for weight maintenance. Discretionary calories are usually between 100 and 300 calories/day and depend on a person's physical activity level (DHHS and USDA, 2005). A major challenge for food manufacturers has been to develop low energy-dense but palatable food and beverage products that help consumers to achieve dietary diversity and diet quality and to use their discretionary calories wisely to achieve energy balance at a healthy weight.

The committee recognizes that among food and beverage manufacturers and the restaurant sector, there are examples of those who have under-taken important changes that collectively can contribute to reversing the epidemic of childhood obesity. As discussed later in the chapter, it is impor-tant to identify specific criteria, key performance indicators, and outcome measures that the public health sector and industry can mutually agree upon, and to use that information to make evidence-based changes to improve the public's health. Specific criteria upon which positive industry changes can be evaluated may include: changes in a company's product portfolio and marketing resources to develop, package, and promote prod-ucts that contribute to healthy lifestyles; reducing the portion sizes of food and beverage products; designing initiatives that easily convey information to consumers about food, beverage, and meal products that meet estab-lished nutrition criteria; the provision of information that promotes regular physical activity; and developing partnerships with government and non-profit organizations to increase the number and quality of programs that promote healthful eating and active lifestyles for children, youth, and their families.

Product Reformulation and New Product Innovations

Subsequent to the release of the *Health in the Balance* report (IOM, 2005), many companies have made efforts to implement the recommenda-tions pertaining to the development of product and packaging innovations that consider energy density, nutrient density, and standard serving sizes to help consumers make healthful choices. The committee also acknowledges that making a substantial change in their product portfolios toward healthier options is an evolving process that will require sufficient time and resources to conduct marketing research and market testing to determine the level of consumer demand and support for these products over the long term.

The Grocery Manufacturers Association's (GMA) Health and Wellness Survey was conducted in 2004 and 2005 with 43 GMA member companies with total sales representing about half of the U.S. food and beverage industry sales. Forty-two of the companies reported introducing 4,496 new or reformulated products into the marketplace since 2002. These products were intended to improve consumer health. Based on information from 38 companies, 67 percent of the new or reformulated products had less satu-rated fat or *trans* fat content, 21 percent of these products had reduced calorie content, 20 percent of these products had reduced added sugar and carbohydrate contents, 12 percent of these products had increased vitamin or mineral content, and 8 percent of these products had reduced sodium content (Kretser, 2006).

Although it is still too early to comprehensively evaluate the rate and extent of healthy new product innovations across the food and beverage industry, there are encouraging signs, with leading food and beverage companies (e.g., General Mills, PepsiCo/Quaker Oats, and Kraft Foods) responding with product innovations targeting healthier nutrition profiles. Many of these products are designed to help consumers meet the Dietary Guidelines for Americans 2005 and offer other benefits, such as increasing whole-grain consumption, encouraging low-fat dairy consumption, and reducing calorie consumption to help consumers balance their calorie intake with their energy expenditure (GMA, 2006). Increases in promotional spending by the larger produce brands (e.g., Dole, Chiquita, and Sunkist) are also apparent, and there has been a leveraging of both private-sector resources (e.g., public service announcements produced through in-kind media, food retailer, and other producer support or commodity board in-kind support) and public-sector resources (e.g., USDA and National 5 a Day partner support) to create an awareness among consumers about the need to increase fruit and vegetable intake through a multisectoral national action plan (PBH, 2005a,c). Many of their activities are targeted to children and youth.

In an effort to overcome the taste barrier, which consumers often provide as a reason for their lower than recommended levels of vegetable consumption, companies such as General Mills' Green Giant brand are packaging frozen vegetables with sauces that complement the vegetables and make their taste more desirable (General Mills, 2006a). As the parent company for Cascadian Farm®, General Mills is expanding efforts to provide organic fruits and vegetables to the mainstream marketplace by meeting the demand of a growing segment of consumers for organic and natural foods (General Mills, 2006a).

The senior-level management of PepsiCo has committed to the goal of having 50 percent of its revenues from new products come from its healthful branded product category. According to the company representative who made a presentation at the IOM symposium on industry, the rate of sales of these products is growing at approximately three times the rate for the rest of the company's product portfolio. Kraft Foods has set similar goals for its business and is also seeing strong growth in demand for its healthier products in the marketplace. This demand may serve to drive competition further and may result in innovation within companies to reformulate existing products or to develop new products such that they can be tagged with the healthy icon or logo. The increased demand may also reaffirm the commitments by corporations to supply healthful products in the marketplace (Appendix H).

These examples highlight the type of leadership required to stimulate broader change within the food, beverage, and restaurant industries. If the largest global companies make these types of commitments and implement them, smaller companies are more likely to follow. It may also influence the house brands or "value" brands of leading food retailers so that they emulate the changes made to the brands of the more recognized companies. This process could lead to a chain of events that has the potential to substantially shift the product portfolios of food, beverage, and restaurant companies and influence how companies, food retailers, and trade associations conduct business. However, these changes need to be evaluated to assess the extent of the changes that companies have made, the impact of these changes on consumers' response and dietary behaviors, as well as business impact.

Food Retailers

The food retailer is an important stakeholder in childhood obesity prevention because it serves as the interface between manufacturers and consumers. Industry stakeholders and public health practitioners often overlook this untapped setting as a means of reaching young consumers with healthful products and health-promotion initiatives. Supermarkets, grocery stores, and other food retail outlets are venues for product selection, merchandising and product promotion, and consumer education. Opportunities exist to make the products selected in these settings more healthy. Such opportunities include identifying for children branded products that have healthier profiles; developing healthier private-label products for young consumers as well as the entire family; introducing portion-controlled, packaged foods and beverages; and increasing the convenience of purchasing fresh fruits and vegetables. A variety of in-store merchandising and promotion activities can bring healthier choices to the attention of consumers. These include shelf markers, package icons or logos, and special displays that can be used to flag healthier products for children, youth, and family meals. Cross-merchandising, premiums, product sampling, in-store promotional entertainment, and price promotions can also be used to highlight healthier options (Childs, 2006).

Expanding Consumer Demand for Healthful Products

A substantial barrier to this progressive shift in the food, beverage, and meal product landscape is the continuous need to build consumer demand for healthful products. The new products must have an appealing taste, look appealing, be convenient, and represent value to consumers compared with those of the products that they will replace. Although health is an important driver of the food industry, consumers are less willing to trade taste for health (Sloan, 2006). Taste is consistently identified as a key driver of consumption, followed by price, convenience, ease of preparation, and freshness (Yankelovich, 2006). This process will require continued investment in improved technologies that can make healthier foods and beverages taste better, that can improve convenience (e.g., longer shelf life and reduced preparation time) and that can offer high value (e.g., low cost products with innovative packaging). This investment can emerge from consumer demand and the success of early versions of these products in the marketplace.

Many full serve restaurants and QSRs are expanding the availability of healthier items on their menus; establishing their own guidelines for advertising and marketing of food, beverages, and meals; and educating their customers by providing nutrition information and product labeling. For example, Burger King provides a nutrition guide online; Denny's has the D-Zone Kids' Menu; Pizza Hut has the Fit 'N Delicious menu; and Chick-fil-A advertises The Trim Trio™, a combination meal with 330 calories, less than 4 grams of fat, and no *trans* fat (Cohn, 2006).

These efforts are now beginning to get some recognition through innovative awards programs that are being established to highlight restaurants that offer healthier choices. Arkansas Governor Mike Huckabee established an awards program for restaurants under his Healthy Arkansas initiative (2006). This program was developed to recognize restaurants that assist Arkansas residents to make healthy choices when they eat away from home. Three categories of awards (gold, silver, and bronze) are given to restaurants that meet specified standards established for food safety; provide healthier menu options, such as at least one fruit and vegetable without added sugar or fat, and nutrition information and education about the their meals; and have designated smoke-free areas. Restaurants may show Healthy Arkansas Restaurant logos to promote their receipt of the award. Currently, 138 restaurants across the state have applied for the designation as a Healthy Arkansas establishment. Among the QSRs that have received the designation are McDonald's Corporation, Subway, and a variety of Yum! Brands chains including Burger King and Pizza Hut.

The restaurant sector's previous attempts to change products and sell healthier menu items, such as McDonald's Corporation's McLean Deluxe burger and Taco Bell's lower-fat Border Lights menu, launched in the 1990s, have received mixed results (Collins, 1995; Ramirez, 1991). The reasons for their low profitability are complex and not well documented. McLean Deluxe may have benefited from a more creative presentation and promotional effort while Border Lites may have had less appeal to their teenage customer base. The new menu introductions may have been too early for consumers to perceive them as necessary, as the obesity epidemic has only recently been raised to the level of broad public awareness.

Alternatively, these early attempts to sell healthier options may have been unprofitable because the main consumer benefit that was marketed was health instead of taste or convenience. As Wansink and Huckabee (2005) suggest, most consumers generally equate healthful foods with compromised taste, especially since healthier choices are generally marketed as new and different, as well as healthier, which may raise consumer concern about how the new product will taste. If the product is more expensive than the alternative and often less healthy choice, it will not be appealing or affordable to a large segment of consumers.

Building and sustaining consumer demand for reformulated food and beverage products and restaurant meals is an important strategy for helping Americans to consume more healthful diets. Achieving this goal will require continued innovation around the composition and packaging of foods, beverages, and meals; improvements in the taste of healthier products; and making them convenient and affordable for consumers. Innovative approaches are needed to change consumers' perceptions of the taste and desirability of healthier products. Similarly, it is important to highlight the changes in consumer expectations that are needed and the trend toward eating more of their meals outside of the home. As consumers' incomes increase, they eat away from home more frequently and spend a greater proportion of their food dollar on meals consumed away from home (NRA, 2006). Making healthy choices at such meals also needs to be viewed as integral to healthful eating and not as a treat or a special occasion.

Product Packaging and Meal Presentation

Food and Beverage Companies

Package size, plate shape, restaurant ambiance, and lighting are environmental factors that can influence the volumes of food, beverages, and meals consumed. Small changes in these factors can be instrumental in reducing the overconsumption of foods (Wansink, 2004). According to the GMA Health and Wellness Survey, conducted with 42 GMA members, 50 percent had either changed or initiated a change in multiserving packaging, and 56 percent of 41 companies had created special package sizes for children and youth (GMA, 2006; Kretser, 2006). Specific packaging innovations have included changing single-serving milk from unresealable cartons to resealable plastic bottles that have up to a 3-month shelf-life; replacing aluminum cans that contain meals such as chili with shelf-stable, single-serving carton packaging or plastic cupped or bowled packages; and using portable and resealable pouches that can contain a variety of products including beverages, snacks, candy, cereals, meats, soups, and sauces (Fusaro, 2004).

In addition, other recent new packaging initiatives by Kraft Foods and PepsiCo have introduced 100-calorie packages of popular snack food brands.

The single-serving, calorie-controlled packages can potentially meet consumer demand for convenience, establish a new and acceptable portion size standard for consumers (Sloan, 2006), and assist consumers with limiting their consumption of snacks at a single eating occasion. However, evaluations of these initiatives are needed to demonstrate that consumers do not overcompensate by consuming more of the calorie-controlled packages or consuming more calorie-dense foods or beverages at other times of the day.

Restaurants

The *Health in the Balance* report recommended that full serve restaurants and QSRs expand their healthier food options and provide families with the calorie content and general nutrition information of their meals at the point of purchase (IOM, 2005). The restaurant industry estimates that the full serve restaurant and QSR sector will have provided approximately 70 billion meals or snacks to U.S. consumers in 2006 (NRA, 2006). More than 925,000 commercial restaurants are projected to generate an estimated $511 billion in annual sales in 2006, an increase from $42.8 billion in 1970. The restaurant industry's share of American's food dollar is approximately 47.5 percent (NRA, 2006) and is projected to increase to 53 percent by 2010 (Cohn, 2006).

In this report, the term *fast food* is used to describe the foods, beverages, and meals designed for ready availability, use, or consumption and that are sold at eating establishments for quick availability or takeout (Appendix B). This definition is similar to that provided by the North American Industry Classification System (NAICS), which defines fast food restaurants as the U.S. industry sector that "comprises establishments primarily engaged in providing food services where patrons generally order or select items and pay for them before eating. Food and drink may be consumed on the premises, taken out, or delivered to the customer's location" (NAICS, 2002).

It has been suggested that researchers have no universally accepted definition of fast food, which may present methodological challenges for accurately describing the characteristics of the foods, beverages, and meals obtained at these establishments (Kapica et al., 2006). However, a robust evidence base from over the past 25 years is available and documents that a large proportion of foods, beverages, and meals purchased from fast food restaurants or QSRs tend to have larger portion sizes and are higher in total calories (from fat and added sugars) and energy density than foods, beverages, and meals prepared and consumed at home (IOM, 2005, 2006).

The percent of total calorie intake of children and adolescents ages 12 to 18 years obtained from foods purchased and consumed away from home increased from 26 to 40 percent between 1977–1978 and 1994–1996

(Nielsen et al., 2002b). Trends in the calorie intakes of children and adolescents ages 2–18 years by selected eating locations showed a substantial increase in away-from-home calories obtained from restaurants, especially QSRs, from 5 percent in 1977–1978 to 15 percent in 1994–1996 (Nielsen et al., 2002a). Data for more recent trends in young peoples' calorie intake from foods and beverages obtained at restaurants are not available. A review of the available literature finds that nearly one-half of away-from-home calories obtained at full serve restaurants and QSRs were higher in fat content (IOM, 2006). Although healthier menu options are gaining attention, most QSRs continue to offer choices that are predominantly high in total calories, saturated fat, sugar, and salt. Many QSRs indicate that sustained consumer demand is inextricably related to a broader sustained societal effort focused on promoting healthier choices (IOM, 2006).

Restaurants are important venues for increasing fruit and vegetable consumption. A recent survey, combined with menu trend research, found that although 67 percent of consumers reported visiting a QSR at least once every 2 weeks, only 18 percent reported regularly consuming fruits or vegetables from such restaurants. Additionally, whereas 13 percent of all meals are eaten at or carried out from a commercial restaurant (including casual dining and QSRs), only 7 percent of total fruit and vegetable servings were consumed at restaurants. Many opportunities exist to use plate presentation, promote convenience, and use limited-time offers and incentives to promote produce consumption when consumers eat out at restaurants (PBH, 2005b).

The growing public concern about obesity presents certain marketing risks—such as increased costs associated with developing, reformulating, packaging, test marketing, and promoting food and beverage products, as well as uncertainty related to creating and sustaining consumer demand for these new products. However, the public's interest and concern also present potentially profitable marketing opportunities not yet fully explored: food and beverage manufacturers can compete for and expand their market share for healthier food and beverage product categories, serve as role models for the industry by substantially shifting overall product portfolios toward healthier products, and engage in socially responsible corporate behaviors in the response to the childhood obesity epidemic. Despite the challenges of market forces and the marketplace, companies can make positive changes that expand consumers' selection of healthier products, as well as to reduce the risks of government regulation or litigation (Mello et al., 2006).

Physical Activity Opportunities

The *Health in the Balance* report recommended that the leisure, entertainment, and recreation industries develop products and opportunities that promote regular physical activity and reduce sedentary behaviors (IOM, 2005). Although some efforts are under way to develop products that enhance opportunities for physical activity, additional investment in both the development and the promotion of products that support increased physical activity levels is needed.

Using home videogame systems is a sedentary activity that has been associated with a higher body mass index (BMI) level in children who spend more time engaging in such activities (Stettler et al., 2004; Vandewater et al., 2005). Recently, the videogame industry has used its creativity to increase children's awareness about obesity. The annual Games for Health (2006), a conference produced by The Serious Games Initiative, convenes game manufacturers to focus on health-related issues. Such products as a fantastic voyage-style adventure called Escape from Obeez City have been developed in which children explore the impact of obesity on the human body (Big Red Frog, 2006; Brown, 2006). Another example is the videogame Squire's Quest!, which is designed to allow children to earn their way to knighthood through such tasks as creating fruit- and vegetable-containing recipes. Two separate evaluations of this videogame found that children playing the game increased their fruit and vegetable consumption by one serving compared with the levels of fruit and vegetable consumption of children who did not play the game (Baranowski et al., 2003; Cullen et al., 2005).

Interactive videogames, also called physical gaming, are electronic games that use the players' physical activity as input in playing the game. The media has paid special attention to physical games such as *Dance Dance Revolution*®, in which players use a floor pad to mimic dance moves shown on a screen. The most recent version of this videogame informs players about how many calories they burn in each dance session (Brown, 2006). Interactive videogames for the PlayStation2® computer entertainment system use the EyeToy™, a tiny camera that projects an image of the game player directly onto the screen. These methods of physical gaming, however, often require the purchase of an additional piece of equipment, such as a dance pad or a camera, which adds to the cost of the system, thereby limiting the potential audience. Nevertheless, innovative approaches to physical gaming are being developed and offer promising possibilities.

Some companies are beginning to produce branded physical activity equipment for children and youth. For example, McDonald's Corporation has started a new multicategory licensing initiative called McKIDS™ that unifies its branded product line including toys, interactive videos, books, and DVDs to reflect active lifestyles (McDonald's Corporation, 2003). The McKIDS™ line of products offers branded bikes, scooters, skateboards, outdoor play equipment, and interactive DVDs. There is a need for evaluations that assess how these products are promoted to children and youth and whether use of the branded equipment promotes desirable behavioral and health outcomes.

Advertising and Marketing Communications

The media and entertainment industries have a tremendous reach into the lives of the American public. These industries have important opportunities and responsibilities to depict and promote healthful diets and physical activity among children and youth (IOM, 2006). Among the many challenges in addressing the reach and the influence of paid media and marketing communications in the lives of children and youth are the multiple venues and vehicles that can be used to deliver consistent messages that promote healthy lifestyles (IOM, 2006).

Advertising and Marketing Strategies, Venues, and Vehicles

Today's paid media and marketing strategies, tactics, and messaging extend beyond traditional print and broadcast or cable television advertising, which is relatively easy to monitor and control, to newer forms of interactive media and marketing communications such as product placement across multiple media platforms, Internet marketing, and mobile or wireless telephone marketing. Two recent studies that examined Internet marketing designed by food and beverage companies for children and youth documented a range of techniques used to engage and immerse children in company brands. These techniques include advergames, brand identifiers, brand characters, brand benefit claims, customized Internet visits, viral marketing, cross-promotional paid media tie-ins, and on-demand access to television advertisements (Moore, 2006; Weber et al., 2006).

Companies advertise and market to children and youth through a variety of venues and use many strategies to develop brand awareness and brand loyalty at an early age. One company that made a presentation at the industry symposium, Kraft Foods, announced in 2005 that it would advertise to children ages 6 to 11 years only those food and beverage products meeting the company's healthful criteria, during children's broadcast television, radio programming, and in paid print media geared toward this age group. The company indicated that by the end of 2006, it will redesign its websites intended for viewing by children ages 6 to 11 years so that they feature only products that meet the Sensible Solution™ nutrition standards of their more healthful product line (Gorecki, 2006; Kraft Foods, 2005). However, these proposed guidelines will not apply to products promoted on television during prime-time programs viewed primarily by adults or coviewed by children and youth with their parents.

In accordance with this marketing trend, the entertainment media, particularly television programs and broadcast and cable television networks targeting children and youth, have begun to promote fruit and vegetable consumption and other healthful behaviors. They have also entered into partnerships that feature product cross-promotions, which market new products or products related to those already used by consumers. Certain media outlets use approaches that are based on the finding that children often view food as having physical characteristics as well as social constructs. Sesame Workshop, in partnership with the Produce for Better Health Foundation (PBH), uses its characters to model fun ways to move and play as well as ways to encourage snacks that support a healthful diet (PBH, 2005a). Additionally, PBH is also partnering with Wal-Mart, the nation's largest retailer, to conduct a series of in-store marketing activities using Shrek, Charlie Brown, Spiderman®, Curious George®, and Peter Rabbit™ to promote fruit and vegetable consumption (Childs, 2006; PBH, 2005a). Evaluations of the partnerships, policies, and outcomes related to these interventions are needed.

The Cartoon Network has initiated a healthy lifestyles program called Get Animated that uses celebrity endorsements and partnerships to extend its outreach to children and families to encourage physical activity and making choices that contribute to a healthful diet. In conjunction with its cable television campaign, the network sponsors a nationwide tour of cartoon-based spokescharacters that involve children in various activities to show that fruits, vegetables, and physical activity can be fun and cool (Time Warner, 2006) (Appendix H).

Univision Communications is the leading Spanish-language media company in the United States. (The company's television operations include the Univision Network, TeleFutura Network, Galavisión, and the Univision and TeleFutura Television Groups. Univision also owns and operates Univision Radio, Univision Music Group, and Univision Online.) The company's multimedia obesity-related initiatives focus on promoting healthy lifestyles by educating and engaging the Hispanic and Latino communities and engaging individuals in these communities in ways to be healthy. By collaborating with health care organizations, community groups, and allied health professional societies and organizations, the network created several public service announcements, special programs, commercials, and news segments that it regularly features to promote health and nutrition among its primarily Spanish-speaking viewers (Univision Communications, 2003). It also partners with the National Institutes of Health (NIH) initiative We Can! to inform parents about ways to help them encourage their children to maintain a healthy weight (NHLBI, 2006) (Appendix D).

Some efforts are underway to use storylines and programming that promote healthy lifestyles. Media messages regarding healthy lifestyles are facilitated by organizations such as Hollywood, Health, and Society, an organization based at the University of Southern California that focuses on linking television writers with health experts so that accurate health and nutrition information can be integrated into their television program scripts. This program was formed with support from the Centers for Disease Control and Prevention (CDC) and the NIH. The organization facilitated the incorporation of a storyline about diabetes into a popular television show on a major Hispanic network. An evaluation of the impact of this effort included tracking of the numbers of individuals who accessed diabetes information that was linked through the network's website and promoted on the television show (Appendix H).

In 2004, the Ad Council, a private nonprofit organization that provides public service advertising, with support from the Robert Wood Johnson Foundation (RWJF), formed a public-private partnership, the Coalition for Healthy Children, to formulate research-based messages targeted to parents, children, and youth through the collective strength of the food, beverage, restaurant, and marketing industries; the media; nonprofit organizations; foundations; and government agencies. The coalition members work to provide consistent messages about physical activity, food choices, portion sizes, the balancing of food and physical activity, and parental role modeling across multiple media platforms. They also work to incorporate consistent messages into their internal communications programs as well as their advertising, packaging, websites, community-based programs, and marketing events (Ad Council, 2006b). In 2005, an evaluation of the coalition activities concluded that although consumer awareness is relatively high for healthy messages about diet and activities, the attitudes and behaviors of children and parents do not reflect this heightened awareness (Yankelovich, 2005). An evaluation is under way to assess how the effectiveness of the Ad Council's obesity prevention messages compare with the effectiveness of other advertising and marketing messages of food and beverage companies within the advertising information environment (Berkeley Media Studies Group, 2005).

Spokescharacters are a particularly important marketing strategy used to reach young children. In 1963, the McDonald's Corporation created Ronald McDonald as a spokescharacter who appealed to children, with the purpose of promoting the foods, beverages, and meals served and consumed at the QSR franchise (Enrico, 1999). In 2005, Ronald McDonald became the company's spokesperson to advocate "balanced active lifestyles" (McDonald's Corporation, 2005). His image was changed to emphasize physical activity and to introduce and promote some healthier options. Although a relatively recent development, publicly available information about the outcomes and impact of this change on children's diets and physical activity behaviors would be useful.

In 2005, Nickelodeon—a company of Viacom International, which is a leading entertainment company for American children—announced that it would begin licensing several of its popular cartoon spokescharacters, including SpongeBob SquarePants® and Dora the Explorer®, to produce companies to promote fruit and vegetable consumption (Smalls, 2005). In 2006, Nickelodeon announced plans to license the use of images of these characters to promote the consumption of apples, pears, cherries, and soybeans (Horovitz, 2006). Other characters are being used to promote fruit consumption, including the Warner Brothers characters Bugs Bunny™ and Tweety™ Bird and the Sesame Workshop's characters Elmo™ and Cookie Monster™ (Horovitz, 2006; Sunkist, 2005). Independent evaluations that assess these characters' appeal and influence on children's food preferences, product sales, and the levels of consumption of fruits and vegetables are needed.

Self-Regulatory Guidelines: Children's Advertising Review Unit

The industry-supported, self-regulatory Children's Advertising Review Unit (CARU) was formed in 1974 as an industry self-regulatory mechanism to promote responsible advertising and promotional messages for children and youth under 12 years of age. The purpose of industry self-regulation is to ensure that advertising messages directed to young children are truthful, accurate, and sensitive to this audience (CARU, 2003a,b). CARU works with food, beverage, restaurant, toy, and entertainment companies, as well as advertising and marketing agencies, to ensure that advertising messages directed at children younger than 12 years adhere to these guidelines (CARU, 2003a,b) (Box 5-5).

An assessment conducted by the National Advertising Review Council (NARC, 2004), which establishes policies and procedures for CARU, suggests that within its designated technical purview, the CARU guidelines have generally been effective in enforcing voluntary industrywide standards for traditional forms of advertising and that the number of advertisements that contain words and images that directly encourage children to consume excessive amounts of food has been reduced (IOM, 2006). Nevertheless, CARU reviews advertisements for accuracy and to reduce deceptive advertising, but it does not have the ability to monitor or regulate the nutrition information provided by commercials. Implicit in the NARC review findings is the limited scope of authority of CARU. The guidelines do not address issues related to the volume of food, beverage, and meal advertising targeted to children and youth; the broader marketing environment; or the many integrated marketing strategies that have increased to reach young people since CARU's inception in 1974 (IOM, 2006).

BOX 5-5
Groups Relevant to Advertising and Marketing Practices
Affecting Children and Youth

National Advertising Review Council
The National Advertising Review Council (NARC) was established to provide guidance and develop standards for truth and accuracy in national advertising through a voluntary self-regulation system. NARC sets the policies for the National Advertising Division, National Advertising Review Board, Children's Advertising Review Unit, and the Electronic Retailing Self-Regulation Program.

Children's Advertising Review Unit
The Children's Advertising Review Unit (CARU) promotes responsible children's advertising as part of a strategic alliance with the major advertising trade associations through NARC, including the American Association of Advertising Agencies, the American Advertising Federation, the Association of National Advertisers, and the Council of Better Business Bureaus. CARU is the children's arm of the advertising industry's self-regulation program and evaluates child-directed advertising and promotional material in all media to advance truthfulness, accuracy, and consistency with its *Self-Regulatory Guidelines for Children's Advertising* and relevant laws.

American Association of Advertising Agencies
The American Association of Advertising Agencies (AAAA) is the national trade association representing the advertising agency business in the United States. Its membership produces approximately 80 percent of the total advertising volume placed by agencies nationwide. It provides to its members guidance on strengthening their advertising practices.

American Advertising Federation
The American Advertising Federation (AAF) is an industry trade association that works to protect and promote advertising practices through a nationally coordinated grassroots network of members that include advertisers, advertising agencies, media companies, local advertising clubs, and college chapters.

Consumer advocacy groups have expressed growing concern about CARU's ability to effectively monitor children's food and beverage advertising, given the newer forms of marketing across multiple forms of media (e.g., broadcast and cable television; and print, electronic, and wireless media) that are often difficult to monitor and regulate. In response to this concern, the industry trade association, GMA, proposed a seven-point plan to strengthen CARU's enforcement capacity to effectively self-regulate the industry. These suggestions also provided guidance on enhancing CARU's visibility, resources, transparency, and public accessibility (GMA, 2005).

At the IOM industry symposium in Irvine, California, the director of NARC announced that in response to these requests, CARU had appointed

Association of National Advertisers
The Association of National Advertisers (ANA) provides leadership to drive marketing communications, media and brand management excellence, and to promote and defend industry interests.

Council of Better Business Bureaus
The Council of Better Business Bureaus (CBBB) is the parent organization for the Better Business Bureau (BBB) system, which is supported by more than 300,000 local business members nationwide, and works to foster fair relationships between businesses and consumers. The CBBB and all local Better Business Bureaus are private, nonprofit organizations funded by membership dues and other support.

American Marketing Association
The American Marketing Association (AMA) is a professional association for individuals and organizations involved in the practice, teaching, and study of marketing worldwide. It serves to advance marketing competencies, practice, and leadership; to advocate for marketing efficacy and ethics; and as a resource for marketing information, education, and training.

Ad Council
The Ad Council is a private, nonprofit organization that mobilizes volunteer talent from the advertising and communications industries, the facilities of the media, and the resources of the business and nonprofit communities to deliver messages to the American public. The Ad Council produces, distributes, and promotes thousands of public service advertising campaigns annually in such areas as improving the quality of life for children, preventive health care, education, community well-being, environmental preservation, and strengthening families.

SOURCES: AAAA (2006); AAF (2006); Ad Council (2006a); AMA (2006); ANA (2006); CARU (2003a,b); CBBB (2005).

a new director of communications, added two child nutritionists to its advisory group, and established three task forces to examine the need for expanding the group's purview (e.g., websites and interactive media, paid product placement in children's programming, and the appropriate use of licensed characters in food and beverage promotion). It was also reported that CARU has built a closer relationship with the U.S. Department of Health and Human Services (DHHS) and the Federal Trade Commission (FTC) to strengthen the voluntary industry self-regulatory approach (Appendix H), which is acknowledged and encouraged by these federal government agencies (FTC and DHHS, 2006). Support by these federal agencies is essential to assist the industry with defining advertising and marketing guidelines appropriate for each sector (e.g., foods, beverages, restaurants, leisure, and entertainment). CARU also reported that companies appear to be incorporating the CARU guidelines into their own advertising review systems and request that CARU conduct prescreening of their advertisements (CBBB, 2006).

The *Health in the Balance* report recommended that industry develop and strictly adhere to marketing and advertising guidelines that minimize the risk of obesity in children and youth (IOM, 2005). To reach this goal, the IOM committee recommended that DHHS convene a national conference to develop new guidelines for the advertising and marketing of foods, beverages, and sedentary entertainment directed toward children and youth, with attention given to product placement, promotion, and content. The IOM committee also recommended that industry implement the advertising and marketing guidelines, and that FTC be given the authority and resources to monitor compliance with these practices and guidelines (IOM, 2005).

The IOM report *Food Marketing to Children and Youth: Threat or Opportunity?* provides three additional recommendations related to advertising and marketing to children and youth (IOM, 2006). First, it recommends that industry work through CARU to revise, expand, apply, enforce, and evaluate explicit industry self-regulatory guidelines beyond traditional advertising to include evolving vehicles and venues for marketing communication (e.g., the Internet, advergames, and branded product placement across multiple media platforms). Second, the report recommends that industry ensure that licensed characters[6] are used only for the promotion of foods and beverages that support healthful diets for children and youth. Third, it recommends that industry foster cooperation between CARU and FTC to evaluate and enforce the effectiveness of the expanded self-regulatory guidelines (IOM, 2006).

In July 2005, FTC and DHHS held a joint workshop, Marketing, Self-Regulation, and Childhood Obesity, that provided a forum for industry, academic, public health advocacy, and government stakeholders, as well as consumers, to examine the role of the private sector in addressing the rising childhood obesity rates. A summary of the workshop contains recommendations and next steps for industry stakeholders, including a request that industry strengthen self-regulatory measures to advertise responsibly to children through CARU. FTC and DHHS both indicated that these institu-

---

[6]Licensed characters are branded cartoon characters or other animal or human spokescharacters that are easily recognized by children. A third-party licensing agreement allows the copyright holder of the branded character to loan its intellectual property to another company in exchange for payment. In the children's media industries, companies can license the characters and images to food, beverage, and restaurant companies for a fee (IOM, 2006).

tions plan to closely monitor the progress made on the recommendations in the joint FTC and DHHS summary report (FTC and DHHS, 2006). Moreover, through Public Law 109-108, FTC has requested public comment and information on food industry marketing activities targeted to children and adolescents and expenditures for those activities. The public comments and information will be submitted in a report to Congress (FTC, 2006).

CBBB has recognized the need to consider changes in the self-regulatory advertising guidelines to respond appropriately to new marketing techniques and also to the knowledge about children's cognitive abilities in understanding marketing messages (CBBB, 2006). Children younger than 7 to 8 years of age lack the cognitive skills to discern commercial from non-commercial content—that is, they are unable to attribute persuasive intent to advertising and other forms of marketing. Children usually develop these skills at about the age of 8 years; however, children as old as 11 years of age may not activate these cognitive defenses, especially with embedded forms of marketing, such as product placement in commercials and programs, unless they are explicitly cued to activate these skills (IOM, 2006).

In early 2006, CBBB announced plans to review the CARU guidelines for advertising to children. As part of the CARU review process, an industry working group that receives input from a diverse group of CARU advisers has been established. The industry working group is currently engaged in an ongoing process to consider whether and how the industry self-regulatory guidelines should be revised and has indicated that the scope of the review will be broad. After the review, the industry working group will make recommendations to the board of directors of NARC, CBBB, and the Electronic Retailing Self-Regulatory Program. Once the NARC board has given approval, the recommendations will be posted for public comment and the NARC board will consider implementing the recommendations (CBBB, 2006).

Information and Education

Information and education are necessary but not sufficient factors to promote behavioral changes in young consumers and their parents. The recommended items should be available, accessible, affordable, appealing, and sufficiently promoted to consumers. One of the approaches that has been adopted by food and beverage manufacturers to help consumers make healthier product choices is to highlight the existing products in their portfolios that meet certain nutrition standards that are based on recommendations by FDA, the IOM's Dietary Reference Intakes, and the Dietary Guidelines for Americans 2005. Such nutrition standards include limits for the percentage of calories derived from fat, saturated fat, and *trans* fat; sugar, sodium, and fiber content; the reduction of calories and fat compared with those of other brands; or food-based guidelines that support the 2005 Dietary Guidelines for Americans. One way to assist consumers in recognizing these products is to put a branded icon or logo on the front label of the product package to indicate that these items meet established nutrition criteria.

PepsiCo uses the SmartSpot™ logo to distinguish "good for you" and "better for you" products from their other portfolio products, and Kraft Foods uses the Sensible Solution™ logo to identify products whose nutrient contents meet specific nutrient criteria according to the guidelines of FDA and IOM. General Mills promotes 14 different Goodness Corner™ icons (e.g., "whole grain" symbol) that meet specific nutrient criteria according to FDA guidelines that define limits for calories, total fat, saturated fat, *trans* fat, cholesterol, added sugars, and sodium; identify products that are high in fiber, vitamins, and minerals; and meet the 2005 Dietary Guidelines for Americans food-based guidelines.

This type of product branding enables consumers to identify healthful products as determined and conveyed by the company that makes and promotes the products. The healthy logos or icons may serve to build brand awareness and brand loyalty among consumers by making it easier for them to identify healthier products. The icons have the potential to provide clear and positive messages, demonstrate the companies' efforts toward expanding the healthier product portfolios, and providing healthful solutions to customers. Because the proprietary logos or icons that food companies have introduced to communicate the nutritional qualities of their branded products to consumers have not been evaluated, it is not yet known how consumers understand them. There may also be great variations in the consistency, accuracy, and effectiveness of these logos or icons (IOM, 2006). Furthermore, these icons may be useful for a company but do not broadly encourage the consumption of fruits and vegetables or allow comparison among brands (Appendix H).

As a means of addressing these concerns, in 2007, PBH—in partnership with the government and nonprofit organizations—plans to launch a new brand, The Fruits and Veggies—More Matters!™, and an icon that is intended to be easily recognized by consumers to promote the greater consumption of produce. The brand is designed to communicate the higher recommendations for produce put forward by the Dietary Guidelines for Americans 2005 (PBH, 2006).

As noted at the IOM industry symposium, a standard industrywide logo or icon may be more useful to consumers. All corporations could then use such a standard to designate products that meet agreed-upon nutrition and health standards. The present IOM committee encourages the pilot testing and formative evaluation of the feasibility of implementing an industrywide logo and icons that promote fruit and vegetable consumption.

Some leading food and beverage manufacturers are also providing consumers with educational information about healthful eating and active living. The GMA Health and Wellness survey found that 90 percent of its 42 members used multiple media channels (e.g., the product label, websites, brochures, and educational kits) to provide educational information. Approximately 25 member companies reported plans to use the USDA MyPyramid to promote healthy lifestyle messages (GMA, 2006). For example, General Mills provides on its cereal boxes information about the 2005 Dietary Guidelines for Americans and the website MyPyramid.gov as well as other resources to help consumers achieve a more healthful lifestyle (General Mills, 2005a,b). Evaluations that assess whether consumers apply the information to dietary changes are needed. Consumer and marketing research has demonstrated that although consumers say they are familiar with the food guidance system, fewer actually incorporate the guidance into their diets (IRI, 2006; Yankelovich, 2006). If current means of distributing information do not accomplish the desired changes in consumers' behaviors, further research into behavior change methodologies is recommended.

Several companies have developed programs and tools to assist families and parents in planning healthy meals or engaging in regular physical activity (Chapter 8). For example, parents and a group of food companies and food retailers including Annie's Homegrown, Applegate Farms, Horizon Organic, Newman's Own, Newman's Own Organics, and Whole Foods Market, initiated the Eat Smart, Grow Strong[SM] campaign in 2005. The campaign is focused on encouraging families to consume foods that contribute to a healthful diet and promoting healthy eating habits at home (Public Interest Media Group, 2005). The campaign's interactive website offers parents a range of ideas for healthy recipes and includes games that teach children about healthy eating habits.

Food retailers also offer several opportunities for educating young consumers about nutritious product choices and physical activity. They can conduct educational tours for school groups and provide nutrition information for teachers and students, as well as providing print and Internet-based information and menu planning ideas for families (Childs, 2006). The International Food Information Council (IFIC) Foundation, the Food Marketing Institute (FMI), and USDA have collaborated on developing a consumer brochure, Your Personal Path to Health, which offers nutrition information based on MyPyramid, as well as on portion sizes; making healthful selections when eating out at restaurants; and budgeting discretionary calories for sweets, fats, and caloric beverages (IFIC Foundation et al., 2006). The brochures will be distributed throughout supermarkets and other food retail outlets. An evaluation of the effectiveness of the brochures in food retail settings would be useful.

Hannaford is a food retailer that has recently embarked on developing a weighted rating system called Guiding Stars[SM], which was developed by analyzing the nutritional value of more than 27,000 food items sold in their grocery stores. The score determines whether an item receives one, two, three or no stars. The more positive nutritional attributes that a product has will give it a higher score. The system is designed to help consumers to make wise choices quickly while shopping (Hannaford Bros., 2005). An evaluation of consumers' understanding and use of the system is needed.

The *Health in the Balance* report recommended that full serve and fast food restaurants or QSRs should expand their healthier options and provide calorie content and general nutrition information at the point of purchase (IOM, 2005). Additionally, the FDA's Obesity Work Group has encouraged the restaurant industry to launch a nationwide voluntary point-of-sale nutrition information campaign for consumers (FDA, 2004) (Appendix D). Although the number of QSRs, full serve, and family style restaurants that provide nutrition information has increased over the past decade, the committee finds that more industrywide adoption is needed to make nutrition information more accessible at point of choice and relevant to consumers, including for children's menu items.

One evaluation of 287 of the largest chain restaurants across the nation found that 54 percent provided some type of nutrition information to consumers. Of those that provided information, 86 percent offered it through a company website. However, 46 percent of restaurants did not provide any type of nutrition information (Wootan and Osborn, 2006). A second evaluation was conducted to assess the availability of nutrition information for menu items at 15 of the highest-ranking full serve restaurant chains by sales volume. Of the 10 restaurants that offered nutrition information on their standard menus, 9 restaurants provided information for only menu items with specific health claims, such as "heart healthy" or "low fat," For selected items. Among 15 restaurants, only 4 provided a children's section in the main menu, 9 restaurants provided a separate children's menu, and only 1 restaurant provided nutrition information about the children's menus (Harnack, 2006). Given the increased trend in eating meals away from home, it is important that major chain restaurants of all types provide consumers with information on healthful choices, especially for children (Harnack, 2006; Wootan and Osborn, 2006).

As the leading QSR in sales, McDonald's Corporation began providing nutrition information on its food packaging in 2006. The new packaging displays nutrient content information through the use of easily understood icons—representing calories, protein, fat, carbohydrates, and sodium—and a bar chart format to convert scientific information into customer-oriented information about a product's nutritional value and how it relates to daily nutrition recommendations. Independent evaluations of the consumer use of restaurant nutrition labeling are needed to assess consumers' behavior changes with respect to industry's changes.

Recent actions by FDA are providing steps toward improving the availability of consumer nutrition information to assist with point-of-purchase choices (Chapter 4). In April 2005, FDA released two advance notices of proposed rule making to elicit stakeholder and public input on two recommendations of the FDA Obesity Working Group: to make calorie information more prominent on the Nutrition Facts label and to increase information about serving sizes on packaged foods (FDA, 2005b,c). In September 2005, FDA issued a final rule on the nutrient content claims definition of sodium levels for the term "healthy" (FDA, 2005a). The committee awaits further progress that FDA can make toward finalizing the rule making and exploring the use of evidence-based nutrient and health claims regarding the link between the nutrition properties or biological effects of foods and a reduced risk of obesity and related chronic diseases.

Public-Private Partnerships

Creating and maintaining public-private partnerships that support community-based health and wellness initiatives are essential components of childhood obesity prevention. Many of these partnerships involve corporate or private foundations, which are becoming important leaders in the response to childhood obesity. Private foundations, such as RWJF, sponsor significant national and regional initiatives and research. The Kansas Health Foundation, the Missouri Foundation for Health, Healthcare Georgia Foundation, and The California Endowment co-sponsored the regional symposia, while the Henry J. Kaiser Family Foundation, the Sunflower Foundation, the William J. Clinton Foundation, and the California Wellness Foundation participated in one or more of the symposia (Appendixes F to H). The community-based organizations attending the symposia reported that they seek funds from many sources to operate obesity prevention programs for children.

Leading food and beverage companies, such as PepsiCo, General Mills, and Kellogg, have established corporate foundations that are involved in partnerships focused on nutrition and physical activity. In 2005, General Mills reported that it contributed $78 million to communities across the United States, $20 million of which was awarded by the General Mills Foundation as grants for promoting child nutrition and fitness, social services, education, and arts and culture (General Mills, 2005b). Since 2002, the General Mills' Champions for Healthy Kids[SM] grants program has invested more than $6 million in nutrition and fitness programs that have reached approximately 100,000 children and youth (primarily racial/ethnic minority populations) throughout the United States (General Mills, 2006a).

The goal of the grant program is to promote healthy eating choices and active lifestyles among children and adolescents. The populations served include preschoolers enrolled in the Head Start Program in Connecticut, low-income African-American teens in Chicago, Alaska Native children and youth participating in the community-based Camp Fire USA Alaska Council, and 21,000 elementary and middle-school children in North Carolina (General Mills, 2006a).

Many company and corporate foundations have initiatives to address health, physical activity, and obesity prevention issues, many of which focus on improving opportunities for healthy lifestyles in low income African-American and Hispanic/Latino communities. PepsiCo has partnered with America on the Move, a nonprofit organization that promotes the implementation of small lifestyle changes to increase physical activity and reduce calorie intake (America on the Move, 2006). General Mills has partnered with the Black Entertainment Television (BET) Foundation to launch A Healthy BET, which provides information and advice to African-American women on eating healthy and staying physically fit (General Mills, 2006b). Kraft Foods has a partnership with the National Latino Children's Institute to promote *Salsa Sabor y Salud* (Food, Fun, and Fitness) (Kraft Foods, 2006). PepsiCo partners with the National Urban League, a leading advocacy group for African Americans and the National Council of La Raza, a leading advocacy group for Latinos (PepsiCo, 2006a). PepsiCo also provided an $11.6 million grant to support the YMCA to implement activities through the YMCA Activate America™ initiative across the nation (PepsiCo, 2006b). Other corporate foundations have formed partnerships with DHHS and the Boys and Girls Clubs of America to create initiatives that support young people in making informed decisions about their physical, mental, and social well-being (Appendix H).

Strong public-private partnerships need to involve multiple sectors—local businesses, local and state government, and industry—in order to leverage the strength needed to stimulate changes in the current childhood obesity epidemic. Partnerships are useful in that they provide a network of support, bring increased credibility to each partner, use limited resources for mutual benefit, and create networking advantages through diverse and shared communication channels (Chapter 6; Appendix H).

In 2005, Nickelodeon and the Alliance for a Healthier Generation (the latter of which is a joint initiative of the American Heart Association and the William J. Clinton Foundation) announced that it had entered into a public-private partnership to reach children and youth with the goal of promoting a healthy future generation (Alliance for a Healthier Generation, 2005). The collaboration launched the television program, Let's Just Play® Go Healthy Challenge, which focuses on children's real-life struggles to engage in healthy lifestyles over a 5-month period. Evaluation of the reach and impact of this type of programming on young viewers' eating patterns and physical activity behaviors is needed. Although Nickelodeon has publicly committed more than $28 million and 10 percent of its air time to messages that promote health and wellness (Alliance for a Healthier Generation, 2005), there is a need to independently evaluate the outcomes of this and similar commitments made by industry stakeholders.

A second initiative of the Alliance for a Healthier Generation is the Healthy Schools Program,[7] which was established in 2005 with funding from RWJF. The purpose of this program is to foster healthful environments that support efforts to reduce obesity in school-aged children and youth (Alliance for a Healthier Generation, 2006c) (Chapter 7). In May 2006, the Alliance announced a new initiative, along with representatives from Cadbury Schweppes, The Coca-Cola Company, PepsiCo, and the American Beverage Association to establish new guidelines in schools that will limit portion sizes; prohibit the sale of sweetened beverages and high-calorie, low-nutrient foods; and offer calorie-controlled servings of beverages to children and adolescents in the school environment. This is the Alliance's first industry agreement as part of the Healthy Schools Program and has the potential to affect 35 million students throughout the United States (Alliance for a Healthier Generation, 2006a,b) (Chapters 2, 7). The Alliance plans to conduct an in-depth and multistage evaluation is planned with quantifiable and measurable outcomes to assess the effectiveness of the changes resulting from this public-private partnership.

In 2006, Aetna and the Aetna Foundation announced that it will award up to $2.9 million through its Regional Community Health Grants Program. The program will fund efforts to ensure the healthy development of children from birth through elementary school, with an emphasis on obesity (and diabetes) as it relates to family and caregiver involvement; pediatric care; school-based implementation of the program; and integrated care delivery for obesity and diabetes and will provide links to ongoing preventive and sustainable care (Aetna, 2006).

Corporate Social Responsibility

Corporate social responsibility is commonly defined as the "obligation of a company to use its resources in ways to benefit society, taking into account the society at large and improving the welfare of society, independent of direct gains of the company" (Kok et al., 2001). Some of the specific

---

[7]The Healthy Schools Program is one of four initiatives of the Alliance for a Healthier Generation, which has set the goal to halt the increase in U.S. childhood obesity rates within 5 years and reverse the childhood obesity trend within 10 years.

ways in which companies demonstrate their social responsibility are to provide health care insurance, to provide work site health promotion and wellness services for their employees and their employees' family members, and to fund and support community activities and services (GMA, 2006; Kreuter, 2005; Snider et al., 2003). Work sites are also an important venue for reaching parents with messages and educational materials about childhood obesity prevention.

A number of corporations are actively involved in community initiatives related to obesity prevention and increasing the levels of physical activity among adults and young people, often through the public-private partnerships discussed above. Examples include NikeGO (sponsored by Nike, Inc.); Girls on the Run (2006) (sponsored by New Balance and Kellogg's); PE4Life (2006) (sponsored by multiple companies including New Balance, Reebok, Russell Athletic, Dick's Sporting Goods, and the National Sporting Goods Association, and several PepsiCo companies [Quaker, Gatorade, and Tropicana]); and America on the Move (including *Latinos en Movimiento*). These partnerships have multiple sponsors including the PepsiCo Corporate Fund and Cargill (America on the Move, 2006; National Council of La Raza, 2006). These are all examples of corporate-sponsored public-private partnerships that focus on increasing physical activity in adults and young people. Further efforts are needed to effectively engage the food, beverage, and restaurant industries in supporting community-based initiatives that focus on increasing access to healthful and affordable foods, such as the promotion of farmers' markets and new food retail establishments in low-income communities.

Corporate social reporting, the public reporting of socially responsible activities and behaviors, has grown considerably in recent years. Public reporting of nonfinancial performance is driven by public relations, competition, greater attention to the role of companies in promoting health by the nonprofit sector, and the growing presence and influence of institutional investors (Lang et al., 2006). An analysis of 25 of the leading global food manufacturers, retailers, and restaurants was conducted to examine the companies' corporate responsibility documents to explore their position on recommendations relevant to the World Health Organization's (WHO's) Global Strategy on Diet, Physical Activity, and Health (WHO, 2004). The analysis found that although 23 of the 25 companies had corporate social responsibility reports or statements of purpose and values related to nonfinancial company goals, only 11 of the companies made reference to health in their reports (e.g., Kraft Foods, PepsiCo, Kroger, McDonald's Corporation, and Yum! Brands). Additionally, the meaning of "health" in the company reporting varied from being broad and vague to more specific and measurable (Lang et al., 2006). The researchers concluded that the companies can do much more to elevate diet, health, and physical activity to the same priority as environmental and social justice issues and activities summarized in their corporate social responsibility reports.

APPLYING THE EVALUATION FRAMEWORK TO INDUSTRY

What Constitutes Progress for Industry?

To evaluate whether industry changes are shifting in a desirable direction to promote healthier diets and lifestyles, one must examine multiple types of available evidence to assess whether industry stakeholders are acting as collaborators and partners with other sectors and stakeholders in addressing childhood obesity prevention.

As described above, a systematic evaluation of the progress made by the leading 25 global food manufacturers, retailers, and restaurants in responding to the recommendations of the WHO's Global Strategy on Diet, Physical Activity, and Health was conducted (Lang et al., 2006). U.S. food and beverage manufacturers evaluated were The Coca-Cola Company, Kraft Foods, Masterfoods/Mars, and PepsiCo; U.S. food retailers evaluated were Kroger and Wal-Mart; and the QSRs evaluated were McDonald's Corporation, Burger King, and Yum! Brands. These companies are global marketplace leaders and have the ability to influence their entire sectors as role models for leadership and corporate social responsibility. The findings of the evaluation were based on the companies' self-reporting systems, which had limitations because of the variable quality of the information that was publicly available. Additionally, independent assessments of the efforts by these companies are needed to enhance transparency and public accountability.

The categories of activities that were examined in the evaluation included the company's business objectives and strategy; company operations; sales and market-share data; research and development and new product development; the company's published policies and spending on advertising, marketing, promotion, and sponsorship; company's position on corporate responsibility; the company's position on diet, nutrition, physical activity, and commitment to changing product portfolios to increase the number and proportion of healthy products; the company's position on product formulation and portion size, labeling, product nutrition information, and nutrition claims; stakeholder engagement; and whether the company promotes healthy lifestyles and physical activity internally and externally (Lang et al., 2006). The evaluation had four major conclusions. The food industry (e.g., manufacturers, retailers, and restaurants) should give higher priority to improve the profile of diet, physical activity, and health issues in corporate and sectoral business strategies; establish strategies, objectives, and indicators to internalize a health-promotion culture throughout the company; enhance the company's reporting systems to track and make available the company's impact on diet, physical activity, and health; and strengthen existing self-regulatory advertising codes (Lang et al., 2006).

The International Business Leaders Forum and Insight Investment (2006) have released a proposed draft framework that describes potential components of a comprehensive response to preventing obesity and chronic diseases. These components include undertaking an assessment of health-related business benefits and risks, establishing business objectives in response to obesity and health issues, and developing a companywide strategy for reaching the objectives. Furthermore, the framework suggests that companies establish relevant governance mechanisms at the highest levels (e.g., shareholders and company boards) so that the need for responsibility and accountability to address consumer health issues and integrate healthy lifestyle principles and objectives into their annual corporate reporting process is transmitted through the company.

Both qualitative and quantitative indicators can be used to assess industry initiatives and effectiveness. Qualitative measures include changes in the food industry management structure, and establishing senior-level positions or divisions that oversee a company's nutrition, health, and wellness activities. This serves as an indicator that health and obesity prevention are being given special attention and are an integral part of the business plan. Establishment of external advisory panels to advise the company about their products, marketing, and other activities is another indicator that a company is serious about the issue. Participating in and convening stakeholder dialogues addressing childhood obesity are also signals that a company is seeking to better understand the issue and is interested in taking action to address it.

Indicators of progress for food and beverage manufacturers include changes in product content (e.g., the development of new products or the reformulation of existing products) and packaging (e.g., the creation of calorie-controlled packages and containers) that support consumers' efforts to reduce excess energy consumption. Increasing the numbers of packaged or restaurant food items that meet the Dietary Guidelines for Americans 2005, reducing the package sizes for products high in energy density and total calories, providing more prominent label information conveying the total calorie content of a typical serving, and providing nutrition information for restaurant foods, beverages, and meals are all important steps in childhood obesity prevention efforts. Changes in marketing and advertising practices are also essential so that children and youth are not the focus of efforts to promote foods and beverages of poor nutritional quality and high energy density.

Quantitative measures include the number of new healthful product introductions over a specified time period and the sales and market shares of these new products. Additionally, the percentage of a company's sales portfolio devoted to healthful foods and beverages could be a publicly accessible means to track progress. As discussed below, industry and marketing firms consider much of the quantitative and qualitative information to be proprietary. Therefore, innovative approaches that provide information to the public while preserving the privacy and sale of commercial data are needed.

Challenges to Accurate Measurement of Progress

Public and Proprietary Data Sources

Most commercial marketing research data are obtained by private companies, marketing research and public relations firms, or companies that are associated with the marketing industry. The data that are collected and analyzed are generally proprietary and not publicly available. These data are retained for internal use or are expensive to purchase, thereby preventing widespread access to the data by the public health community or general public. These data are needed to better understand how marketing influences young people's behaviors, and to help assess the direct relationship between advertising and marketing activities and sales (IOM, 2006). The IOM report, *Food Marketing to Children and Youth: Threat or Opportunity?*, recommended that a means should be developed to make commercial marketing data available, if possible, as a publicly accessible resource (IOM, 2006). These data could help enhance understanding of the dynamics that shape the health and nutrition attitudes and the behaviors of children and youth at different ages and in different circumstances. They could also be used to inform a multifaceted social marketing program that would target parents, caregivers, and families to promote healthful diets and lifestyles for children and youth. Other groups have concurred with this recommendation to increase the public availability of commercial data. There is a particular need to improve the government's access to data on consumer attitudes and behaviors. Expanding government's access to syndicated commercial databases was a specific recommendation of the Keystone Forum on Away-From-Home Foods. Government agencies could establish in their annual budgets recurring line items for funds to ensure the continuous and timely access to commercial data sets (Keystone Center, 2006).

Supermarket scanner point-of-sale data are another useful form of marketing research data that are collected but which are difficult or expensive to access (NRC and IOM, 2004). Researchers could purchase these data from marketing and media companies, analyze them, and then publish the results of their analyses in peer-reviewed publications. The ACNielsen Fresh

Foods Homescan data uses a consumer panel that comprises 15,000 randomly selected households across the United States. Among these data are purchase data and demographic information for all households in the sample. The USDA Economic Research Center has used these data to obtain purchase information for random-weight, non-uniform product code (UPC)-coded food purchases such as fruit and vegetables, in addition to the standard fixed-weight UPC-coded products. A special feature of the Fresh Foods Homescan data is that the panelists record their food purchases from all retail outlets that sell food for home consumption, including grocery stores, drug stores, mass merchandisers, supercenters, and convenience stores. Information about where the purchase was made and whether it was made with a promotion, sale, or coupon is also tracked (Leibtag, 2005). These types of commercial data may be used for longitudinal epidemiological studies or for surveillance of national food- and nutrient-purchasing patterns within and between countries and segments of populations (Van Wave and Decker, 2003).

Tracking of Media Advertising and Marketing Promotion

Marketers pay to advertise and promote branded products through a variety of media channels, referred to as measured media and unmeasured media. The spending categories for measured media correspond to the categories that are tracked by media research companies such as Nielsen, TNS Media Intelligence/Competitive Media Reporting, and Forrester. Commonly tracked measured media includes television (e.g., network, spot, cable, syndicated, and Spanish-language networks), radio (e.g., network, national spot, and local radio), magazines (e.g., local and Sunday magazines), business publications, newspapers (e.g., local and national), outdoor advertising, telephone directory advertising, and the Internet. Spending on unmeasured media (including sales promotions, coupons, direct mail, catalogs, and special events) is not systematically tracked. Therefore, to be able to assess changes in spending on advertising and marketing for healthier food and beverage products consumed by children and youth, there must be a way to assess spending across all media categories (measured and unmeasured).

Applying the Evaluation Framework

This section illustrates how the evaluation framework described earlier in this report (Chapter 2) can be applied to two specific examples—industry's collective efforts to develop and promote the consumption of low-calorie and high nutrient-density beverage products by children and youth and efforts by corporations to promote physical activity among children and youth. Figures 5-1 and 5-2 provide examples of the types of resources and inputs and the types of strategies and actions that can be evaluated to determine if desirable short-term, intermediate, and long-term outcomes are being achieved.

Figure 5-1 focuses on key components in developing and promoting low-calorie and nutrient-dense beverage products for sale in the marketplace and settings where they are available to children and youth. The three key resources and inputs highlighted in the evaluation framework are the leadership and commitment by companies, retailers, and trade associations to develop consistent health promotion policies; the strategic planning of companies that reflect substantial investments and growth in healthier beverage product portfolios (e.g., low-calorie and calorie-free beverages, such as bottled water) over a specific time frame; and funding (evidence that companies are dedicating substantial resources to develop and promote affordable, calorie-free, or low-caloric and nutrient-dense beverage products in smaller serving sizes (e.g., 8- or 12-ounce servings for reduced-calorie beverages and larger portions for calorie-free beverages). To assess whether individual companies and the industry sector as a whole are moving toward the goal of developing and promoting low-calorie and nutrient-dense beverage products, companies and industry can be evaluated on the strategies and actions they employ, which can include:

(1) Company development of programs and policies to reflect healthier beverage product portfolios and integrated marketing plans that emphasize low-calorie or noncalorie beverages.

(2) Marketing and promotions that reflect responsible advertising and marketing guidelines—including advertising, public relations, promotion and pricing—particularly for children younger than 8 years of age, who do not understand the meaning of the persuasive intent of commercial messages. These guidelines are especially relevant to evolving forms of marketing vehicles and venues that are not systematically tracked, such as product placement across multiple forms of media, spokescharacter endorsement of products, Internet marketing, and mobile marketing.

(3) Education through a variety of methods, including general educational materials, product labeling, proprietary icons or logos, and health claims to assist young consumers and their parents with making informed decisions about purchases at food retail outlets and restaurants.

(4) Active collaborations with other sectors by individual companies or collectively by the industry sector. Collaboration may be assessed through company membership in trade associations, coalitions, and involvement in public-private partnerships that support obesity prevention and health promotion, particularly with an emphasis on consumption of healthier beverages by children and youth.

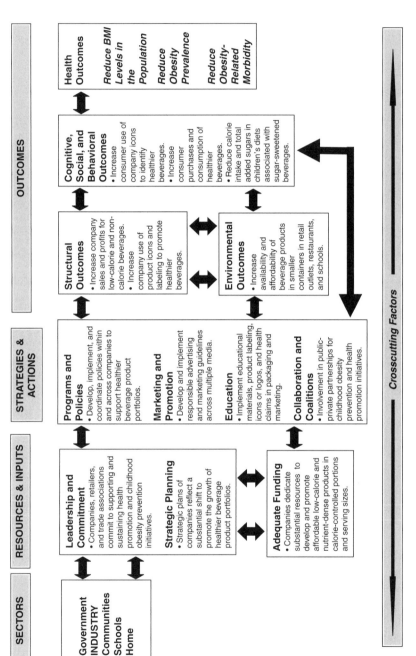

FIGURE 5-1 Evaluating industry efforts to develop low-calorie and nutrient-dense beverages and promote their consumption by children and youth.

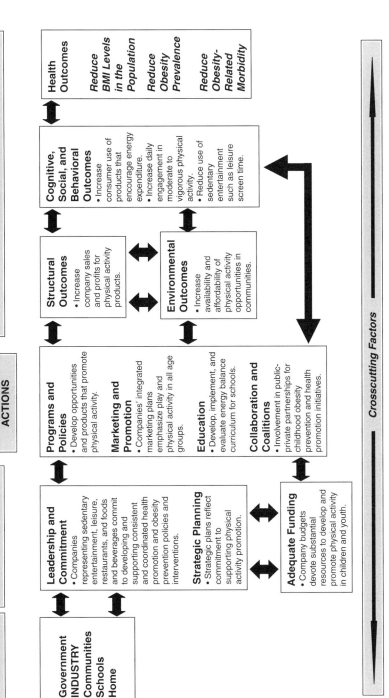

FIGURE 5-2 Evaluating industry efforts to support increased play and physical activity among children and youth.

Selected outcomes are illustrated in Figure 5-1, including institutional outcomes (e.g., increased company sales and profits for low-calorie and nutrient-dense or noncalorie beverages) and environmental outcomes (e.g., the increased availability and affordability of beverage products in smaller containers in retail outlets, restaurants, and schools). A variety of behavioral outcomes could be assessed, including whether a company's use of its branded icon or logo to highlight the healthier choices for consumers has increased and whether company-specific market research demonstrates an increase in consumer purchases and consumer consumption of low-calorie and nutrient-dense beverages. It will also be important to assess changes in calorie intake attributed to sugar-sweetened beverages and the impact on young peoples' diets and body mass index (BMI) levels. These changes can contribute to desirable health outcomes: reduced mean population BMI levels, a reduced prevalence of obesity among children and youth, and reduced rates of obesity-related morbidity.

NEEDS AND NEXT STEPS IN ASSESSING PROGRESS

Promote Leadership and Collaboration

Evidence of leadership and sustained commitment to childhood obesity prevention by multiple corporations in the various relevant sectors of industry is vital to achieving progress in obesity prevention. It is also important that the relationship between industry and the public health community be collaborative and not adversarial. Bringing the skill sets, the strengths, and the resources of both the public health sector and industry, as well as other stakeholders, together to build and sustain collaborative childhood obesity prevention efforts will require leadership and commitment from all sectors. Progress is being made in achieving increased numbers of healthful product options and providing responsible marketing and media messages for children and youth. The transition to social norms that support healthy choices may take years or may occur more rapidly. Corporations can also show leadership in the organizational modeling of physical activity and fitness and nutrition practices and policies.

Develop, Sustain, and Support Evaluation and Evaluation Capacity

As corporations continue to develop initiatives and make changes aimed at improving the dietary quality of foods and beverages or increasing physical activity, independent evaluations of these efforts are needed. An important component of the evaluation is the tracking of key performance indicators to assess industry progress. Examples of indicators that could be used to evaluate all industry sectors include the number of new health promotion programs or initiatives launched within a specific time frame; the rate of compliance with stated commitments, such as the implementation of calorie-controlled portions of product lines, enhanced labeling, or the provision of more nutrition information (e.g., on the basis of statistically relevant samples of products or the numbers of consumers reached); and the percentage of the corporate product portfolio that comprises healthful products (UNESDA, 2005).

Evaluations of healthier options at full serve restaurants and QSRs are challenging but are certainly needed, given that consumers are eating out more frequently. Glanz and colleagues (2005) propose four indicators that may be useful as a means of assessing the availability of healthier choices: healthy main dish options (e.g., low-fat, low-calorie, and healthy salads as main dishes); the availability of fruit (without added sugar or sauce); the availability of nonfried vegetables (and vegetables without high-fat sauces); and portion sizes (e.g., the availability of small portions and the absence of supersizing). Other data useful for the assessment of changes in the restaurant sector include the expansion of healthier menu options, visual assessments of how nutrition information is provided at restaurants, and interviews with restaurant staff (Glanz et al., 2005).

Food retailers could be evaluated on the basis of such outcomes as the nutritional contents of their packaged and processed foods, whether food retailers have made label information more accessible and understandable for consumers, the proportion of in-store promotions and shelf space devoted to healthful snack foods, reductions in the extent of display area for sweets and other foods that do not contribute to a healthful diet at the check-out counter, and increases in the amount of in-store information and advice about healthful eating made available to customers (Dibb, 2004).

Public-sector initiatives need to be explored at the federal, state, and local levels that would support industry efforts and may include public recognition, company awards for excellence, competitions, and performance-based tax breaks (IOM, 2006). The committee concludes that it is essential for government and nonprofit organizations to encourage and incentivize companies to support the evaluation of obesity prevention interventions. Government and nonprofits should acknowledge the companies that demonstrate leadership and strategic commitment and collaborate with the public health community on undertaking evaluations. Government agencies could also provide technical assistance to ensure the consistency of these efforts with evidence-based nutrition guidelines and assistance with the monitoring of compliance and the dissemination of the results. Similarly, industry trade associations, such as GMA, could work with government or nonprofit partners to develop or institutionalize formal guidelines, promising practices, competitions, incentives, or recognition programs that encourage its corporate members to develop and promote food and beverage products that support a healthful diet and reward them for doing so (IOM, 2006). This approach has been taken with the National 5 a Day partnership. Analogous efforts are needed for the restaurant and food retailer sectors, as well as the entertainment, leisure, and recreation industries.

After reviewing the evidence, the committee concludes that adequate funds should be made available to support independent and periodic evaluations of industry's progress toward making changes that support childhood obesity prevention goals. It is also important that resources be increased to support the evaluation capacity of industry, researchers, and other relevant stakeholders.

Enhance Surveillance, Monitoring, and Research

As discussed earlier in the chapter, efforts are under way to review the appropriateness and adequacy of the CARU guidelines for advertising to children. As part of the CARU review process, an industry working group has been established and is considering whether and how the industry self-regulatory guidelines should be revised. The committee supports assessment efforts of NARC, CBBB, CARU, and the companies that adhere to CARU guidelines as part of the review process. The committee also recommends an expeditious review.

Adequate funds are needed to support not only an internal review process but also independent and periodic evaluations of industry's efforts to promote healthier lifestyles. After the recommendations have been developed, CARU and the companies will be evaluated on the basis of what they have publicly committed to and how quickly they put their public commitments into action. It is important for companies to develop their own guidelines, in addition to adhering to the CARU guidelines, because internal guidelines can facilitate the creation of an internal corporate culture that proactively protects children, whereas external guidelines may be perceived as being optional.

Given that the industry working group recommendations were not available for the committee's review, the committee offers several areas in which revisions to the CARU guidelines would be beneficial and that deserve serious consideration. These recommendations build on the relevant recommendations in the IOM report, *Food Marketing to Children and Youth: Threat or Opportunity* (IOM, 2006), and are organized around specific themes relevant to marketing to children and youth and desirable evaluation outcomes (i.e., structural, institutional, and systemic outcomes) (Table 5-2). The committee recommends that Congress designate a responsible agency to conduct the periodic monitoring and evaluation of the self-regulatory guidelines of CARU. Such evaluations should include an assessment of CARU's effectiveness, impact, and enforcement capacity. Fur-

TABLE 5-2 Areas Relevant to the CARU Guidelines Assessment and Review Process

Themes	Evaluation Outcomes
Children's health	CARU and adhering industry stakeholders (e.g., food, beverage, restaurant, toy, and entertainment companies, and advertising and marketing agencies) should broaden their involvement in matters of children's health (e.g., through expanded board and advisory group membership and the establishment of health and wellness advisory boards and committees).
Healthful eating and lifestyle messages	CARU and adhering industry stakeholders should work closely with advertisers and public health professionals to develop strategies for the delivery of consistent healthy lifestyle messages by diverse companies (e.g., food, beverage, restaurant, leisure, and entertainment companies) and multiple forms of media (e.g., broadcast, cable, print, electronic, wireless media) to which children, youth, and their parents are exposed.
Expansion of self-regulatory guidelines for newer forms of marketing	CARU should expand its guidelines beyond those for the traditional broadcast and cable television media to address food, beverage, meal, and sedentary entertainment advertising and promotion to children and youth to include guidelines for newer forms of electronic media (e.g., videogames, interactive websites, advergames, mobile phones, and text messaging).
	Industry stakeholders (e.g., food, beverage, restaurant, toy, and entertainment companies, and advertising and marketing agencies) should develop within their own companies guidelines beyond those for the traditional broadcast and cable television to address food, beverage, meal, and sedentary entertainment advertising and promotion to children and youth to include guidelines for newer forms of electronic media.
Predissemination review of advertisements and commercial content	CARU should encourage and strengthen the voluntary predissemination review process of company advertisements before public dissemination through diverse communication channels.
Product placement	CARU should consider measures to monitor paid and in-kind product placement on children's programming, including broadcast and cable television, children's films, music, books, and mobile marketing, such as commercial content of cell phone advertising, to ensure that the products are consistent with healthy lifestyle messages.
Use of third-party licensed characters	CARU should ensure that third-party licensed characters (e.g., cartoon spokescharacters) are used to promote low-calorie and high-nutrient foods and beverages that support a healthful diet and healthy lifestyles.
Collaboration with the federal government	CARU and adhering industry stakeholders should work closely with and foster cooperation with FTC to monitor, evaluate, and enforce the effectiveness of the expanded self-regulatory guidelines.

thermore, the committee also recommends that the government and academic institutions work with industry to review efficacy and effectiveness research and evaluations to determine the best methods for demonstrating measurable changes in behavioral outcomes. Finally, the committee encourages NARC and the industry working group to examine the self-regulatory guidelines for marketing to children that exist in other countries, including specific commitments that are being made to address the childhood obesity epidemic, to inform its assessment and review process (FIAB, 2005; Hawkes, 2004; IOM, 2006; WFA, 2006).

The committee also recommends that FDA be given the authority to evaluate the efforts undertaken by full serve restaurants and QSRs to expand healthier food, beverage, and meal options to consumers and evaluate the effectiveness of providing nutrition labeling and general nutrition information at the point of choice on consumers' purchasing behaviors. CDC should evaluate the effectiveness of corporate-sponsored physical activity programs, energy balance education programs, and the use of branded physical activity equipment (e.g., physical videogaming) on children's leisure-time preferences and physical activity behaviors.

The IOM report *Food Marketing to Children and Youth: Threat or Opportunity?* (IOM, 2006) recommended that the federal research capacity, supported by DHHS (e.g., National Institutes of Health, CDC, FDA), the USDA, the National Science Foundation, and FCC and FTC), should be expanded to study the ways in which marketing influences children's and adolescents' attitudes and behaviors. Of particular importance is research related to newer promotion techniques and venues: healthier foods, beverages, and portion sizes; product availability; the impact of television advertising on diet and diet-related health; diverse research methods that systematically control for alternative explanations; stronger measurement techniques; and methods with high relevance to detect changes that occur as part of daily life.

The present IOM committee concurs with this research recommendation. To support the recommendation, the committee suggests that the food retail sector, the restaurant sector, and relevant trade associations and companies collaborate with USDA and DHHS to provide data on pricing strategies, consumer food purchases, and consumption trends from proprietary retail scanner systems, household scanner panels, household consumption surveys, and marketing research. The collaborative work should examine the quality of the data, consider reducing the cost of the data to increase accessibility, and establish priorities for using the information to promote healthful diets and physical activity.

Corporate responsibility can be demonstrated by sharing marketing research findings, to the greatest extent possible, that will assist the public health sector to develop, implement, and evaluate more effective childhood obesity prevention policies, programs, and interventions. Data sharing will need to balance many considerations including transparency, public accessibility, the demands of the competitive marketplace, and legal issues. In certain cases, it might be appropriate for the data to be released after a time lag to keep the public informed with relatively recent data. The committee recommends that the public and private sectors engage in a collaborative process that will assist relevant stakeholders in sharing proprietary data for the public good.

SUMMARY AND RECOMMENDATIONS

Changes in the development and promotion of products and services that contribute to healthy lifestyles are under way. However, much remains to be done. Most of the attention to date has focused on changes in the food and beverage industries. Indeed, changes in product formulations, packaging, labeling, and marketing are occurring as the result of corporate initiatives and government efforts, as well as through collaborations between industry and community partners. Independent evaluations of these changes are critical, as is the broader engagement of a wider array of relevant industries. In addition to the changes made by the food and beverage industries, innovative approaches to encouraging and promoting physical activity are being explored, however further efforts and creative advances are greatly needed in this area. Strengthening the alliances between the public health community and industry will bring the strengths of all groups to bear on preventing childhood obesity.

Recommendation 1: Government, industry, communities, schools, and families should demonstrate leadership and commitment by mobilizing the resources required to identify, implement, evaluate, and disseminate effective policies and interventions that support childhood obesity prevention goals.

Implementation Actions for Industry
Industry should use the full range of available resources and tools to create, support, and sustain consumer demand for products and opportunities that support healthy lifestyles including healthful diets and regular physical activity.

To accomplish this,
- Industry should continue to support and market product innovations and reformulations that promote energy balance at a healthy weight for children and youth and that are compatible with obesity prevention goals.

- Industry should support the review of the existing self-regulatory guidelines for advertising directed to children. It should also expand the guidelines to advertising vehicles beyond those used in traditional advertising to include evolving vehicles and venues for marketing communication and apply and enforce the guidelines for the traditional and expanded vehicles. Companies should consider developing their own advertising and marketing guidelines for children that are consistent with the industry-wide guidelines.

Recommendation 2: Policy makers, program planners, program implementers, and other interested stakeholders—within and across relevant sectors—should evaluate all childhood obesity prevention efforts, strengthen the evaluation capacity, and develop quality interventions take into account diverse perspectives, that use culturally relevant approaches, and that meet the needs of diverse populations and contexts.

Implementation Actions for Industry
Industry should partner with government, academic institutions, and other interested stakeholders to undertake evaluations to assess its progress in preventing childhood obesity and promoting healthy lifestyles.

To accomplish this,
- Industry should evaluate its progress in developing and promoting affordable foods, beverages, and meals that support a healthful diet; physical activity products and opportunities; storylines and programming that promote healthy lifestyles; and advertising and marketing practices directed to children and youth.
- Industry should provide resources and expertise to local businesses and community-based organizations to implement and evaluate initiatives that provide opportunities for consumers to engage in healthful eating and regular physical activity, especially for children and youth in racially and ethnically diverse groups and high-risk populations.

Recommendation 3: Government, industry, communities, and schools should expand or develop relevant surveillance and monitoring systems and, as applicable, should engage in research to examine the impact of childhood obesity prevention policies, interventions, and actions on relevant outcomes, paying particular attention to the unique needs of diverse groups and high-risk populations. Additionally, parents and caregivers should monitor changes in their family's food, beverage, and physical activity choices and their progress toward healthier lifestyles.

Implementation Actions for Industry
The U.S. Congress, in consultation with industry and other relevant stakeholders, should appropriate adequate funds to support independent and periodic evaluations of industry's efforts to promote healthier lifestyles.

> *To accomplish this,*
> - The FDA should be given the authority to evaluate full serve and quick serve restaurants' expansion of healthier food, beverage, and meal options; the effectiveness of the restaurant sector in providing nutrition labeling and nutrition information at the point of choice; and the effect of this information on consumers' purchasing behaviors.
> - The CDC should evaluate the effectiveness of corporate-sponsored physical activity programs, energy-balance education programs, and the use of branded physical activity equipment (e.g., physical videogames) on children's leisure-time preferences and physical activity behaviors.
> - The U.S. Congress should designate a responsible agency to conduct the periodic monitoring and evaluation of the self-regulatory guidelines of CARU, which should include an assessment of CARU's effectiveness, impact, and enforcement capacity.
> - The food retail sector, the restaurant sector, and relevant trade associations should collaborate with the USDA and DHHS to provide marketing data on pricing strategies, consumer food purchases, and consumption trends from proprietary retail scanner systems, household scanner panels, household consumption surveys, and marketing research. The collaborative work should examine the quality of the data, consider reducing the cost to make the data more accessible, and establish priorities for applying the information to promote healthful diets.
> - Industry should demonstrate corporate responsibility by sharing marketing research findings that may help public health professionals and community-based organizations develop and implement more effective childhood obesity prevention messages, policies, and programs.

Recommendation 4: Government, industry, communities, schools, and families should foster information-sharing activities and disseminate evaluation and research findings through diverse communication chan- nels and media to actively promote the use and scaling up of effective childhood obesity prevention policies and interventions.

Implementation Actions for Industry
Industry should collaborate with the public sector and other relevant stakeholders to develop a mechanism for sharing proprietary data and a sustainable funding strategy that can inform and support child- hood obesity prevention interventions.

To accomplish this,

- The private sector (e.g., industry and foundations) and the public sector (e.g., government and nonprofit organizations) should partner to develop a mechanism for the sharing propri- etary data (e.g., product sales information, marketing research data, and the results of evaluations of industry-supported pro- grams) that can inform research efforts and assist in developing a healthy lifestyles social marketing campaign. A long-term funding strategy should be established to sustain the campaign. Such a strategy should include a dedicated government appro- priation and a dedicated set-aside from relevant industries.
- Government and other interested stakeholders should develop incentives and rewards for industry stakeholders that collabo- rate on this endeavor.

REFERENCES

AAAA (American Association of Advertising Agencies). 2006. *Inside the AAAA: About Us.* [Online]. Available: http://www.aaaa.org/eweb/Dynamic Page.aspx?Site=4A_new&Web Key=d94ac5ca-e68d-4587-be89-5a8e7ea82e39 [accessed August 1, 2006].

AAF (American Advertising Federation). 2006. *About AAF.* [Online]. Available: http://www. aaf.org/about/index.html [accessed July 24, 2006].

Ad Council. 2006a. *About Ad Council.* [Online]. Available: http://www.adcouncil.org/ default.aspx?id=68 [accessed July 24, 2006].

Ad Council. 2006b. *Coalition for Healthy Children: Combating Childhood Obesity.* [Online]. Available: http://healthychildren.adcouncil.org/about.asp [accessed July 24, 2006].

Aetna. 2006. *2006 Regional Community Health Grants Program.* [Online]. Available: http:// fconline.fdncenter.org/pnd/10001192/aetna [accessed March 13, 2006].

Alliance for a Healthier Generation. 2005. *Nickelodeon, Clinton Foundation and American Heart Association Announce Partnership to fight Childhood Obestiy* [Online]. Avail- able: http://www.healthiergeneration.org/docs/afhg_nr_lets_just_play_10-20-05.pdf / [ac- cessed August 3, 2006].

Alliance for a Healthier Generation. 2006a. *Alliance for a Healthier Generation and Industry Leaders Set Healthy School Beverage Guidelines for U.S. Schools.* [Online]. Available: http://www.healthiergeneration.org/docs/afhg_ nr_school_beverage_5-3-06.pdf [accessed May 8, 2006].

Alliance for a Healthier Generation. 2006b. *School Beverage Guidelines.* [Online]. Available: http://www.healthiergeneration.org/engine/renderpage.asp?pid=s017 [accessed July 31, 2006].

Alliance for a Healthier Generation. 2006c. *What is the Health Schools Program?* [Online]. Available: http://www.healthiergeneration.org/docs/afhg_sp_ healthy_schools_qa.pdf [accessed August 3, 2006].

AMA (American Marketing Association). 2005. *Marketing Definitions.* [Online]. Available: http://www.marketingpower.com/content4620.php [accessed August 4, 2005].

AMA. 2006. *Mission Statement.* [Online]. Available: http://www.marketingpower.com/content424.php [accessed July 26, 2006].

America on the Move. 2006. *America on the Move Sponsors.* [Online]. Available: http://aom.americaonthemove.org/site/c.hiJRK0PFJpH/b.1311205/k.DED2/sponsors.htm [accessed July 19, 2006].

ANA (Association of National Advertisers). 2006. *ANA Mission.* [Online]. Available: http://www.ana.net/about/mission/mission.htm [accessed July 24, 2006].

Baranowski T, Baranowski J, Cullen KW, Marsh T, Islam N, Zakeri I, Honess-Morreale L, deMoor C. 2003. Squire's Quest! Dietary outcome evaluation of a multimedia game. *Am J Prev Med* 24(1):52–61.

Berkeley Media Studies Group. 2005. *The Advertising Story: A Study of the Context of the Ad Council/Coalition for Healthy Children's Obesity Prevention Messages in TV and Web-Based Advertising.* Berkeley, CA: Public Health Institute.

Beverage Digest. 2006. *Special Issue: All-Channel Carbonated Soft Drink Performance in 2005.* [Online]. Available: http://www.beverage-digest.com/pdf/top-10_2006.pdf [accessed July 11, 2006].

Big Red Frog. 2006. *BodyMechanics: Putting a Little Superhero in All of Us.* [Online]. Available: http://www.bodymechanics.com [accessed July 27, 2006].

Blake M. 2006. *Innovation in Healthy Convenience Food and Drinks.* Business Insights. Brief summary. [Online]. Available: http://www.globalbusinessinsights.com/report.asp?id=rbcg0149 [accessed July 13, 2006].

Boone LE, Kurtz DL. 1998. *Contemporary Marketing Wired.* 9th ed. Orlando, FL: The Dryden Press.

Brown D. 2006. Playing to win: Video games and the fight against obesity. *J Am Diet Assoc* 106(2)188–189.

Brown K, Endicott RC, MacDonald S, Schumann M, Macarthur G, Sierra J, Matheny L, Green A, Ryan M. 2005. 50th annual 100 leading national advertisers. *Advertising Age* June 27. Pp. 1–84. [Online]. Available: http://www.adage.com/images/random/lna2005.pdf [accessed June 17, 2006].

Business Insights. 2005. *New Profit Opportunities in Health and Nutrition to 2009.* Brochure. [Online]. Available: http://www.globalbusinessinsights.com/etwodir/mailings/rc445/rc445pdfs/rc445e-brochure.PDF [accessed March 10, 2006].

Business Insights. 2006. *Innovative Trends in Kids' Food and Drinks.* Brochure. [Online]. Available: http://www.globalbusinessinsights.com/etwodir/mailings/rc608/rc608pdfs/rc608a-brochure.pdf [accessed March 13, 2006].

CARU (Children's Advertising Review Unit). 2003a. *Self-Regulatory Guidelines for Children's Advertising.* 7th ed. New York: Council of the Better Business Bureaus, Inc.

CARU. 2003b. *About the Children's Advertising Review Unit (CARU).* [Online]. Available: http://www.caru.org/ [accessed November 10, 2005].

CBBB (Council of the Better Business Bureaus). 2005. *About Us.* [Online]. Available: http://www.narcpartners.org/about/index.asp [accessed July 24, 2006].

CBBB. 2006. *CARU Launching Complete Review of Children's Advertising Guidelines.* February 6. [Online]. Available: http://www.caru.org/news/2006/caru.pdf [accessed June 15, 2006].

Childs NM. 2006 (January 24). *Obesity—What Are We Doing About It? Informing the Consumer: The Retail Interface.* Presentation at the Institute of Food Technologists Symposium, Washington, DC. [Online]. Available: http://www.ift.org/divisions/food_law/Slides_200601/CHILDS.pdf [accessed March 13, 2006].

Cohn SR. 2006 (January 24). *Away From Home Dining.* Presentation at the Institute of Food Technologists Symposium, Washington, DC. [Online]. Available: http://www.ift.org/divisions/food_law/Slides_200601/COHN.pdf [accessed March 13, 2006].

Collins G. 1995. From Taco Bell, a healthier option. *The New York Times.* February 9. [Online]. Available: http://query.nytimes.com/gst/fullpage.html?res=990CE7D81F3FF93 AA35751C0A963958260&sec=health&pagewanted=print [accessed July 24, 2006].

Cullen KW, Watson K, Baranowski T, Baranowski JH, Zakeri I. 2005. Squire's Quest: Intervention changes occurred at lunch and snack meals. *Appetite* 45(2):148–151.

DHHS (U.S. Department of Health and Human Services) and USDA (U.S. Department of Agriculture). 2005. *Dietary Guidelines for Americans 2005.* [Online]. Available: http://www.healthierus.gov/dietaryguidelines [accessed December 29, 2005].

Dibb S. 2004. *Rating Retailers for Health: How Supermarkets Can Affect Your Chances of a Healthy Diet.* London, United Kingdom: National Consumer Council. [Online]. Available: http://www.ncc.org.uk/food/rating_retailers.pdf [accessed January 4, 2006].

Dorfman L, Wallack L, Woodruff K. 2005. More than a message: Framing public health advocacy to change corporate practices. *Health Educ Behav* 32(3):320–336.

Enrico D. 1999. Top 10 advertising icons. The Advertising Century: Special Issue. *Advertising Age* vol 43. [Online]. Available: http://www.adage.com/century/century.html [accessed July 12, 2006].

ERS, USDA (Economic Research Service, U.S. Department of Agriculture). 2006. *Food CPI, Prices, and Expenditures.* [Online]. Available: http://www.ers.usda.gov/Briefing/CPI FoodAndExpenditures/ [accessed June 18, 2006].

Evans WD, Price S, Blahut S. 2005. Evaluating the truth® brand. *J Health Commun* 10(2): 181–192.

FDA (U.S. Food and Drug Administration). 2004. *Calories Count: Report of the Working Group on Obesity.* [Online]. Available: http://www.cfsan.fda.gov/~dms/owg-toc.html [accessed May 17, 2006].

FDA. 2005a. Food labeling; nutrient content claims, definition of sodium levels for the term "healthy." Final Rule. *Fed Regist* 70(188): 56828–56849.

FDA. 2005b. Food labeling; Prominence of calories. *Fed Regist* 70(63).

FDA. 2005c. Food labeling; nutrient content claims, definition of sodium levels for the term "healthy" *Fed Regist* 70(63).

FIAB (Federation of Food and Drink Industries). 2005. *Code of Self-Regulation of the Advertising of Food Products Directed at Minors, Prevention of Obesity and Health.* Spanish Ministry of Health and Consumer Affairs. [Online]. Available: http://www.aesa.msc.es/aesa/web/FileServer?file=PAOS_ING.pdf&language=en_US&download=yes [accessed June 22, 2006].

Freudenberg N. 2005. Public health advocacy to change corporate practices: Implications for health education practice and research. *Health Educ Behav* 32(3):298–319.

FTC (Federal Trade Commission). 2006. Request for information and comment: Food industry marketing practices to children and adolescents. *Fed Regist* 71(4):10535–10536. [Online]. Available: http://a257.g.akamaitech.net/7/257/2422/01jan20061800/edocket. access.gpo.gov/2006/06-1931.htm [accessed March 6, 2006].

FTC and DHHS. 2006. *Perspectives on Marketing, Self-Regulation, and Childhood Obesity: A Report on a Joint Workshop of the Federal Trade Commission and the Department of Health & Human Services, April 2006.* [Online]. Available: http://www.ftc.gov/os/2006/05PerspectivesOnMarketingSelfRegulation&ChildhoodObesityFTCandHHSReportonJoint Workshop.pdf [accessed May 3, 2006].

Fusaro D. 2004. Packages that are changing the face of food processing. *Food Processing Magazine* [Online]. Available: http://www.foodprocessing.com/articles/2004/68.html [accessed January 4, 2006].

Games for Health. 2006. *Games for Health.* [Online]. Available: http://www.gamesforhealth. org/index2.html [accessed July 27, 2006].

General Mills. 2005a. *General Mills Announces Major Nutrition Education Initiative in Conjunction with New Food Guide Pyramid.* News release. April 19. [Online]. Available: http://www.generalmills.com/corporate/health_wellnessin_the_news_detail.aspx?item ID= 10561&catID=7586&section=news [accessed May 16, 2006].

General Mills. 2005b. *General Mills Community Action. 2005 Report.* Minneapolis, MN: General Mills Foundation.

General Mills. 2006a. *Champions for Healthy Kids*^{SM}. Minneapolis, MN: General Mills Foundation.

General Mills. 2006b. *Nourishing Lives.* Minneapolis, MN: General Mills Foundation.

Girls on the Run. 2006. *Our Sponsors.* [Online]. Available: http://www.girlsontherun.org/ oursponsors.html [accessed July 28, 2006].

Gladwell M. 2000. *The Tipping Point: How Little Things Can Make a Big Difference.* Boston, MA: Back Bay Books.

Glanz K, Sallis JF, Saelens BE, Frank LD. 2005. Healthy nutrition environments: Concepts and measures. *Am J Health Promot* 19(5):330–303.

GMA (Grocery Manufacturers of America). 2005. *GMA Statement Regarding Proposals to Strengthen Advertising Self-Regulation.* News release. July 15. [Online]. Available: http:// www.gmabrands.com/news/docs/NewsRelease.cfm?DocID=1542& [accessed January 5, 2006].

GMA. 2006. *Industry Report on Health and Wellness.* [Online]. Available: http://www. gmabrands.com/publications/docs/hwreport.pdf [accessed June 22, 2006].

GMA Forum. 2005. *Cannondale Trade Promotion Study 2005. Saying No to the Status Quo.* Second Quarter. Washington, DC. Pp. 72–84.

Gorecki S. 2006. *Food Industry Uses Internet to Reach Kids. United Press International News Release.* July 20. [Online]. Available: http://www.upi.com/ConsumerHealthDaily/ view.php?StoryID=20060719-104259-5440r [accessed July 24, 2006].

Hannaford Bros. 2005. *Guiding Stars.*^{SM} [Online]. Available: http://www.hannaford.com/ Contents/Healthy_Living/Guiding_Stars/gs_how_guidingstars_works.shtml [accessed September 6, 2006].

Harnack L. 2006. Availability of nutrition information on menus at major chain table-service restaurants. *J Am Diet Assoc* 106(7):1012–1015.

Harris JM. 2002. Food manufacturing. In: Harris J, Kaufman P, Martinez S, Price C, eds. 2002. *The U.S. Food Marketing System, 2002.* Economic Research Service, U.S. Department of Agriculture. Agricultural Economic Report No. (AER811). Pp. 3–11. [Online]. Available: http://www.ers.usda.gov/publications/aer811/aer811.pdf [accessed June 21, 2006].

Hawkes C. 2004. *Marketing Food to Children: The Global Regulatory Environment.* Geneva, Switzerland: World Health Organization. [Online]. Available: http://whqlibdoc.who.int/ publications/2004/9241591579.pdf [accessed June 21, 2006].

Healthy Arkansas. 2006. *Healthy Restaurant Awards.* [Online]. Available: http://www. arkansas.gov/ha/healthy_restaurant.html [accessed March 13, 2006].

Holt DB. 2004. *How Brands Become Icons: The Principles of Cultural Branding.* Boston, MA: Harvard Business School Press.

Horovitz B. 2006. Nickelodeon beefs up fruit partnership; some say SpongeBob, Dora plans aimed at public relations. *USA Today* July 19. [Online]. Available: http://www.usa today.com/money/ industries/food/2006-07-18-nickelodeon-usat_x.htm [accessed July 20, 2006].

IBLF (International Business Leaders Forum) and Insight Investment. 2006. *A Proposed Framework for the Corporate Response to Addressing Consumer Health and Obesity.* London, United Kingdom: IBLF and Insight Investment.

IFIC (International Food Information Council) Foundation, FMI (Food Marketing Institute), USDA (U.S. Department of Agriculture). 2006. *Your Personal Path to Health: Steps to a Healthier You!* [Online]. Available: http://www.ific.org/publications/brochures/upload/MyPyramidBrochure.pdf [accessed July 24, 2006].

Insight Investment. 2006. *Investor Responsibility Briefing. Obesity: How is the Food Industry Responding?* London, UK. [Online]. Available: http://www.insightinvestment.com/Documents/responsibility/Articles/obesity.pdf [accessed July 29, 2006].

IOM (Institute of Medicine). 2005. *Preventing Childhood Obesity: Health in the Balance.* Washington, DC: The National Academies Press.

IOM. 2006. *Food Marketing to Children and Youth: Threat or Opportunity?* Washington, DC: The National Academies Press.

IRI (Information Resources, Inc.). 2006. Healthy eating trends: Innovative solutions to evolving consumer needs. *Times & Trends* Jan:1–19.

JPMorgan. 2006. *Obesity: Re-Shaping the Food Industry.* Global Equity Research. January 24.

Kaiser Permanente. 2006. *Kaiser Permanente's Comprehensive Approach to the Obesity Epidemic: Bringing Expertise and Resources to Bear at Every Level.* [Online]. Available: http://www.calwic.org/docs/kaiserbroch_feb06.pdf [accessed June 20, 2006].

Kapica CM, Alexander D, Mink P, Butchko H. 2006. The definition of fast food in published studies. Experimental Biology Meeting, San Francisco, April 1–5. *Experimental Biology 2006 Meeting Program.* Abstract 139.9. P. 48.

Kennedy E. 2004. Dietary diversity, diet quality, and body weight regulation. *Nutr Rev* 62(7):S78–S81.

Keystone Center. 2006. *Keystone Forum on Away-From-Home Foods: Opportunities for Preventing Weight Gain and Obesity.* Washington, DC: The Keystone Center. [Online]. Available: http://www.keystone.org/spp/documents/Forum_Report_FINAL_5-30-06.pdf [accessed June 3, 2006].

Kok P, van der Wiele T, McKenna R, Brown A. 2001. A corporate social responsibility audit within a quality management framework. *J Business Ethics* 31(4):285–297.

Kraft Foods. 2005. *Kraft Foods Announces Marketing Changes to Emphasize More Nutritious Products.* January 12. [Online]. Available: http://www.kraft.com/newsroom/01122005.html [accessed July 24, 2006].

Kraft Foods. 2006. *Contributions and Communities.* [Online]. Available: http://www.kraft.com/responsibility/cc_salsa_sabor_salud.aspx [accessed July 19, 2006].

Kretser AJ. 2006 (January 24). *The Packaged Food Industry.* Presentation at the Institute of Food Technologists Symposium, Washington, DC. [Online]. Available: http://www.ift.org/divisions/food_law/Slides_200601/KRETSER.pdf [accessed February 20, 2006].

Kreuter MW. 2005. Commentary on public health advocacy to change corporate practices. *Health Educ Behav* 32(3):355–362.

Lang T, Rayner G, Kaelin E. 2006. *The Food Industry, Diet, Physical Activity and Health: A Review of the Reported Commitments and Practice of 25 of the World's Largest Food Companies.* Centre for Food Policy, City University, London, United Kingdom. [Online]. Available: http://www.city.ac.uk/press/The%20Food%20Industry%20Diet%20Physical %20Activity%20and%20Health.pdf [accessed June 17, 2006].

Ledikwe JH, Blanck HM, Khan LK, Serdula MK, Seymour JD, Tohill BC, Rolls BJ. 2006. Low-energy-density diets are associated with high diet quality in adults in the United States. *J Am Diet Assoc* 106(8):1172–1180.

Leibtag ES. 2005. Where you shop matters: Store formats drive variation in retail food prices. *Amber Waves* 13–18. Economic Research Service, U.S. Department of Agriculture. [Online]. Available: http://www.ers.usda.gov/AmberWaves/November05/Features/Where YouShop.htm [accessed June 21, 2006].

Lichtenstein AH, Appel LJ, Brands M, Carnethon M, Daniels S, Franklin B, Kris-Etherton P, Harris WS, Howard B, Karanja N, Lefevre M, Rudel L, Sacks F, Van Horn L, Winston M, Wylie-Rosett J. 2006. Diet and lifestyle recommendations revision 2006. A scientific statement from the American Heart Association Nutrition Committee. *Circulation* 114(1):82–96.

Marketing Intelligence Service. 2005. *ProductScan® Online Database of New Products.* [Online]. Available: http://www.productscan.com [accessed July 31, 2006].

McDonald's Corporation. 2003. *McDonald's™ Introduces New McKIDS™ Multi-Category, Worldwide Licensing Program.* News release. November 13. [Online]. Available: http://www.mcdonalds.com/corp/news/corppr/2003/cpr11132003.html [accessed January 4, 2006].

McDonald's Corporation. 2005. *Ronald McDonald®: Balanced, Active Lifestyles Ambassador.* [Online]. Available: http://www.mcdepk.com/ronald/index.html [accessed July 12, 2006].

McDonald's Corporation. 2006. *Balanced, Active Lifestyles. . .its what I eat and what I do.* [Online]. Available: http://www.rmhc.org/corp/values/balance.html [accessed June 19, 2006].

Mello MM, Studdert DM, Brennan TA. 2006. Obesity—The new frontier of public health law. *N Engl J Med* 354(24):2601–2610.

Moore ES. 2006. *It's Child's Play: Advergaming and the Online Marketing of Food to Children.* Menlo Park, CA: Kaiser Family Foundation. [Online]. Available: http://www.kff.org/entmedia/upload/7536.pdf [accessed July 24, 2006].

NAICS (North American Industry Classification System). 2002. *NAICS Definitions: Limited-Service Restaurants.* [Online]. Available: http://www.naics.com/censusfiles/ND722211.HTM [accessed April 6, 2006].

NARC (National Advertising Review Council). 2004. *Guidance for Food Advertising Self-Regulation.* New York, NY: NARC. [Online]. Available: http://www.narcpartners.org/NARC_White_Paper_6-1-04.pdf [accessed January 5, 2006].

National Council of La Raza. 2006. *Latinos en Movimiento.* [Online]. Available: http://www.nclr.org/section/america_on_the_move/ [accessed July 13, 2006].

NHLBI (National Heart, Lung, and Blood Institute). 2006. *We Can! Media Partners.* [Online]. Available: http://www.nhlbi.nih.gov/health/public/heart/obesity/wecan/news/partners.htm [accessed July 27, 2006].

Nielsen SJ, Siega-Riz AM, Popkin BM. 2002a. Trends in energy intake in U.S. between 1977 and 1996: Similar shifts seen across age groups. *Obes Res* 10(5):370–378.

Nielsen SJ, Siega-Riz AM, Popkin BM. 2002b. Trends in food locations and sources among adolescents and young adults. *Prev Med* 35(2):107–113.

NRA (National Restaurant Association). 2006. *Restaurant Industry Fact Sheet.* [Online]. Available: http://www.restaurant.org/pdfs/research/2006factsheet.pdf [accessed March 12, 2006].

NRC (National Research Council) and IOM. 2004. *Children's Health, The Nation's Wealth.* Washington, DC: The National Academies Press.

Packaged Facts. 2003. *U.S. Market for Kids' Foods and Beverages.* 5th edition. Report summary. [Online]. Available: http://www.marketresearch.com/researchindex/849192.html#pagetop [accessed March 13, 2006].

Packaged Facts. 2006. *Snack Food Trends in the U.S.: Sweet, Salty, and Healthy Kids Snacks.* Brief Summary. [Online]. Available: http://www.packagedfacts.com/pub/1119533.html [accessed July 11, 2006].

Parks SC. 2002. The fractured ant hill: A new architecture for sustaining the future. *J Am Diet Assoc* 102(1):33–38.

PBH (Produce for Better Health Foundation). 2005a. *2004 Annual Report.* Wilmington, DE: PBH. [Online]. Available: http://www.pbhfoundation.org/pdfs/pulse/success/financials/2005_annual_report.pdf [accessed June 21, 2006].

PBH. 2005b. *Closing the Opportunity Gap: Offering More Fruits and Vegetables on the Nation's Menu.* Wilmington, DE: PBH. [Online]. Available: http://www.5aday.org/html/press/pressrelease.php?recordid=90 [accessed June 21, 2006].

PBH. 2005c. *National Action Plan to Promote Health Through Increased Fruit and Vegetable Consumption.* Wilmington, DE: PBH. [Online]. Available: http://www.5aday.org/commcenter/actionplan/pbh_nap_book041905.pdf [accessed June 21, 2006].

PBH. 2006. *PBH Unveils New Brand. . .Fruits & Veggies—More Matters!*™ Wilmington, DE: Produce for Better Health Foundation. [Online]. Available: http://www.pbh foundation. org/pdfs/retail/aisle5/archive/JUNE 2006_RND3.pdf [accessed July 6, 2006].

PE4Life. 2006. *PE4Life Sponsors.* [Online]. Available: http://pe4life.com/sponsors.php [accessed July 24, 2006].

PepsiCo. 2006a. *Health and Wellness.* [Online]. Available: http://www.pepsico.com/PEP_ Citizenship/Contributions/HealthandWellness/index.cfm [accessed June 19, 2006].

PepsiCo. 2006b. *PepsiCo Joins with America's YMCAs to Help Americans Live Healthier Lives.* [Online]. Available: http://www.ymca.net/about_the_ymca/press_release_20060308_pepsico.html [accessed June 19, 2006].

Public Interest Media Group. 2005. *Eat Smart, Grow Strong.* [Online]. Available: http://www.eatsmartgrowstrong.com/ [accessed May 9, 2006].

Ramirez A. 1991. Fast food lightens up but sales are often thin. *The New York Times.* March 19. [Online]. Available: http://query.nytimes.com/gst/fullpage.html?res=9D0CE7DD1430F93AA25750C0A967958260&sec=health&pagewanted=print [accessed July 23, 2006].

Roberts K. 2004. *The Future Beyond Brands: Lovemarks.* New York: PowerHouse Books.

RWJF (Robert Wood Johnson Foundation). 2006. *Active Living by Design.* [Online]. Available: http://www.activelivingbydesign.org/index.php?id=4 [accessed June 19, 2006].

Schor JB. 2004. *Born to Buy: The Commercialized Child and the New Consumer Culture.* New York, NY: Scribner.

Sloan AE. 2006. Top 10 functional food trends. *Food Technology* 60(4):23–40.

Smalls M. 2005 (July 14). *Current Media Efforts to Foster Healthier Choices for Children.* Presentation at the U.S. Department of Health and Human Services–Federal Trade Commission Workshop About Perspectives on Marketing, Self-Regulation, and Childhood Obesity, Washington DC. [Online]. Available: http://www.ftc.gov/bcp/workshops/food marketingtokids/ index.htm [accessed May 29, 2006].

Snider J, Hill RP, Martin D. 2003. Corporate social responsibility in the 21st century: A view from the world's most successful firms. *J Business Ethics* 48:175–187.

Stettler N, Signer TM, Suter PM. 2004. Electronic games and environmental factors associated with childhood obesity in Switzerland. *Obes Res* 12(6):896–903.

Sturm R. 2004. The economics of physical activity. *Am J Prev Med* 27(3S):126–135.

Sunkist. 2005. *"C" Is for Citrus as Sunkist and Sesame Workshop Announce Healthy Habits for Life Partnership.* [Online]. Available: http://www.sunkist.com/press/release.asp?id=72 [accessed November 18, 2005].

Tillotson J. 2006a. The mega-brands that rule our diet, part 2. *Nutr Today* 41(1):17–21.

Tillotson J. 2006b. Whole Foods Market: Redefining the supermarket experience. *Nutr Today* 41(2):67–69.

Time Warner. 2006. *Cartoon Network to Expand GET ANIMATED Healthy Lifestyles Initiative Through Celebrity Endorsements and National Child Advocacy Group Partnerships.* [Online]. Available: http://www.timewarner.com/corp/newsroom/pr/0,20812, 1168816,00.html [accessed July 27, 2006].

UNESDA (Union of European Beverage Associations). 2005. *Contribution by UNESDA and Its Corporate Members to the EU Platform for Action on Diet, Physical Activity and Health.* [Online]. Available: http://www.unesda-cisda.org/linkdocs/commitments.pdf [accessed April 6, 2006].

Univision Communications. 2003. *Univision to Broadcast Public Affairs Series About Health Issues as Part of "Salud es Vida . . . ¡Enterate!" Campaign.* [Online]. Available: http://www.univision.net/corp/en/pr/Miami_11122003-1.html#null [accessed July 27, 2006].

Vandewater EA, Shim MS, Caplovitz AG. 2004. Linking obesity and activity level with children's television and video game use. *J Adolesc* 27(1):71–85.

Van Wave TW, Decker M. 2003. Secondary analysis of a marketing research database reveals patterns in dairy product purchases over time. *J Am Diet Assoc* 103(4):445–453.

Wansink B. 2004. Environmental factors that increase the food intake and consumption volume of unknowing consumers. *Annu Rev Nutr* 24:455–479.

Wansink B, Huckabee H. 2005. De-marketing obesity. *Calif Management Rev* 47(4):6–18.

Weber K, Story M, Harnack L. 2006. Internet food marketing strategies aimed at children and adolescents: A content analysis of food and beverage brand websites. *J Am Diet Assoc* 106(9):1463–1466.

WFA (World Federation of Advertisers). 2006. *Soft Drink Manufacturers Cease Advertising to Children.* News release. January 25. [Online]. Available: http://www.wfanet.org/news/article_detail.asp?Lib_ID=1668 [accessed June 21, 2006].

WHO (World Health Organization). 2003. *Diet, Nutrition and the Prevention of Chronic Diseases.* Technical Report Series No. 916. Geneva, Switzerland: WHO. [Online]. Available: http://www.who.int/hpr/NPH/docs/who_fao_expert_report.pdf [accessed June 8, 2006].

WHO. 2004. *Global Strategy on Diet, Physical Activity, and Health.* Report No. WHA57.17. [Online]. Available: http://www.who.int/gb/ebwha/pdf_files/WHA57/A57_R17-en.pdf [accessed May 23, 2006].

Wilbert C. 2006. Teens back off sugary drinks. *The Atlanta Journal-Constitution.* June 22. News release. [Online]. Available: http://www.ajc.com/business/content/business/coke/stories/0621bizcoke.html cxntnid=amn062206e [accessed July 18, 2006].

Williams J. 2005. *Product Proliferation Analysis for New Food and Beverage Products Targeted to Children 1994–2004.* Working Paper. University of Texas at Austin.

Wong F, Huhman M, Heitzler C, Asbury L, Bretthauer-Mueller R, McCarthy S, Londe P. 2004. VERB™—A social marketing campaign to increase physical activity among youth. *Prev Chron Dis* [Online]. Available: http://www.cdc.gov/Pcd/issues/2004/jul/04_0043.htm [accessed July 23, 2006].

Wootan M, Osborn M. 2006. Availability of nutrition information from chain restaurants in the United States. *Am J Prev Med* 30(3):266–268.

Yach D, McKee M, Lopez AD, Novotny T. 2005. Improving diet and physical activity: 12 lessons from controlling tobacco smoking. *Br Med J* 330(7496):898–900.

Yankelovich. 2005. *Ad Council Obesity Media Initiative Study.* Chapel Hill, NC.

Yankelovich. 2006. *Food for Life: An Attitudinal And Database Perspective On Food, Diet and Preventive Health Care.* [Online]. Available: http://www.yankelovich.com/products/Food%20For%20Life%20Final%20Presentation%2003-27-06.pdf [accessed July 31, 2006].

6

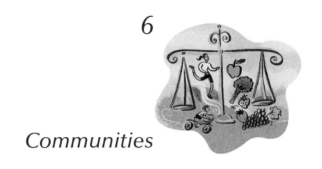

Communities

As noted in the *Health in the Balance* report (IOM, 2005), childhood obesity prevention efforts are ultimately about strengthening community capacity and mobilizing community resources and involvement. Whether the community in question is large or small, rural or urban, or termed a neighborhood or barrio, it will inevitably comprise smaller relational networks that include faith-based organizations; worksites; schools; and a variety of government, nonprofit, and voluntary organizations. This chapter uses the term community to denote a geographic entity but acknowledges the strengths and opportunities brought about by groups of people who are linked by social ties; who share common interests, perspectives, and ethnic or cultural characteristics; and who engage in joint action in particular geographic locations or settings (MacQueen et al., 2001).

Communities across the nation are increasingly aware of the childhood obesity epidemic, and this awareness is being transformed into active efforts to improve community access to foods and beverages that contribute to a healthful diet and increase opportunities for regular physical activity. However, the extent of these changes and the degree to which city councils, local businesses, schools, faith-based organizations, local health departments, and other organizations with a stake in the health and quality of life of children and youth are actively engaged in this issue may vary widely.

The community-based approach to the prevention of childhood obesity builds on the reality that communities have numerous resources and assets that, if they are mobilized strategically, can directly affect the health and well-being of children and adolescents. These resources and assets can be accessed through the nonprofit organizations that work directly with children and youth. Planning and community development agencies that determine the physical design and use of resources in the built environment, such as paths, parks, and neighborhoods, can make the built environment more user-friendly and thus encourage physical activity. Health care professionals and systems through which primary care services are delivered can address childhood obesity as part of their regular delivery of care. Faith-based organizations, community coalitions, foundations, and worksites can address community and family well-being and are increasingly doing so. Schools are also a vital asset that serve as a link between families and communities and have the capacity to strengthen and reinforce childhood obesity prevention strategies and initiatives and will be discussed more thoroughly in Chapter 7.

The present Institute of Medicine (IOM) committee recommends increased efforts to address the community-based recommendations presented in the *Health in the Balance* report (Box 6-1) and to incorporate an evaluation component into all policies, programs, and initiatives. This chapter highlights the key actions that need to be taken to activate a community's assets around the common goal of preventing childhood obesity. It begins with a brief review of key strategies associated with effective community-based prevention efforts. That review is followed by examples of progress that focus on mobilizing communities, improving the built environment, and enhancing the role of health care providers and the health care system in childhood obesity prevention. The chapter concludes with recommendations for guiding communities to assess their progress in establishing promising childhood obesity prevention efforts.

KEY ELEMENTS OF COMMUNITY-BASED STRATEGIES

Although communities may vary widely in their demographics and resources, efforts to engage communities in promoting healthy lifestyles generally involve active grassroots efforts that build on the strengths of the residents and the locale. Mobilizing community participation, developing partnerships, and creating synergistic actions were some of the many themes that emerged from the discussions at the committee's symposium, *Progress in Preventing Childhood Obesity: Focus on Communities*, held in Atlanta, Georgia, on October 6 and 7, 2005, in collaboration with the Healthcare Georgia Foundation and the Robert Wood Johnson Foundation (RWJF) (Appendix G). The key elements of community-based strategies are discussed below.

BOX 6-1
Recommendations for Communities from the 2005 IOM report,
Preventing Childhood Obesity: Health in the Balance

Community Programs
Local governments, public health agencies, schools, and community organizations should collaboratively develop and promote programs that encourage healthful eating behaviors and regular physical activity, particularly for populations at high risk of childhood obesity. Community coalitions should be formed to facilitate and promote crosscutting programs and community-wide efforts.

To implement this recommendation:
- Private and public efforts to eliminate health disparities should include obesity prevention as one of their primary areas of focus and should support community-based collaborative programs to address social, economic, and environmental barriers that contribute to the increased obesity prevalence among certain populations.
- Community child- and youth-centered organizations should promote healthful eating behaviors and regular physical activity through new and existing programs that will be sustained over the long term.
- Community evaluation tools should incorporate measures of the availability of opportunities for physical activity and healthful eating.
- Communities should improve access to supermarkets, farmers' markets, and community gardens to expand healthful food options, particularly in low-income and underserved areas.

Built Environment
Local governments, private developers, and community groups should expand opportunities for physical activity, including recreational facilities, parks, playgrounds, sidewalks, bike paths, routes for walking or bicycling to school, and safe streets and neighborhoods, especially for populations at high risk of childhood obesity.

To implement this recommendation:
Local governments, working with private developers and community groups should
- Revise comprehensive plans, zoning and subdivision ordinances, and other planning practices to increase the availability of and accessibility to opportunities for physical activity in new developments.

Leadership

Committed and sustained leadership is a common and essential element emerging from promising community-based efforts to address childhood obesity. At a minimum, leadership is viewed as the investment of adequate resources and the commitment of the institutions and organizations that engage in obesity prevention efforts. The sustainability of community-improvement initiatives has been attributed to leaders' transition from a

- Prioritize capital improvement projects to increase opportunities for physical activity in existing areas.
- Improve the street, sidewalk, and street-crossing safety of routes to school; develop programs to encourage walking and bicycling to school; and build schools within walking and bicycling distance of the neighborhoods that they serve.

Community groups should
- Work with local governments to change their planning and capital improvement practices to give higher priority to opportunities for physical activity.

The U.S. Department of Health and Human Services and the U.S. Department of Transportation should
- Fund community-based research to examine the impact of changes to the built environment on the levels of physical activity in the relevant communities and populations.

Health Care
Pediatricians, family physicians, nurses, and other clinicians should engage in the prevention of childhood obesity. Health care professional organizations, insurers, and accrediting groups should support individual and population-based obesity prevention efforts.

To implement this recommendation:
- Health care professionals should routinely track body mass indices, offer relevant evidence-based counseling and guidance, serve as role models, and provide leadership for obesity prevention efforts in their communities.
- Professional organizations should disseminate evidence-based clinical guidance and establish programs on obesity prevention.
- Training programs and certifying entities should require obesity prevention knowledge and skills in their curricula and examinations.
- Insurers and accrediting organizations should provide incentives for maintaining a healthy body weight and include screening and obesity preventive services in routine clinical practice and quality assessment measures.

SOURCE: IOM (2005).

focus on projects addressing the symptoms of societal problems (e.g., chronic disease outcomes) to a focus on changing the underlying cultures, incentives, and settings that give rise to these symptoms (Norris and Pittman, 2000). Because of the multiple sectors and stakeholders involved in childhood obesity prevention, leadership on this issue can come from the private or the public sector: from government leaders, health care professionals, school administrators and staff, community residents, and local business leaders. Leaders at the forefront of change in this area are often inspired by a personal health problem or by an interest in health promotion. Individual and organizational leadership are needed as driving forces in sustaining collaborative efforts, dedicating resources, and working to change social norms that support healthier lifestyles.

Building Community Coalitions

Community coalitions consist of public- and private-sector organizations, together with individual citizens, working to achieve a shared goal through the coordinated use of resources, leadership, and action and the provision of direction in these areas. The synergistic effects of these collaborative partnerships result from the multiple perspectives, talents, and expertise that are brought together to work toward a common goal. However, challenges exist in developing and refining appropriate methods to evaluate the impact of coalition efforts on a variety of outcomes (Fawcett et al., 2000; Lasker et al., 2001; Roussos and Fawcett, 2000; Shortell, 2000). The efforts needed to prevent childhood obesity require a diverse set of skills and expertise—from renovating community recreational facilities to developing multimedia campaigns to promote healthy lifestyles. Because childhood obesity prevention is central to the health of the community's children and youth, the development of community coalitions is a particularly relevant means of addressing this issue.

The characteristics of successful coalitions include focusing on a well-defined and specific issue, determining common goals, and keeping the coalition focused on providing leadership and direction rather than micromanaging the solutions (Kreuter et al., 2000). All these characteristics are attainable for community coalitions focused on childhood obesity prevention. The diverse set of community organizations and businesses that need to be involved to address childhood obesity includes more than just those stakeholders in the traditional health-related disciplines. These other organizations and businesses that are stakeholders include the building industry, food and beverage companies, the restaurant and food retail sectors, the entertainment industry and the media, the educational community, the public safety sector, transportation divisions, parks and recreation departments, environmental organizations, community rights advocates, youth-related organizations, foundations, employers, and universities, among others. Many stakeholders who might not have considered childhood obesity prevention as an area of interest now find that they have an important role to play in working toward healthier communities. Nevertheless, these organizations face challenges in developming and maintaining community coalitions. These challenges include effectively addressing competing priorities, transforming organizational cultures, and identifying sustainable funding sources.

Cultural Relevance

Building on a community's cultural assets to enhance childhood obesity prevention efforts is fundamental to the promotion of grassroots involvement and the sustainability of policies, programs, and initiatives. The extent to which culturally competent adaptations are made can greatly affect intervention and policy outcomes (Chapter 3). Culturally appropriate enhancement strategies can be categorized as *peripheral* (developing packaging to appeal to a particular group by using certain colors, images, graphics, pictures of group members, or titles), *evidential* (presenting data and information documenting the impact of the relevant health issue on a specific group), *linguistic* (increasing accessibility by using the preferred language or dialect of the group), *constituency based* (drawing directly on the experiences of group members through their inclusion as project staff or their substantive engagement as decision makers), and *sociocultural* (integrating the group's normative attitudes, values, and practices into messages and approaches) (Hopson, 2003; Kreuter et al., 2003).

Sufficient Resources and Sustained Commitment

Community-wide childhood obesity prevention efforts require careful planning and coordination, well-trained staff, and sufficient resources. Success is greatly enhanced by community engagement in the issue, which can take a great deal of time and effort to achieve. Insufficient resources may result in messages and other planned campaign interventions that are inadequate to achieve the exposure necessary to change the awareness, knowledge, attitudes, beliefs, or behaviors of target groups over time, especially among high-risk populations. Furthermore, a sustained commitment is needed from community leaders, as implementing the changes necessary to alter the physical environment can be both time and resource intensive. For example, the revision of city zoning or planning policies may require extensive time, including the time required to engage community residents, organizations, and businesses in discussions on the proposed changes.

Focus on Safety

Safety is an important construct of the social environment that is likely to influence childhood obesity prevention efforts (Lumeng et al., 2006). Crime rates and residents' perceptions of neighborhood safety will affect the likelihood that people will walk or bicycle in their neighborhoods. These barriers include both "stranger danger" and "traffic danger," which are important influences on the decisions that parents make regarding their children's outdoor play and mode of transportation to school and which also influence the decisions that adolescents make regarding walking or cycling for transport (Carver et al., 2005). Many of the ongoing walk-to-school efforts (e.g., the Safe Routes to Schools program) began as efforts to address child safety concerns. It is anticipated that both community safety and obesity prevention efforts would mutually benefit from attempts to enhance the community environment and that other benefits would also ensue.

Community-Based Participatory Research

Developing effective intervention actions in communities involves the activation of community group members to take ownership and influence the content and implementation of interventions, the evaluation process, and the dissemination of findings. These concepts are often grouped under the rubric *community-based participatory research*. This research paradigm recalls the historical roots of public health, in which problems were identified and addressed through collaboration with the public or community for the common good (Israel et al., 1998). By nature, community-based participatory interventions are culturally competent and congruent with the needs and values of a target group because the methods emerge from affected communities as well as university, government, and foundation partners. As discussed in Chapter 3, this is an area of particular relevance for planning, implementing, and evaluating culturally relevant interventions involving racially, ethnically, and culturally diverse subpopulations at high risk for obesity and related chronic diseases.

Building on Multiple Social and Health Priorities

As discussed in Chapter 3, childhood obesity prevention may not rank high as a priority for some communities and neighborhoods that are facing more immediate concerns such as poverty, crime, violence, underperforming schools, and limited access to health care. The opportunity in these communities is to identify and support efforts that can produce many potential benefits; for example, improving playgrounds and recreational facilities may enhance safety, reduce crime, increase physical activity, and improve quality of life. Finding common ground may serve as a key element in garnering sufficient investment for sustained efforts. The challenge is that many of these efforts are resource intensive and require significant political commitment and social support to be accomplished. Building and strengthening the partnerships between organizations working to empower communities can result in collective efficacy, which has been described as "the willingness of community members to look out for each other and intervene when trouble arises" (Cohen et al., 2006). A recent study found that adolescents living in communities with higher levels of collective efficacy had lower body mass index (BMI) levels than those living in communities without a strong sense of connection. These differences remained significant even while the level of neighborhood disadvantage was held constant. This suggests that even youth living in neighborhoods of higher socioeconomic status may be adversely affected when they lack a connection to their community (Cohen et al., 2006).

EXAMPLES OF PROGRESS IN PREVENTING CHILDHOOD OBESITY IN COMMUNITIES

Given that the United States has approximately 36,000 incorporated cities and towns and many more locales (U.S. Bureau of the Census, 2006), the committee can provide only selected examples of the array of positive changes that are occurring throughout the nation in response to childhood obesity. As sufficient outcome data with which to evaluate the effectiveness of various policies, programs, and interventions are not yet available for most of the efforts, the descriptions provided are intended to highlight the many and varied efforts that have been and that are being made to address the problem of childhood obesity. They are characterized here as promising practices rather than best practices because sufficient evidence to directly link the effort with reducing the incidence or prevalence of childhood obesity and related co-morbidities is lacking.

Mobilizing Communities

Communities that promote healthy lifestyles and that actively engage their citizens in improving access to opportunities for healthful eating and regular physical activity draw on the talents, resources, and energies of multiple community stakeholders. As noted earlier, efforts to prevent childhood obesity compete with many other efforts to address health and social priorities for the scarce resources that are available at the local level. Furthermore, challenges often arise when attempts are made to coordinate programs under completely different administrative structures (e.g., schools and local health departments) within the community, state, and region. However, these challenges can be effectively confronted in many communities. Programs and initiatives at the community level often work to engage children, youth, and adults in obesity prevention efforts focused on all age groups.

Community Programs and Initiatives

The nature and breadth of community-based programs and initiatives vary widely and may involve community youth organizations, voluntary health organizations, and public-private partnerships. Programs may also range from multi-city and well-resourced efforts sponsored by corporations or national organizations to efforts sponsored by individual communities engaging in specific projects or programs such as building a playground or expanding bike trails. Likewise, the scope of the evaluation may be modest or sophisticated, and the outcome indicators or performance measures may differ depending on the purpose for which they are intended (Chapter 2). Evaluation methodologies may range from research-based efforts with multiple comparison groups to assessments using more modest outcome measures, such as implementing a policy that supports a capital improvement project to build a new community playground where parents can engage in physical activity with their children.

A number of national youth-related organizations are working with their multiple local chapters to incorporate obesity prevention efforts and goals into their programs, often with the support of foundation or corporate sponsors. For example, Girl Scout councils have developed partnerships with community parks and recreation departments, sports organizations, as well as schools and colleges for physical activity instruction and facilities. Girl Scout programs that are focused on healthy lifestyles include shape UP! and GirlSports (Girl Scouts, 2006). Additionally, the Girl Scouts organization conducted focus group research with online surveys of more than 2,000 8- to 17-year-old girls to explore how they view obesity, how they define health, and what motivates them to lead a healthy lifestyle (Girl Scout Research Institute, 2006).

Other examples are also available. The YMCA has instituted YMCA Activate America™, a long-term commitment to obesity prevention that focuses on improving their programs; providing community leadership; and developing strategic partnerships with universities, government, and corporations (YMCA, 2006). The Boys and Girls Clubs of America feature a number of fitness-related programs, including Triple Play: A Game Plan for the Mind, Body and Soul. The Coca-Cola Company and Kraft Foods Inc. have sponsored that program with the goal of increasing healthy habits and physical activity, and promoting healthful diets (BGCA, 2006). At the IOM committee's symposium in Wichita, Kansas, students presented a local 4-H-sponsored mentoring program, Kansas Teen Leadership for Physically Active Lifestyles, in which high school students engage with elementary school children in after-school and summer programs focused on promoting physical activity and healthful eating (Sparke et al., 2005).

Community centers, after-school programs, and summer camps are often used as sites for obesity prevention interventions. For example, the GEMS (Girls Health Enrichment Multisite Studies) set of research-based studies has examined a variety of approaches (e.g., dance, team building, games, aerobics, nutrition education, and reduced television viewing) that are being implemented in community settings to engage 8- to 10-year-old African-American girls in obesity prevention and management (Baranowski et al., 2003; Beech et al., 2003; Robinson et al., 2003; Story et al., 2003).

Faith-based organizations are also becoming more engaged in promoting healthy lifestyles. The leaders of many faiths are realizing that messages about physical health and spiritual health are congruent. Indeed, participants at the IOM committee's symposium on healthy communities in Atlanta described several efforts being undertaken by different faith-based groups to promote health (Appendix G). This process often starts with the minister addressing his or her own health concerns as well as encouraging congregation members to make healthful nutrition and physical activity choices as a way of demonstrating their concern for others and the church family. Congregations are encouraging members to bring healthier meals to church potluck gatherings and are sponsoring health fairs, cooking and exercise demonstrations, physical activity classes, and informational sessions on how to improve the health of the congregation. Others are partnering with local health departments or other health care providers to offer health screenings at places of worship, a setting where people may feel more comfortable than they would in a health clinic. Some congregations have parish nurses or ministers who provide health information, facilitate health promotion activities, and conduct health screenings for congregational members (Brudenell, 2003; Chase-Ziolek and Iris, 2002). Research-based efforts are evaluating the effectiveness of faith-based approaches to obesity prevention; for example, a program called Healthy Body Healthy Spirit is an intervention funded by the National Heart, Lung, and Blood Institute to increase physical activity and the levels of consumption of fruits and vegetables among African Americans recruited through churches (Resnicow et al., 2005).

National efforts that work at the community level often involve successful collaborations among federal agencies, corporations, and community-based, youth-related organizations (Chapters 4 and 5). The numerous ongoing public-private collaborations include Action for Healthy Kids (a collaborative public-private effort focused on changes in schools and involving a number of partners including Aetna Foundation, the American Public Health Association, Centers for Disease Control and Prevention [CDC], the Department of Education, the Kellogg's Fund, the National Dairy Council, the National Football League, the National PTA, the Robert Wood Johnson Foundation, and USDA) (Action for Healthy Kids, 2006) and the 5 A Day for Better Health Program (a national public-private partnership with multiple collaborators including the American Heart Association, American Cancer Society, Association of State and Territorial Directors of Health Promotion and Public Health Education, CDC, National Alliance for Nutrition and Activity, National Cancer Institute, Produce for Better Health Foundation, Produce Marketing Association, United Fresh Fruit and Vegetable Association, and USDA (PBH, 2006) (Chapter 4). Other national initiatives include NikeGO, sponsored by Nike, Inc. (Nike, 2006); Girls on the Run, sponsored by New Balance and the Kellogg Company (Girls on the Run, 2006); America on the Move® (2006), a nonprofit organization that promotes small lifestyle changes to increase physical activity and reduce calorie intake, with multiple sponsors including PepsiCo and Cargill; and the Women's National Basketball Association's Be Smart - Be Fit - Be Yourself program for youth (WNBA, 2005).

Evaluations of these programs vary in scope. For example, the America On the Move Foundation's assessment strategy includes scientific research in clinical environments of America On the Move programs conducted through the University of Colorado's Center for Human Nutrition; evaluation of the national online program for individuals and groups based on pre- and post-intervention data and on programs customized for specific settings; and survey data collection through national and state-based instruments of individuals' health-related knowledge, beliefs, and behaviors, including actual physical activity levels (through the use of stepometer data) (Wyatt et al., 2004).

Numerous state and federal programs operate at the local level. For example, six cities, five counties, and three American Indian tribes have received funding through the STEPS to a HealthierUS Cooperative Agreement Program (Steps Program) that enables communities to develop an action plan, a community consortium, and an evaluation strategy that supports chronic disease prevention and health promotion (DHHS, 2006) (Chapter 4). Cooperative extension services are another example of federal, state, and local partnerships that work through land-grant universities and local extension offices to disseminate information to families and individuals and engage communities to work on a range of nutrition- and agriculture-related issues (CSREES, 2006). Additionally, federal food and nutrition programs, such as the Special Supplemental Nutrition Program for Women, Infants, and Children (WIC), provide opportunities to convey information about dietary and physical activity changes to the parents of young children and to the employees working in these programs (Box 6-2; Chapters 4 and 8). Furthermore, work site efforts focused on improving employee health often have direct and indirect benefits for children and youth by providing parents with information that they can use to influence the nutrition and physical activity behaviors of their children. For example, the National Business Group on Health has developed a tool kit for employers and fact sheets for parents focused on healthy weight for families (NBGH, 2006).

BOX 6-2
Engaging Adult Health and Social Services Providers
as Vehicles for Social Norm Changes

In 1999, the U.S. Department of Agriculture (USDA) funded a childhood obesity prevention initiative called Fit WIC to support and evaluate social and environmental approaches to preventing and reducing obesity in preschool children (USDA, 2005). California was one of the four state Special Supplemental Nutrition Program for Women, Infants, and Children (WIC) programs that participated in the pilot program evaluation. The Fit WIC program, implemented through California WIC clinics and evaluated by the University of California at the Berkeley Center for Weight and Health (Crawford et al., 2004), compared six WIC sites (three of which served as intervention groups and three of which served as control groups) that participated in a pilot staff wellness intervention program to improve staff effectiveness in preventing childhood obesity. The intervention approaches focused primarily on supporting beneficial behaviors rather than on weight loss and on motivating staff members to eat healthfully and to be more physically active throughout the work day. Among the organizational changes at WIC sites were healthy food choices (e.g., fresh fruit or vegetables) when refreshments were served at meetings or celebrations and integrating 10-minute physical activity breaks into regular staff meetings or at certain times of the work day. Compared with the staff at the control site, the staff in the intervention group perceived greater support for their efforts to make healthful food choices available at the worksite and to engage in physical activity and reported substitutions in the types of foods served during meetings and the placement of a priority on physical activity in the workplace. Staff members at the intervention site were also more likely to counsel WIC participants to engage in physical activity with their children and reported that they believed that they had greater sensitivity in handling weight-related issues. This study underscores the potential reach of fitness promotion (Glasgow et al., 1999) in organizations serving high-risk groups, given the multiplier effect, that is, the positive influence of healthy provider behavior on clients.

SOURCES: Abramson et al. (2000); Frank et al. (2000); Lewis et al. (1986); Thompson et al. (2003).

Foundations

Foundations are active partners in many community-based obesity prevention efforts. As the funding sources for grantees at the community and grassroots levels, foundations may require that an evaluation plan be submitted with the grant application. For example, The California Endowment's Healthy Eating/Active Communities (HEAC) initiative funds several community demonstration projects to implement programs promoting physical activity and healthful eating in six low-income communities throughout California (California Endowment, 2006). As part of the HEAC initiative, adolescents involved in the Youth Study are using digital cameras to provide images of their physical activity and eating environments and will engage in discussions about evaluating the need for environmental changes (Craypo et al., 2006).

Active Living by Design and Active Living Leadership initiatives, through the support of RWJF are using the expertise of a diverse group of professionals—such as urban planners and designers, environmentalists, asthma control activists, leisure and travel industry specialists, economists, and public policy advocates and decision makers—to explore the possibilities for greater community efforts to increase the levels of physical activity among children and youth (Active Living Leadership, 2004). Recently, RWJF launched the Healthy Eating Research initiative, which places special emphasis on building a field of research that will benefit children in low-income and different racial/ethnic populations at the highest risk for obesity by improving their eating habits (RWJF, 2006). Some foundations coordinate their efforts with those of industry, government, and other sectors to fully leverage resources and scale up programs and initiatives. For example, the Alliance for a Healthy Generation, described in Chapters 2, 5, and 7 is designed as an extensive collaborative effort involving foundations, non-profit organizations, industry, and state government leadership. However, evaluations are needed to assess the effectiveness of the Alliance.

One of the strengths of local, statewide, and regional foundations is their familiarity with the cultural assets and demographic characteristics of the areas they serve and their ability to focus grants and funding opportunities on innovative projects that build on local assets. The committee, through its three regional symposia, had the opportunity to learn more about the community-based obesity prevention programs and initiatives funded by the Kansas Health Foundation, the Sunflower Foundation, the Healthcare Georgia Foundation, the Missouri Foundation for Health, the Robert Wood Johnson Foundation, and the W. K. Kellogg Foundation. Some corporate foundations are also active partners in childhood obesity prevention efforts at the community level (Chapter 5).

As foundations across the nation continue in their commitment to childhood obesity prevention, it is important to build on their strengths and to identify the ways in which foundations can be most effective. For example, foundations often have greater flexibility in their funding mechanisms than government agencies so that they can more quickly explore untested or promising approaches or respond more rapidly to evaluations of natural experiments (discussed later in this chapter). Further, foundations are often effective in partnering with organizations that can sustain the activity if it is proven efficacious, efficient, and culturally and socially appropriate.

Evaluating the efforts of foundations will include consideration of the long-term sustainability of funding for projects related to obesity prevention and the extent to which obesity prevention initiatives are a funding priority.

Developing and Strengthening Community Coalitions

As noted earlier, the development of community coalitions is a particularly relevant approach to the prevention of childhood obesity. The efforts of groups and individuals with many diverse areas of expertise are needed to move obesity prevention efforts forward and can have a synergistic effect when coordinated. Community coalitions relevant to childhood obesity prevention often focus on broader but related issues, such as encouraging healthy lifestyles or preventing chronic diseases, such as type 2 diabetes, in children, youth, and adults. The healthy communities movement, and its outgrowth, the Coalition for Healthier Cities and Communities, provide an example of an initiative focused on health promotion and disease prevention that measures community-based outcomes including improved cardiovascular health, reductions in crime, reduction of the rates of teen pregnancy, and declines in the numbers of new human immunodeficiency virus (HIV) infections (Norris and Pittman, 2000).

Another example is the Border Health Strategic Initiative (Border Health ¡SI!), a diabetes prevention intervention that involves several communities along the Arizona–Mexico border, which developed community coalitions focused on building partnerships with local universities, community health workers (*promotores de salud*), and other community stakeholders. The initiative used the REACH 2010 community-based participatory research model to focus on implementing policy changes in schools, involving planning and zoning commissions, in long-range community planning, and organizing an annual community forum for elected and appointed local officials to discuss policy changes to promote health (Meister and de Zapien, 2005) (Chapter 3).

Examples of community coalitions and initiatives (Boxes 6-3 and 6-4) highlight the range of stakeholders and the importance of leadership in initiating and sustaining community efforts. Often, the mayor or another key community leader can galvanize the political will and multistakeholder support that is needed to build a coalition focused on improving the health of the community. Generally, these efforts focus on all citizens, including children and youth.

Community coalitions often conduct local surveys and assessments as they get under way to provide baseline information; follow-up assessments can then be performed during the course of the coalition's work to assess progress. The Bexar County (Texas) Community Health Collaborative be-

---

BOX 6-3
Sonoma County (California) Family Activity and Nutrition Task Force

In 1998, the Sonoma County Family Activity and Nutrition Task Force was initiated to bring together individuals, professionals, and community-based organizations to focus on the health, nutrition, and physical activity levels of children in the county. The task force works through four subcommittees:

- **The farm-to-school subcommittee** promotes increased fruit and vegetable availability in the local schools.
- **The direct service subcommittee** promotes prevention and treatment options in the community.
- **The community outreach and advocacy subcommittee** works to increase public awareness of obesity-related issues and solutions.
- **The child-care subcommittee** works with Head Start and the Community Child Care Council to educate parents and care providers about nutrition and obesity-related issues.

In February 2006, the Task Force received a five-year grant from Kaiser Permanente to implement the Healthy Eating Active Living-Community Health Initiative in two local communities, South Park and Southwest Santa Rosa. Phase 1 of the project will involve the development of a community action plan, and Phase 2 will implement and evaluate the plan over four years.

SOURCE: Sonoma County (2006).

---

gan with a baseline health needs assessment in 1998. That assessment was followed up by a comparable assessment effort in 2002 (Health Collaborative, 2003). The assessments, conducted in collaboration with the University of Texas Health Science Center, provided detailed information on a range of health issues in various areas of the county. Follow-up plans have involved the use of the community health planning tool MAPP (Mobilizing for Action through Planning and Partnerships) (NACCHO, 2004) to develop and implement a strategic plan for next steps in improving the county's health status (Health Collaborative, 2003; San Antonio Metropolitan Health Department, 2006).

Because childhood obesity may be a vast and complex issue for a community organization with limited time and resources, it may be necessary for a community group to focus on a single, manageable project to yield tangible results and measurable outcomes. For example, a number of community initiatives are focused on building a playground or changing a local school district's policies related to the availability and sale of competi-

---

BOX 6-4
Examples of Community Initiatives and Coalitions

- **Health and Wellness Coalition of Wichita:** Partners in this community coalition in Wichita, Kansas include nonprofit organizations, local businesses, city and county agencies, and local academic institutions.
- **Fit City Madison:** The mayor of Madison, Wisconsin, began this initiative in response to concern about city-wide obesity rates. Fit City is now a coalition effort involving more than 50 community organizations that schedule health-related and active living events, including regular walks with the mayor.
- **ACT!vate Omaha:** This program is a partnership in Omaha, Nebraska, of local health and city governments officials, health educators, health care providers, workplace wellness organizations, architects, and community groups aimed at fostering active living.
- **Bexar County (Texas) Community Health Collaborative:** This community coalition began with a community health needs assessment sponsored as a joint effort by San Antonio area health care organizations. It has since expanded to include numerous other partners, including the YMCA of Greater San Antonio, and has launched Fit City and Walk San Antonio initiatives.
- **Consortium to Lower Obesity in Chicago Children (CLOCC):** The consortium began as a community-based effort of Children's Memorial Hospital focused on obesity prevention in children ages 3 to 5 years. CLOCC now involves multiple community partners and provides resources and connections for children, their caregivers, and those who work with their parents and caregivers.

SOURCES: ACT!vate Omaha (2006); CLOCC (2006); Fit City Madison (2006); Health and Wellness Coalition of Wichita (2005); Health Collaborative (2006).

---

tive foods in schools (Chapter 7). Even if the group disbands after a project is completed, progress has been made and awareness has increased among all of the stakeholders involved. Although the progress that results from a collaboration is difficult to measure, collaborations have important benefits such as empowering community residents and local organizations and increasing the community's capacity to address a problem (Kreuter et al., 2000).

Enhancing the Built Environment

The built environment represents the human-made elements of the physical environment (e.g., the buildings, the infrastructure, and arrangements in space and the aesthetic qualities of these elements). Over the past 50 years, the physical environment has changed dramatically, and it is increasingly recognized as a factor contributing to the obesity epidemic

(Brownson et al., 2005; IOM, 2005; Sallis and Glanz, 2006). Relevant features of the built environment include land use patterns and the paths, roads, and other means of transport that link one location with another. Additionally, the built environment encompasses the way in which the interiors of buildings are structured to accommodate or necessitate movement, as well as the structure of the community food environment, which plays a role in determining access to fruits, vegetables, and other foods and beverages that contribute to a healthful diet (Brownson et al., 2006; Gordon-Larsen et al., 2006; Handy et al., 2002; Kahn et al., 2002; TRB and IOM, 2005; Zimring et al., 2005).

Local zoning boards, city planning commissions, capital improvement committees, and many other entities are involved in decisions regarding land use, transportation, building development, and the locations of sidewalks and bicycle and pedestrian paths (TRB and IOM, 2005). Organizations and movements such as Smart Growth and New Urbanism work to facilitate and implement active travel, livable and sustainable communities, mixed land use (e.g., residential, office, and retail space), and the preservation of open space (New Urbanism, 2006; Smart Growth Network, 2003). Latino New Urbanism (2006) is a recent outgrowth of these efforts and involves the consideration of Latino culture in the development of urban properties and land use plans.

Promoting Physical Activity

Communities are becoming more aware of the need to enhance healthy lifestyles for children and youth by offering safe and attractive places in neighborhoods for recreation and play and by promoting active travel. Numerous issues related to the built environment are particularly important for populations at high risk for obesity. In addition, in many locales, fewer recreational facilities are present in low-income neighborhoods than in more affluent areas (Cradock et al., 2005; Sallis and Glanz, 2006). It is thus important to identify the extent of the disparities in access to opportunities for physical activity so that these issues can be addressed. For example, in Boston, Massachusetts, the nonprofit organization Play Across Boston conducted a needs assessment with funding from CDC, that involved a census of the public recreational facilities, as well as the collection of data on the physical activity programs available to children and youth outside of school hours (Hannon et al., 2006). Combining this information with household income and population census data provided insights into the areas where recreational opportunities needed to be enhanced.

Many communities are expanding and improving their playground and gymnasium facilities; adding and restoring walking and biking trails; taking pedestrian issues into consideration when they plan for new road construction; and involving children, youth, and families in a variety of physical activity-related programs (Sallis and Glanz, 2006). For example, voters in Los Angeles have approved a major bond issue that will support the upgrading of urban parks, and some public school playgrounds in downtown Denver have been converted into community parks (Brink and Yost, 2004).

Examples of nation-wide efforts to change the built environment to encourage physical activity are also available: the PedNet Coalition in Columbia, Missouri (Box 6-5); the work of the PATH Foundation and partners to develop a metrowide trail system for Atlanta and DeKalb County in Georgia (PATH Foundation, 2006); the 1000 Friends of New Mexico initiative that promotes smart growth in Albuquerque (1000 Friends of New Mexico, 2006); and the efforts by the Winnebago Tribe's (Nebraska) efforts to increase physical activity and develop plans to improve the built environment (Box 6-6). The Partnership for a Healthy West Virginia offers Walkable Communities Workshops that aim to bring together community stakeholders and help them organize their efforts to improve pedestrian safety and the walkabilities of their communities (Partnership for a Healthy West Virginia, 2006).

BOX 6-5
PedNet Coalition, Columbia, Missouri

The PedNet Coalition is a group of individuals, businesses, and nonprofit organizations working in Columbia, Missouri, to develop and restore a network of nature trails and urban "pedways" to connect residential subdivisions, worksites, shopping districts, parks, schools (including local colleges and the University of Missouri–Columbia), public libraries, recreation centers, and the downtown area. The coalition has developed a plan for a 20-year effort to fully implement the network of trails and paths. Additionally, the coalition sponsors the Walking School Bus program and a number of citywide biking and walking events.

Co-founded in April 2000 by the City of Columbia Disabilities Commission and the City of Columbia Bicycle and Pedestrian Commission, the coalition now has more than 5,000 individuals and 75 organizations, businesses, and government agencies as participants. In July 2005, Columbia was selected by the Federal Highway Administration to receive a Non-Motorized Transportation Pilot Program grant, and the PedNet Coalition is providing input into the planning process.

The evaluation methods that the PedNet Coalition uses include tracking of the travel mode to school at four elementary schools (twice a year for the past 2.5 years) and tracking of the number of participants at the annual Bike, Walk, and Wheel Week events.

SOURCE: PedNet Coalition (2006).

BOX 6-6
Winnebago Tribe
Winnebago, Nebraska

The Winnebago Tribe, a Native American tribal community in Nebraska, is working to enhance the opportunities for physical activity and improved nutrition in the residential and commercial areas of the community. The nonprofit development arm of the Winnebago Tribe has worked with other community and foundation partners to develop a five-year plan, establish biking and walking support groups, develop community gardening programs, and conduct active living events. One of the goals is to create pedestrian-friendly crossings on a highly traveled highway that separates housing from other areas of the community. The community is involved in planning for mixed-use land development and in implementing other active transport changes.

SOURCE: Winnebago Tribe (2006).

The daily trips that children and youth make to and from school have received considerable attention in many communities as a way to increase students' physical activity levels (WHO, 2002). Community efforts to increase walking and bicycling to and from school focus on improvements to the built environment—intersections, sidewalks, and bike paths—accompanied by programs to encourage parents and children to consider non-motorized methods of travel. For example, urban design changes resulting from California's Safe Routes to Schools legislation (e.g., additions and rebuilding of sidewalks and bike paths and improvements in pedestrian crossings) have been found to increase the rates of walking or bicycle travel by children in a survey of parents at 10 elementary schools (Boarnet et al., 2005).

Schools and communities are also promoting walk- or bike-to-school days through programs such as Safe Routes to Schools and CDC's Kids Walk-to-School program. In Hinsdale, Illinois, a walk-to-school day in 2000 was the beginning of citywide efforts to build new sidewalks and repair existing sidewalks; provide public education on traffic safety issues; and work with transportation engineers, the police force, and others to improve the walkability of the town (Active Living Network, 2005). The federal Safe Routes to School Program, initiated in August 2005 through the transportation reauthorization legislation, provides funds for states and, subsequently, communities to build safer street crossings and establish programs that encourage walking and bicycling to school (FHWA, DoT, 2006).

Enhancing the Community Food Environment

Although information about how the community environment affects the eating patterns of children and youth is limited and more evaluation is needed, efforts are underway to better understand these relationships (Glanz et al., 2005; Moore and Diez Roux, 2006). For example, the RWJF Healthy Eating Research Program mentioned earlier is encouraging solution-oriented research that explores the environmental and policy determinants of healthy eating as strategies for addressing childhood obesity (Story and Orleans, 2006).

Through community advocacy, several cities have shown that it is possible to locate supermarkets in low-income neighborhoods to enhance the neighborhood population's access to fresh fruits and vegetables (Sallis and Glanz, 2006). The Pennsylvania Fresh Food Financing Initiative—a public-private partnership of the Food Trust of Philadelphia, the Greater Philadelphia Urban Affairs Coalition, the Reinvestment Fund, and the Commonwealth of Pennsylvania—provides financing through grants and loans to increase the numbers of supermarkets and grocery stores in underserved communities in Pennsylvania (Food Trust, 2006). The outcomes of this initiative are being evaluated with funding from the National Institutes of Health.

Alternative strategies are also being developed to increase the availability, affordability, and access to foods, beverages, and meals that contribute to healthful diets throughout neighborhoods and communities. Community gardens are moving beyond rural and suburban communities into urban areas. For example, the Harlem Children's Zone, a program and facility designed to provide safe and healthful educational, social, and recreational activities for children and youth, has transformed a vacant lot in New York City into a garden where children work alongside older residents to cultivate and harvest fresh produce and share it with other members of their community (Garden Mosaics, 2006) (Chapter 3).

Mobile markets, such as People's Grocery in West Oakland, California, sell produce in urban neighborhoods and involve youth interns in selling local produce (Flournoy and Treuhaft, 2005). Neighborhood bus systems have also been developed to link residents with supermarkets. In East Austin, Texas, a bus route provides transportation from a low-income Latino community to two supermarkets (Flournoy and Treuhaft, 2005). Evaluations of these initiatives are needed to determine whether access to healthier foods has increased and, if it has, whether the consumption of these foods replaces less healthful alternatives and the effects of these more healthful food alternatives on long-term behavioral and health outcomes.

The creation of local food policy councils is another strategy that can be used to prevent childhood obesity. A food policy council brings together community stakeholders—including consumers, farmers, food processors, distributors, food security advocates, educators, and governmental units— to develop policies and projects to improve access to foods that contribute to a healthful diet while also supporting local farmers (Borron, 2003; McCullum et al., 2005; Webb et al., 1998). Municipal or regional food policy councils have been established across the country including in Santa Cruz, California; New Haven, Connecticut; Knoxville, Tennessee; Portland/ Multnomah, Oregon; and Seattle/King County, Washington. Some states also have active food policy councils (McCullum et al., 2005).

The range of issues on which food policy councils or coalitions may focus include the creation and maintenance of farm-to-school programs (e.g., fresh produce from local farms is used in school salad bars and lunches, and school field trips to local farms are promoted); the creation of youth leadership programs that help youth develop skills in gardening and marketing, for example, through projects to develop school-based edible landscaping and produce stands; improvement of the availability of healthful and affordable foods in low-income communities (e.g., the creation or expansion of farmers markets); working on issues related to land use policies and local or regional food production and consumption (e.g., community gardens, community-supported agriculture, seasonal eating plans, and food system education); and the support of legislation, such as zoning laws, that either ban or regulate the location, number, and densities of fast food outlets, quick serve restaurants, and drive-through establishments in cities and municipalities (Borron, 2003; Cohen et al., 2004; Hamilton, 2002; Mair et al., 2005a,b).

Tool kits are available that provide guidance on conducting a community food assessment, defined as "a participatory and collaborative process that examines a broad range of food-related issues and assets in order to inform actions to improve the community's food system" (CFSC, 2004). These include the U.S. Department of Agriculture's *Community Food Security Assessment Toolkit* (Cohen, 2002) and the Community Food Security Coalition's *Community Food Project Evaluation Handbook* and *Community Food Project Evaluation Toolkit* (National Research Center, Inc., 2004a,b).

A distinction is made between program-level tools, which are used to measure the changes in individuals who participate in or receive direct services from a community food project, and system-level tools, which measure changes in the food system of a community, city, state, region, or the nation. System-level tools (e.g., community mapping and geographic information systems [GIS]) can be used to inventory and identify the types and ranges of local food resources, such as supermarkets, corner grocery stores, full serve and quick serve restaurants, food banks, food pantries, farmers markets, and community gardens (Algert et al., 2006; McCullum et al., 2005; Pothukuchi et al., 2002). System-level tools can also be used to assess changes in the food system that will increase the availability of locally grown food in retail stores, increase the availability of supermarkets within walking distance of residents, and increase the presence of or expand the activities of food policy councils (National Research Center, 2004a,b).

Engaging Health Care Providers and the Health Care System

The *Health in the Balance* report's discussion of the role of health care professionals and organizations focused on providing counseling, leadership, advocacy, and training (IOM, 2005). A systematic assessment of the progress by the health care sector regarding childhood obesity prevention efforts has not yet been conducted. Such an assessment is one component of the larger effort that is needed to engage health care providers in fostering healthy behaviors in their patients (Green, 2005). Nevertheless, there are examples of how certain components of the health care sector have begun to take a more visible role in formulating policies and implementing innovative programs to prevent childhood obesity.

Efforts are ongoing to explore the factors that may encourage pediatricians in counseling their patients on overweight or obesity or that may hinder them from doing so. A survey of North Carolina pediatricians found that those who classified themselves as thin or overweight had greater difficulty providing their patients with weight counseling than pediatricians who classified themselves as average weight (Perrin et al., 2005). A survey of nurse practitioners in the intermountain area of Utah found that barriers to implementing childhood obesity prevention strategies included perceived parental attitudes regarding a lack of motivation to implement healthful changes; difficulties for families to overcome social norms regarding television viewing, videogame playing, and carbonated soft drink and snack foods consumption; and a lack of time and reimbursement for adequate counseling and patient education (Larsen et al., 2006).

Individual physicians and professional organizations have become involved in promoting and implementing obesity prevention programs at the community and state levels (Box 6-7). The IOM committee noted at the symposia in Wichita and Atlanta that physicians who have been elected as state legislators or who hold leadership positions in the state executive branch are often vocal proponents of obesity prevention measures and actively work to propose relevant legislation. Many professional organizations, such as the American Academy of Family Physicians and the American Academy of Pediatrics, provide evidence-based, online patient and provider tool kits and informational websites that help them prevent and manage obesity in children and youth (AAFP, 2004; AAP, 2006) (Chapter 8).

Obesity-related initiatives by major health plans initially focused on treatment options for adults (such as coverage for weight loss drugs or bariatric surgery) but are now increasingly emphasizing obesity prevention

---

BOX 6-7
Physicians as Advocates for Healthy Communities

The California Medical Association (CMA) Foundation began its Physicians for Healthy Communities initiative in 2005 to coordinate the obesity prevention efforts of California's physicians with the healthy eating and physical activity programs run by the California Nutrition Network in schools, community organizations, and local and state government. The California Nutrition Network for Healthy, Active Families is a project of the California Department of Health Services funded by the Food Stamp Program. The CMA Foundation enlisted the support of 40 county medical societies, 37 ethnic physician organizations, and several specialty medical societies. During the first year of the project nearly 150 "physician champions" were identified. In 2006, 250 physician champions were being trained to become educators and advocates for healthy eating and physical activity in schools and communities throughout the state. The CMA Foundation provides physicians with training opportunities, tool kits for working with schools and underserved populations, and guidelines for talking about obesity prevention with patients during patient visits (www.calmedfoundation.org). The CMA Foundation's Physicians for Healthy Communities Initiative is supported by the California Department of Health Services, Kaiser Permanente, Blue Shield of California, and LA Care Health Plan.

SOURCE: CMA Foundation (2006).

---

and ofen include a specific focus on children and youth (Kertesz, 2006b; NIHCM Foundation, 2006). A new effort by America's Health Insurance Plans includes a focus on mini-grants that are awarded to further research on obesity-related interventions. Health plans are developing educational materials and programs for patients and clinicians. For example, CIGNA has developed an online tool kit for physicians to assist them with counseling parents and older youth about childhood obesity (Kertesz, 2006a). Kaiser Permanente has recently instituted BMI as a vital sign that is assessed during clinical visits and as an outcome measure that can be tracked as part of the electronic medical record system (Box 6-8).

Health plans are also involved in community- and school-based programs. In 1998, Blue Cross Blue Shield of Massachusetts began a youth wellness program, Jump Up and Go!, which involves developing partnerships with community-based organizations to provide physical activity programs, school initiatives, health professional educational components, and educational materials to assist pediatric clinicians with counseling children and their parents (Jump Up and Go!, 2006). Other innovative approaches include the Kaiser Permanente worksite farmers markets in California that offer patients and employees the opportunity to purchase fresh fruits, vegetables, and other foods and beverages that contribute to a healthful diet

---

BOX 6-8
Kaiser Permanente's Healthy Eating, Active Living Initiative

Kaiser Permanente's Healthy Eating, Active Living (HEAL) initiative is a multifaceted approach to promoting a healthy lifestyle that integrates prevention-oriented delivery system interventions, community-based initiatives, organizational practice changes, and a media campaign.

Delivery system interventions. In 2002, Kaiser Permanente launched the Weight Management Initiative to introduce and evaluate evidence-based clinical practice changes to support prevention and treatment of overweight. Key elements of this initiative include assessment of BMI as a vital sign, physician training programs on counseling strategies, and point-of-care prompts in examination rooms.

Community health initiatives. The multisectoral HEAL initiatives bring together community-based organizations, schools, public health departments, and the health sector to work together on change strategies, with an emphasis on making changes in institutional practices, public policy, and the built environment.

Organizational practice changes. Efforts are also focused on increasing access to opportunities for physical activity and offering low-calorie high nutrient foods and beverages within Kaiser Permanente medical facilities by sponsoring farmers markets at hospitals and medical office buildings, significantly changing the contents of the vending machines, ensuring that a minimum of 50 percent of vending machine slots supply food and beverages that contribute to a healthful diet, and improving the nutritional quality of foods offered in hospital and medical center cafeterias.

Public policy advocacy. Kaiser Permanente has also funded public health advocacy organizations and has backed legislation designed to make it easier for people to be more physically active and have increased access to foods that contribute to a healthful diet.

Media campaign. In 2004, Kaiser Permanente launched its Thrive advertising campaign. Intended principally to communicate the organization's philosophy of prevention and health promotion to current and prospective members, it has also sought to influence social norms with billboards, television advertisements, and radio spots.

SOURCES: Kaiser Permanente (2006); Loel Solomon, Kaiser Permanente, personal communications, June 2006.

(Kaiser Permanente, 2004) (Box 6-8). Kaiser Permanente has also expanded its Community Benefit Program to focus on obesity prevention efforts through its Healthy Eating, Active Living (HEAL) initiative (Kaiser Permanente, 2006).

Coordinating the community benefit efforts of health care organizations within the community are important, as is concerted involvement in community coalition efforts. Health care organizations can also demonstrate leadership by serving as organizational role models for physical activity and healthful eating practices, which include expanding the availability of low-calorie and high-nutrient foods in worksite vending machines and cafeterias as well as creating incentives for employees to engage in physical activity.

Efforts are under way to consider the types of information that clinicians and other stakeholders need to effectively address childhood obesity (Public Health Informatics Institute, 2005). An example is the All Kids Count program, a national technical assistance program to improve child health and the delivery of immunizations and preventive services through the development of integrated health information systems (Saarlas et al., 2004). Furthermore, regional health networks and electronic health records, which are increasingly being used, may provide sources of data relevant to childhood obesity that would also protect patient confidentiality. For example, western North Carolina Health Network's Data Link Project provides access to electronic health information for health care providers caring for the same patients across multiple health care institutions. Although this system is not being designed to provide regional aggregate health data search capabilities, such capabilities could be incorporated into the network's data linkages with the agreement of the participating entities.

Few mechanisms exist to provide accountability for the various components of the health care system in obesity prevention efforts. The committee encourages health care providers and organizations to provide greater leadership in addressing issues related to promoting healthful eating and regular physical activity. The National Initiative for Children's Healthcare Quality is in the process of developing a national program for recognizing promising clinical practices and clinical partnerships whose efforts have contributed to reducing childhood obesity (NICHQ, 2006).

APPLYING THE EVALUATION FRAMEWORK TO COMMUNITIES

What Constitutes Progress for Communities?

Individual communities across the nation are at different stages of engagement and action in addressing childhood obesity. The committee recognizes that it is not possible to obtain an accurate and systematic assessment of how many communities are fully engaged, how many are only beginning to initiate changes, how many recognize the problem but have not begun to address it comprehensively, and how many have not yet prioritized this issue. It is likely that the attention that childhood obesity is being paid in schools has alerted most communities to this issue. However, it remains to be determined how many communities have recognized that community stakeholders need to take additional actions.

It is important to emphasize the short-term and intermediate outcomes that can be examined in evaluating changes at the community level. It is not realistic for each community program to reduce children's BMI levels in a short time frame, nor is this expected; instead, the focus should be on assessing progress toward short-term outcomes (e.g., changing institutional, local, or state policies to support obesity prevention) and intermediate outcomes such as increasing the proportion of children or youth involved in physical activity on a daily basis, increasing the percentage of physical education or recess periods that children or youth spend in moderate or vigorous physical activity, increasing the number of miles of bicycle and walking trails, and increasing access to affordable fresh fruits and vegetables for families (e.g., through the provision of farmers markets in low-income communities and community or school gardens).

Furthermore, communities need to take full advantage of their racial/ethnic diversity and cultural assets by developing programs and opportunities culturally relevant to the children and adolescents in their communities. Sports activities, dance, foods, and beverages all have distinct cultural relevance that reflect community strength and provide an infrastructure for promoting healthful eating and active living.

The committee identified several important elements in assessing progress in childhood obesity prevention in communities:

- Collect, analyze, and present specific data for the community to make the case for action to local decision makers. Challenges include knowing how and from where to gather community-level data.
- Assess interventions that have evidence of effectiveness, and select promising initiatives that can be implemented by programs in the community.
- Identify funding sources for a new intervention or program; and have the time and the knowledge to identify, apply, and manage the required reporting for external grants.
- Design an evaluation plan and have sufficient numbers of knowledgeable staff with the skills and time available to measure and document the outcomes of an intervention.
- Sustain the intervention, particularly after external grant funding has ended.

Applying the Evaluation Framework

The evaluation framework introduced in Chapter 2 can be used to evaluate community policies and interventions. Two examples of the use of the framework are provided here: one focuses on active transport to school (Figure 6-1), and the other focuses on community gardens (Figure 6-2). Because of the diverse stakeholders involved in community-level changes, the responsibility for implementing, evaluating, and sustaining an intervention at any point in the framework can rest with a number of different organizations or entities. Indicators of progress in the community are varied and usually focus on short-term or intermediate outcomes that can be addressed by creating a community environment that facilitates physical activity and encourages healthful eating (Box 6-9).

Applying the framework in evaluating community interventions includes multiple components:

- The leadership, commitment, political will, financial resources, and capacity development, which are crucial as starting points for community change, can come from a variety of public- and private-sector sources at the national, state, regional, and community levels.
- The strategies and actions needed for community change can involve policy and legislative action, coalition building and collaboration, and program implementation.
- Structural, institutional, and systemic outcomes for communities include changes in policies and regulations by the local government to improve and invest in active transport and improved access to foods that contribute to a healthful diet (e.g., smart growth initiatives and incentives for the establishment of farmers markets).
- Environmental outcomes include the addition or enhancement of bicycle or walking paths or playgrounds, changes in traffic intersections or other road-related efforts to improve the walkability of community thoroughfares, as well as increased access to fruits and vegetables.
- Cognitive, behavioral, and social outcomes relevant to the community sector include the formation of relevant community coalitions, the acquisition of information gained on how to engage in healthy lifestyles by families, increases in the levels of physical activity, and improved nutritional intake.
- The health outcomes at the community level, as in other sectors, are focused on healthy children and youth and reductions in the prevalence of obesity and its associated morbidities.

NEEDS AND NEXT STEPS IN ASSESSING PROGRESS

Although a number of communities around the country are actively involved in improving opportunities for physical activity and healthful eating, there is an urgent need to scale up these efforts and to mobilize many

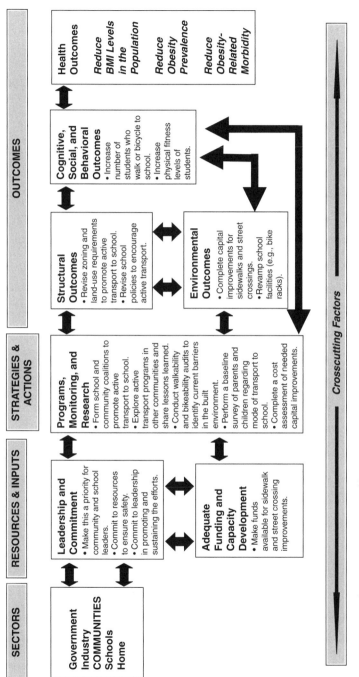

FIGURE 6-1 Evaluating community efforts to increase active transport to school for children and youth.

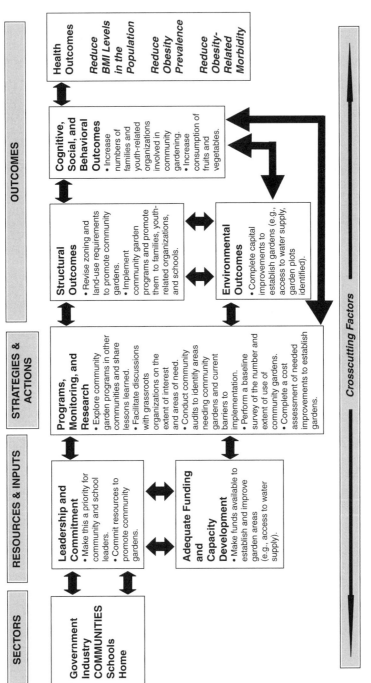

FIGURE 6-2 Evaluating community efforts to increase community gardening.

BOX 6-9
Examples of Community Indicators

- Food banks and emergency food outlets actively provide and promote high-quality fruits, vegetables, and other foods that contribute to a healthful diet.
- Billboard and outdoor advertising and transit companies restrict advertisements for high-calorie, high fat foods and beverages in neighborhoods, particularly around schools, playgrounds, and other youth-oriented facilities.
- Convenient access to high-quality free-for-use parks, playgrounds, outdoor sports facilities (e.g., tennis courts and basketball courts) and green space exists in low-income neighborhoods.
- Zoning and land use requirements promote mixed-use and mandate sidewalks, trails, recreation facilities, and safe pedestrian and bicycle access to schools, shopping (including food), parks, recreation centers, and worksites, particularly in low-income neighborhoods.

SOURCES: California Department of Health Services (2006); Chapter 4.

---

more towns, cities, and counties to become actively involved in childhood obesity prevention. The following sections detail the next steps and implementation actions for communities.

Promote Leadership and Collaboration

Civic, social, and faith-based leaders in a community can galvanize action by local residents, businesses, schools, and organizations to improve the quality of life and the focus on nutrition and physical activity in the community. Often, many community groups may be working independently on individual projects and initiatives. A greater coordination of efforts and communication about the range of efforts has the potential to leverage these efforts to reach more individuals and families and can also encourage other groups to initiate nutrition and physical activity interventions. Leadership can also be shown in the organizational modeling of fitness and nutrition policies and practices. In all of these efforts, it is important that evaluation be a priority. Indeed, leadership is demonstrated in the resources and emphasis that are placed on evaluation and on the dissemination of the results of those evaluations.

Develop, Sustain, and Support Evaluation Capacity and Implementation

Increase Funding and Technical Assistance Support for Evaluation

Evaluation at the program level often takes a backseat to implementing the intervention itself. Therefore, it is necessary for programs to design evaluation components into the implementation plan from the outset of the effort.

Programs may be overwhelmed by the concept of evaluation, which may seem to involve complex and time-consuming tasks, especially given quality assurance reports or grant reporting requirements that they must fulfill. Evaluations are often directed at assessing the process, that is, quantifying the service or program delivery efforts (such as the number of units or clients) rather than at the more important questions regarding an assessment of the influence of the program or service.

Evaluation needs to be an essential component of community actions. Clear requirements for evaluation as well as strong technical assistance should be included as part of the grant application process in government agencies and private foundations. Funding agencies should provide technical assistance to grantees as they develop an evaluation component or establish guidelines and selection criteria requiring community-based organizations to subcontract with academic institutions or other trained and experienced professionals for evaluation services. This was the model that CDC's Racial and Ethnic Approaches to Community Health (REACH) initiative used and is consistent with a community-based participatory research model in that the resources are controlled by the community-based organization rather than the academic institution.

Increasingly, it is recognized that tools are needed to assist communities with conducting their evaluations. For example, CDC's *Physical Activity Evaluation Handbook* is based on other program evaluation efforts in public health and on the work of the Task Force on Community Preventive Services (CDC, 1999, 2002; Martin and Heath, 2006). Additional straightforward evaluation tools for community-based programs need to be developed and disseminated.

Many organizations can barely summon the resources to implement new efforts and so do not include funds for evaluations in their budget planning. In addition to requiring that evaluations be included as an integral component of the program or intervention from the outset, there is a need for foundations, states, federal agencies and others to provide the funding and resources needed to ensure that evaluation efforts are implemented. The Healthy Carolinians community microgrants program, for example, provides funds to encourage and catalyze health promotion activities. Organized at the county level, Healthy Carolinians, a state-wide network of public-private partnerships, awarded small grants (approximately $2,000 each), collected final reports, and conducted surveys to evaluate the program and collate the lessons learned (Bobbitt-Cooke, 2005).

Develop and Widely Disseminate Training Opportunities

The formal training of individuals working in public health at the local level is highly variable (IOM, 2003). For example, in the United States, less than half of the 500,000 individuals in the public health workforce have had formal training in a public health discipline, such as epidemiology or health education (Baker et al., 2005; Turnock, 2001). An even smaller percentage of these professionals have formal graduate training from a school of public health or other public health program. At the local level the public health capacity for chronic disease control is also often low (Frieden, 2004). These findings suggest that there is a significant need for on-the-job training for public health practitioners, including a significant focus on evaluation of chronic disease interventions that address obesity.

Several practitioner focused training programs are promising. CDC has developed a useful six-step evaluation framework that can guide the process of conducting program evaluation (CDC, 1999, 2002). The Evidence-Based Public Health course, developed in Missouri, trains professionals to use a comprehensive approach for program development and evaluation from a scientific perspective (Brownson et al., 2003; Franks et al., 2005; O'Neall and Brownson, 2005). Each year CDC also sponsors a set of physical activity and public health courses operated by the University of South Carolina Prevention Research Center.

The committee encourages existing training programs to assess their focus on chronic disease and childhood obesity prevention and determine the effectiveness of these programs. Furthermore, federal and state agencies, foundations, and voluntary health organizations should increase the resources needed to widely disseminate and implement effective training programs.

Develop and Support Community-Academic Partnerships

Communities and academic institutions have different knowledge, skills, and strengths that can inform and complement each other when they partner to design, implement, and evaluate interventions to prevent childhood obesity. Academic institutions have strengths in intervention design and evaluation, and familiarity with grant funding, and expertise in writing and disseminating intervention outcomes. Local partners bring indispensable knowledge of their community's issues, cultures, and worldviews, institutions, resources, and priorities. Successful intervention collaborations respect both types of knowledge.

At the committee's Atlanta symposium, a county commissioner in Wilkes County, Georgia, discussed how county officials approached the Medical College of Georgia and the University of Georgia to help them address the county's growing obesity rate. After conducting a community health needs assessment in conjunction with the universities, a community task force developed a Wilkes Wild About Wellness community effort that included activities and interventions at local churches and worksites and in other locations (e.g., health fairs, summer day camps, after-school nutrition programs, faith-based wellness classes, and health screenings). The university was involved with the initial assessment of the community's health needs as well as with the design and evaluation of the intervention components (Hardy, 2005; Policy Leadership for Active Youth, 2005). The outcomes being evaluated include the number of participants, the amount of shelf space in grocery stores devoted to food items that contribute to a healthful diet, the extent of print media coverage of health issues, and the addition of walking paths and other environmental changes.

Other examples of successful partnerships can also be found. A community-based intervention in Florida with multiple collaborators (including the American Heart Association, Boys and Girls Clubs of Central Florida, the Food and Drug Administration, and Albertsons, Inc.) used the expertise of nursing students and faculty at the University of Central Florida to assist with the implementation of the intervention and to help plan and carry out the evaluation (DeVault and Watson, 2005). In Tarrant County, Texas, a partnership of Texas Christian University and community participants (including partners from the Cornerstone Community Center, the Tarrant Area Food Bank, and the Texas Cooperative Extension Tarrant County) worked together to design a program, Table Talks, that was presented in English and Spanish. The program provided information on family meal preparation and physical activity and nutrition classes. The pre- and post-intervention measures of that program included knowledge about nutrition and exercise, physical activity patterns, and dietary intake recall (Frable et al., 2004).

Key components of university-community partnerships that address childhood obesity prevention include participatory processes that engage key community members and that structure the partnership to ensure that equal attention and weight are given to the contributions of both the university and the community (Greenberg et al., 2003; Thompson and Grey, 2002). Many communities with diverse populations are cautious about the research conducted with the members of those communities. However, if the intervention is designed and implemented with the community as a partner, this community reluctance can be reduced (Chapter 3). Mechanisms to encourage these types of community-academic partnerships are needed and can be built into federal, state, and foundation grant requirements.

Enhance Surveillance, Monitoring, and Research

The vast numbers of communities, their varied organizational structures, and the independence of each community organization makes it difficult to assess the extent of community change directed toward reducing rates of childhood obesity and the effects of the change on a variety of childhood obesity outcomes. Few national surveys assess community actions, and the tracking of policy changes at the local level is limited. Furthermore, tools that can assist communities with evaluating new programs or conducting self-assessments are only beginning to be fully developed.

Expand Surveillance for Community and Built Environment Outcomes

Only limited national surveys or surveillance systems collect information on community-level outcomes, particularly those relevant to the built environment, community collaborations, and the involvement of the health care system. The National Household Transportation Survey, conducted by the Bureau of Transportation Statistics and the Federal Highway Administration, is one of the few national surveys that collects information on active transport, including daily and long-distance travel, and that measures young people's motorized and non-motorized travel (BTS, 2006) (Chapter 4 and Appendix D).

Metropolitan planning organizations across the country, which have the responsibility for planning and coordinating the use of federal highway and transit funds, often conduct local travel surveys (through travel diaries or other means) that provide valuable local-level details on travel patterns, often including the means of travel to school. For example, the Spokane and Kootenai County (Washington) Regional Travel Survey (2005) reported on the travel patterns of 1,828 households.

Efforts are under way to explore the type of data on the built environment that should be collected. Examples of these data could include the numbers of miles of bicycle lanes per capita; population and employment densities; and the number of recreational facilities, with the locations and conditions of those facilities (Brennan Ramirez et al., 2006). Furthermore, efforts to improve the geographic coding of the data on physical activity and health collected through surveillance systems such as the National Health and Nutrition Examination Survey, could provide further information to assist with examination of the impacts of changes in the built environment (TRB and IOM, 2005) (Chapter 4).

Facilitate Analysis of Local Level Data

Community decision makers need data relevant for their own specific locales to make informed decisions about where and to what extent resources should be devoted to relevant obesity prevention efforts. Funding and implementation priorities are often based on available data; as a result, areas with limited or no data are often overlooked because it is difficult to justify a need or to make a case for investment in intervention efforts without baseline data. Furthermore, the collection of data requires a level of accountability and follow-up, as there is the expectation that data collection will lead to changes and improvements in a community for the public good. Nevertheless, data are often lacking at the community level. Surveys can be expensive to conduct, research and validation of community assessment tools are relatively new, and the intersection of public health and the built environment is only beginning to be explored (Northridge et al., 2003).

Only a limited number of national surveys of childhood obesity prevention efforts have provided data that are aggregated at the regional or city level (Chapter 4 and Appendix D). For example, the CDC's 2004 School Health Profiles survey had weighted data from 11 school districts that enabled analysis of comparison data at the district level (CDC, 2006a) (Appendix C). The Behavioral Risk Factor Surveillance System (BRFSS) conducted by CDC has recently expanded its capabilities to provide local data for several U.S. cities and communities (CDC, 2006b) (Appendix C). The Selected Metropolitan/Micropolitan Area Risk Trends (SMART) BRFSS project provides data for counties, cities, and geographic areas with 500 or more respondents. The SMART BRFSS is a potential model for other systems such as the Youth Risk Behavior Surveillance (YRBS) system, to provide more local level data. Currently, the YRBS system provides data at the national and state levels and has a few specialized data sets, such as data for Bureau of Indian Affairs schools.

Efforts to provide greater specificity at the local level involve increased sample sizes and are therefore more costly to administer and analyze. However, given the need for local-level data for local-level decision making, research efforts focused on accurate methodologies for the extrapolation of state or regional data into meaningful community-level data should be explored.

State, regional, and city surveys are also conducted. The funding sources for these surveys, frequency with which they are conducted, their consistency, and the extent of data that they obtain on topics relevant to childhood obesity prevention are highly individualized. The California Health Interview Survey is one of the more extensive health surveys and provides data for the state and county levels, including representative information for specific racial/ethnic sub-populations. The Indian Health Service can provide tribal and community leaders with local-level data through its electronic health information system (IHS, 2004) (Chapter 3), which in-

---

BOX 6-10
Providing Local Data to Local Decision Makers

Data regarding local constituents often have important impacts on local decision makers; however, local-level measures are frequently not available in many areas of the nation.

Indian Health Service. Because of the Indian Health Service's (IHS's) central role in providing or contracting for health care services for American Indian and Alaska Native populations, it is in a unique situation to serve as a centralized source of data on obesity rates in tribal communities, despite the vast geographic distances between tribal groups. The Resource and Patient Management System is the IHS patient computerized database and contains clinical and demographic information from outpatient and inpatient encounters from more than 300 IHS and tribal health facilities. The result is a measurement and evaluation tool at the local, regional, and national levels that is stronger than the tools generally available for other high-risk groups (IHS, 2004).

California State Assembly Districts. The California Center for Public Health Advocacy compared 2001 and 2004 data on youth fitness and weight status from the California Department of Education's Physical Fitness Test and aggregated the results by state assembly district. The resulting local-level fact sheets organized by county and by assembly district have been instrumental in engaging legislators in obesity prevention issues and in the passage of several assembly bills regarding schools foods and beverages (California Center for Public Health Advocacy, 2005).

---

cludes data from clinic encounters and, frequently, measurements from school health screenings (Box 6-10).

Compilations or surveys of municipal policies regarding healthy communities are only beginning to be explored. Librett and colleagues (2003) conducted a survey of local ordinances in Utah relevant to physical activity levels. Trust for America's Health tracks smart growth initiatives at the state level, with some information available on specific municipalities (TFAH, 2005). An increased emphasis is needed on tracking policy change at the local level that impact access to foods and beverages that contribute to a healthful diet and opportunities for physical activity (Schmid et al., 2006). The committee encourages greater attention and resources to be devoted to local surveillance, monitoring, and data collection efforts. Innovative approaches to collecting and extrapolating data to the local level are also needed.

BOX 6-11
Examples of Community Assessment and Planning Tools

Community Tool Box. Developed by the Kansas University Work Group for Community Health and Development, the Community Tool Box provides an array of planning, assessment, and skill-building resources, including an action planning guide for communities that focuses on strategies and specific community actions for promoting healthy living and preventing chronic disease (Fawcett et al., 2005; University of Kansas, 2006).

Michigan Promoting Active Communities Assessment. In 2000, the Michigan Department of Community Health; the Governor's Council on Physical Fitness, Health, and Sports; the Prevention Research Center of Michigan; and the Michigan State University began recognizing communities that support physical activity. They developed an assessment tool that allows communities to evaluate themselves on a range of policy change and program implementation issues, including policies and planning for non-motorized transportation, zoning policies, bike path availability, sidewalk policies, community resources for physical activity, work sites, schools, and public transportation (Promoting Active Communities, 2006).

MAPP (Mobilizing for Action through Planning and Partnerships). Developed by the National Association of County and City Health Officials in collaboration with CDC, MAPP is a set of strategic planning tools and resources (NACCHO, 2004).

Health impact assessments. Similar to environmental impact assessments, health impact assessments examine the impacts that changes in policies, urban planning, transportation modes, and other alterations to the built and social environments would have on the health of members of the community (Dannenberg et al., 2006). Health impact assessments may also be particularly useful in bringing potential health impacts to the attention of policy makers. These processes have been in fairly wide use in Canada, Australia, and New Zealand and throughout Europe; and interest in such assessments is growing in the United States.

Additional tools. A number of tools that focus on specific attributes of communities have been developed and validated. These include measures of the walkability or bikeability of communities, street and other urban design issues, and assessments of parks and playgrounds (Moudon and Lee, 2003; Williams et al., 2005).

Refine and Disseminate Community Assessment Tools

One of the challenges for communities and community stakeholders is to assess the strengths and gaps in the community environment for encouraging and promoting healthy lifestyles. Certain components of healthy communities (Box 6-11), such as the walkability or the bikeability of community streets, can be assessed through available tools (Emery et al., 2003;

Moudon and Lee, 2003). For example, the prevalence of biking by students at 14 elementary schools in Mesa, Arizona, was assessed using a previously validated bikeability instrument that included average daily traffic, number of through lanes, speed limit, bike-lane width, the quality of the pavement, and other specifics (e.g., intersections, curves, and grades) (Sisson et al., 2006).

Furthermore, several community health report cards and indicators that could serve as a basis for further efforts have been developed. CDC's Healthy Days Measures focus on health-related quality of life and include measures related to physical activity and promoting a healthful diet (CDC, 2000). An example of an innovative approach to community assessment is a community youth-mapping project that involves children and youth in assessing their community's resources and needs regarding, for example, access to opportunities for physical activity and to fruits, vegetables, and other foods and beverages that contribute to a healthful diet (National Community Youth Mapping, 2006).

What is needed is a robust and well-validated tool to promote healthy communities and foster community action. Similar to the School Health Index for schools (Chapter 7), there is a need for CDC, in partnership with other agencies and organizations, to develop a multicomponent well-validated self-assessment tool (or tool kit) that will assist communities with examining multiple factors relevant to healthy communities. This type of community health index tool could include modules on the availability, accessibility, attractiveness, affordability, and safety of places for physical activity and healthier food choices for community members; the involvement of community organizations; and the measurement of the collective efficacy of a community. Adequate funding is needed to develop this tool; and the committee encourages collaborative efforts among U.S. Department of Health and Human Services, the U.S. Department of Transportation, the U.S. Department of the Interior, and other relevant federal agencies and private-sector and nonprofit organizations.

Expand the Use of Spatial Mapping Technologies

Improving the built environment to provide greater access to opportunities for physical activity and to foods and beverages that contribute to a healthful diet involves the identification of underserved areas and the modeling of potential changes to see if more people can be reached or benefit from the proposed interventions. New spatial mapping technologies, known broadly as geographic information systems (GIS), examine different types of datasets that are spatially referenced (such as road and land-use maps, population census data, housing data, and survey data with a corresponding coordinate system) and provide analyses that identify patterns and trends in spatial relationships (Leslie et al., 2005). The use of GIS provides objective measures of the environment and can be used to supplement or replace self-report measures (Porter et al., 2004). GIS technologies are increasingly being used for public health applications and have been used to examine a range of issues of relevance to childhood obesity prevention including the walkability of communities (Handy et al., 2002; Leslie et al., 2005), access to recreational facilities (Gordon-Larsen et al., 2006), and the accessibility of stores that sell fresh produce to food pantry clients who do not have access to fresh fruits and vegetables through most emergency food assistance programs (Algert et al., 2006).

Largely a tool used by researchers, GIS capabilities are now more easily accessible to community organizations, although much remains to be learned about how this technology can be used most effectively at the community level (Porter et al., 2004). A recent CDC and University of New Mexico effort in partnership with American Indian and Alaskan Native communities, Mapping a Shared Vision of Hope, is using GIS technology to provide data and maps relevant to diabetes prevention (Mapping a Vision, 2006). This tool provides spatial distribution data for a range of health and social variables.

As more community information is available in online and mapped formats, increased opportunities become available for mapping multiple facets of community life and identifying strengths and opportunities for promoting physical activity and access to healthful foods in the community (Porter et al., 2004). Presentation of the data visually to community stake-holders has the potential to be an important tool in engaging and tracking community obesity prevention efforts, particularly because they can be focused on a local geographic area. The committee encourages increased exploration and use of GIS and other relevant technologies for the development and evaluation of community-level interventions to promote energy balance in youth.

Develop Rapid Response to Natural Experiments

The realities of the changes that occur in communities pose challenges to the implementation of evaluation research. Often, changes that are relevant to obesity prevention (e.g., a new school policy or a new park or walking path) are not under the control of researchers or are under way before researchers have the time to institute traditional research methodologies or apply for evaluation funding through lengthy funding processes. These events are often called *natural experiments* as they offer a unique opportunity to compare rates of obesity and intermediate indicators before and after the change. To evaluate these natural experiments, mechanisms are needed to quickly allocate resources for evaluation. Quasi-experimental designs (e.g., ecologic studies and time-series designs) are likely to be more useful than randomized approaches for these evaluations (Chapter 2). Funding mechanisms with rapid review cycles, such as those that are often available from foundations, are needed to foster evaluations of these natural experiments.

Encourage the Measurement of Risk and Protective Factors

As discussed in Chapter 3, obesity prevention efforts do not occur in a vacuum, and it is important to consider the larger socioeconomic and cultural contexts in implementing programs and conducting evaluations. These contextual factors (e.g., poverty, extent of social capital, cultural assets and barriers, and mentoring programs) should be considered during the collection and analysis of baseline and outcome data. Interventions could explicitly target some of these factors, such as collective efficacy, which are known to be associated with childhood obesity (Cohen et al., 2006) and other issues of concern to the community, to increase the likelihood of developing effective interventions by engaging community support and developing partnerships. Interventions that strengthen protective factors, in addition to reducing risk factors, will likely have more resonance in diverse communities.

Disseminate and Use Evaluation Results

In addition to the traditional venues of peer-reviewed scientific journals, lessons learned and evaluation results should be disseminated through health education journals and magazines; national organizations including large grant and nonprofit foundations and professional societies; community health center, school, and community action networks; CDC and other commonly accessed websites; community newspapers; and other avenues of communication to reach a wide range of locally based stakeholders. Journals and organizations that represent communities and regions (e.g., the National Association of County and City Health Officials) should seek out new methods to disseminate and promote evaluation results. Action planning guides that are available to assist communities with their planning initiatives that support healthy living (e.g., Fawcett et al., 2005) should be widely disseminated.

A website repository hosted by a credible authority, such as the National Association of County and City Health Officials, should be developed to share community-based evaluation results and lessons learned, as well as links to resources, templates, and evaluation tools. Lessons learned should be shared among communities as should examples of community action plans. For example, in Washington State, the Healthy Communities Tool Kit was developed to share the information gained by two communities, Moses Lake and Mount Vernon, in mobilizing their community in promoting healthy lifestyles (Washington State Department of Health, 2006). Community stakeholders and the relevant government agencies and foundations need to cultivate open communication, identify ways to learn about promising practices in other communities, and focus attention on the lessons learned about the promotion of healthy lifestyles in other locales. The Health and Wellness Coalition of Wichita (2005), for example, commissioned a study to identify obesity prevention efforts in other cities of similar size. Furthermore, focus groups were held with Wichita residents to identify factors that motivate physical activity as well as those that were barriers to physical activity.

SUMMARY AND RECOMMENDATIONS

Communities are where the efforts of government, industry, health care systems, foundations, schools, nonprofit organizations, and many other groups come together to provide increased opportunities for physical activity and enhanced access to foods and beverages that contribute to a healthful diet. Communities differ in the extent of the resources that they have available to devote to childhood obesity prevention efforts. Communities must face the obstacles of limited budgets and competing priorities, and efforts that result in benefits to multiple needs of the community are encouraged.

Each of the report's four recommendations (Chapter 2) is directly relevant to promoting leadership and collaboration and improving the evaluation of community-based interventions, policies, and initiatives. The following provides the report's recommendations and summarizes the specific implementation actions (detailed in the preceding section) that are needed to improve childhood obesity prevention efforts in communities.

Recommendation 1: Government, industry, communities, schools, and families should demonstrate leadership and commitment by mobilizing the resources required to identify, implement, evaluate, and disseminate effective policies and interventions that support childhood obesity prevention goals.

Implementation Actions for Communities
Community stakeholders should establish and strengthen the local policies, coalitions, and collaborations needed to create and sustain healthy communities.

To accomplish this,

- Communities should make childhood obesity prevention a priority through the coordinated leadership of local government, community organizations, local businesses, health care organizations, and other relevant stakeholders. These efforts would involve increased resources, an emphasis on collaboration among community stakeholders, and the development and implementation of policies and programs that promote opportunities for physical activity and healthful eating, particularly for high-risk communities.

Recommendation 2: Policy makers, program planners, program implementers, and other interested stakeholders—within and across relevant sectors—should evaluate all childhood obesity prevention efforts, strengthen the evaluation capacity, and develop quality interventions that take into account diverse perspectives, that use culturally relevant approaches, and that meet the needs of diverse populations and contexts.

Implementation Actions for Communities
Community stakeholders should strengthen evaluation efforts at the local level by partnering with government agencies, foundations, and academic institutions to develop, implement, and support evaluation opportunities and community-academic partnerships.

To accomplish this,
Federal and state agencies, foundations, academic institutions, community-based nonprofit organizations, faith-based groups, youth-related organizations, local governments, and other relevant community stakeholders should

- Increase funding and technical assistance to conduct evaluations of childhood obesity prevention policies and interventions,
- Develop and widely disseminate effective evaluation training opportunities, and
- Develop and support community-academic partnerships.

Recommendation 3: Government, industry, communities, and schools should expand or develop relevant surveillance and monitoring systems and, as applicable, should engage in research to examine the impact of childhood obesity prevention policies, interventions, and actions on relevant outcomes, paying particular attention to the unique needs of diverse groups and high-risk populations. Additionally, parents and caregivers should monitor changes in their family's food, beverage, and physical activity choices and their progress toward healthier lifestyles.

Implementation Actions for Communities
Community stakeholders and relevant partners should expand the capacity for local-level surveillance and applied research and should develop tools for community self-assessment to support childhood obesity prevention efforts.

To accomplish this,
Federal and state agencies, foundations, academic institutions, community-based nonprofit organizations, faith-based groups, youth-related organizations, local governments, and other relevant community stakeholders should

- Expand the surveillance of outcomes of community-level activities and changes to the built environment, as they relate to childhood obesity prevention;
- Facilitate the collection, analysis, and interpretation of relevant local data and information;
- Develop, refine, and disseminate community assessment tools, such as a community health index;
- Develop methods for the rapid evaluation of natural experiments;
- Explore the use of spatial mapping technologies to assist communities with their assessment needs and to help communities make changes that increase access to opportunities for healthy lifestyles; and
- Encourage the evaluation of interventions to examine both the risk and protective factors related to obesity.

Recommendation 4: Government, industry, communities, schools, and families should foster information-sharing activities and disseminate evaluation and research findings through diverse communication channels and media to actively promote the use and scaling up of effective childhood obesity prevention policies and interventions.

Implementation Actions for Communities
Community stakeholders should partner with foundations, government agencies, faith-based organizations, and youth-related organizations to publish and widely disseminate the evaluation results of community-based childhood obesity prevention efforts.

To accomplish this,
- Community stakeholders should publish evaluation results using diverse communication channels and media; and develop incentives to encourage the use of promising practices.

REFERENCES

1000 Friends of New Mexico. 2006. *Grow Smart! 1000 Friends of New Mexico*. [Online]. Available: http://www.1000friends-nm.org/ [accessed June 3, 2006].

AAFP (American Academy of Family Physicians). 2004. *Obesity and Children: Helping Your Child Keep a Healthy Weight*. [Online]. Available: http://www.aafp.org/afp/20040215/928ph.html [accessed June 2, 2006].

AAP (American Academy of Pediatrics). 2006. *Overweight and Obesity*. [Online]. Available: http://www.aap.org/healthtopics/overweight.cfm [accessed June 2, 2006].

Abramson S, Stein J, Schaufele M, Frates E, Rogan S. 2000. Personal exercise habits and counseling practices of primary care physicians: A national survey. *Clin J Sport Med* 10(1):40–48.

Action for Healthy Kids. 2006. *Action for Healthy Kids*. [Online]. Available: http://www.actionforhealthykids.org/ [accessed July 26, 2006].

ACT!vate Omaha. 2006. *Welcome to ACT!vate Omaha*. [Online]. Available: http://www.activateomaha.org/ [accessed July 26, 2006].

Active Living Leadership. 2004. *Healthy Community Design: Success Stories from State and Local Leaders*. San Diego, CA: Active Living Leadership.

Active Living Network. 2005. *Making Places for Healthy Kids*. [Online]. Available: http://www.activeliving.org/downloads/aln_report_final.pdf [accessed May 2, 2006].

Algert SJ, Agrawal A, Lewis DS. 2006. Disparities in access to fresh produce in low-income neighborhoods in Los Angeles. *Am J Prev Med* 30(5):365–370.

America on the Move. 2006. *America on the Move Sponsors*. [Online]. Available: http://aom.americaonthemove.org/site/c.hiJRK0PFJpH/b.1311205/ k.DED2/sponsors.htm [accessed July 23, 2006].

Baker EL, Potter MA, Jones DL, Mercer SL, Cioffi JP, Green LW, Halverson PK, Lichtveld MY, Fleming DW. 2005. The public health infrastructure and our nation's health. *Annu Rev Public Health* 26:303–318.

Baranowski T, Baranowski JC, Cullen KW, Thompson DI, Nicklas T, Zakeri IE, Rochon J. 2003. The Fun, Food, and Fitness Project (FFFP): The Baylor GEMS pilot study. *Ethn Dis* 13(1 Suppl 1):S30–S39.

Beech BM, Klesges RC, Kumanyika SK, Murray DM, Klesges L, McClanahan B, Slawson D, Nunnally C, Rochon J, McLain-Allen B, Pree-Cary J. 2003. Child- and parent-targeted interventions: The Memphis GEMS pilot study. *Ethn Dis* 13(1 Suppl 1):S40–S53.

BGCA (Boys and Girls Clubs of America). 2006. *Sports, Fitness, and Recreation*. [Online]. Available: http://www.bgca.org/programs/sportfitness. asp [accessed June 19, 2006].

Boarnet MG, Anderson CL, Day K, McMillan T, Alfonzo M. 2005. Evaluation of the California Safety Routes to Schools legislation: Urban form changes and children's active transportation to school. *Am J Prev Med* 28(2 Suppl 2):134–140.

Bobbitt-Cooke M. 2005. Energizing community health improvement: The promise of microgrants. *Prev Chronic Dis* [Online]. Available: http://www.cdc.gov/pcd/issues/2005/nov/05_0064.htm [accessed March 4, 2006].

Borron SM. 2003. *Food Policy Councils: Practice and Possibility. Bill Emerson National Hunger Fellow Congressional Hunger Center Hunger-Free Community Report*. Eugene, Oregon. [Online]. Available: http://www.lanefood.org/pdf/food_policy_councils/food_policy_council_report_february_2003.pdf [accessed May 8, 2006].

Brennan Ramirez LK, Hoehner CM, Brownson RC, Cook R, Orleans CT, Hollander M, Barker DC, Bors P, Ewing R, Killingsworth R, Petersmarck K, Schmid T, Wilkinson W. 2006. Indicators of activity-friendly communities: An evidence-based consensus process. *Am J Prev Med* 31(6):515–524.

Brink L, Yost B. 2004. Transforming inner-city school grounds: Lessons from learning land-scapes. *Children, Youth, and Environments* 14(1):208–232.

Brownson RC, Baker EA, Leet TL, Gillespie KN. 2003. *Evidence-Based Public Health*. New York, NY: Oxford University Press.

Brownson RC, Boehmer TK, Luke DA. 2005. Declining rates of physical activity in the United States: What are the contributors? *Annu Rev Public Health* 26:421–443.

Brownson RC, Haire-Joshu D, Luke DA. 2006. Shaping the context of health: A review of environmental and policy approaches in the prevention of chronic diseases. *Annu Rev Public Health* 27(1):341–370.

Brudenell I. 2003. Parish nursing: Nurturing body, mind, spirit, and community. *Public Health Nurs* 20(2):85–94.

BTS (Bureau of Transportation Statistics). 2006. *National Household Travel Survey*. [Online]. Available: http://www.bts.gov/programs/national_household_travel_survey/ [accessed May 16, 2006].

California Center for Public Health Advocacy. 2005. *Rates of Childhood Overweight in California Counties, Cities and Communities*. [Online]. Available: http://www.public healthadvocacy.org/policy_briefs/overweight 2004.html [accessed July 31. 2006].

California Department of Health Services. 2006. *Communities of Excellence in Nutrition, Physical Activity, and Obesity Prevention (CX3)*. [Online]. Available: http://www.ca5aday.org/CX3 [accessed July 14, 2006].

California Endowment. 2006. *Healthy Eating, Active Communities*. [Online]. Available: http://www.calendow.org/program_areas/heac.stm [accessed May 12, 2006].

Carver A, Salmon J, Campbell K, Baur L, Garnett S, Crawford D. 2005. How do perceptions of local neighborhood relate to adolescents' walking and cycling? *Am J Health Promot* 20(2):139–147.

CDC (Centers for Disease Control and Prevention). 1999. Framework for program evalua-tion in public health. *MMWR* 48(RR-11):1–40.

CDC. 2000. *Measuring Healthy Days: Population Assessment of Health-Related Quality of Life*. [Online]. Available: http://www.cdc.gov/hrqol/pdfs/mhd.pdf [accessed July 31, 2006].

CDC. 2002. *Physical Activity Evaluation Handbook*. [Online]. Available: http://www.cdc.gov/nccdphp/dnpa/physical/handbook/pdf/handbook.pdf [accessed May 2, 2006].

CDC. 2006a. *School Health Profiles: Surveillance for Characteristics of Health Education Among Secondary Schools (Profiles 2004)*. Atlanta, GA: CDC. [Online]. Available: http://www.cdc.gov/healthyyouth/profiles/index.htm [accessed May 12, 2006].

CDC. 2006b. *SMART: Selected Metropolitan/Micropolitan Area Risk Trends: Frequently Asked Questions for SMART BRFSS*. [Online]. http://www.cdc.gov/brfss/smart/faqs.htm [accessed July 31, 2006].

CFSC (Community Food Security Coalition). 2004. *Community Food Security News. Special Issue on Community Food Assessments*. Spring. Venice, CA: CFSC.

Chase-Ziolek M, Iris M. 2002. Nurses' perspective on the distinctive aspects of providing nursing care in a congregational setting. *J Community Health Nurs* 19(3):173–186.

CLOCC (Consortium to Lower Obesity in Chicago Children). 2006. *Welcome to CLOCC*. [Online]. Available: www.clocc.net [accessed July 26, 2006].

CMA (California Medical Association) Foundation. 2006. *Physicians for Healthy Communi-ties*. [Online]. Available: http://www.calmedfoundation.org/ projects/phyChampion.aspx [accessed July 26, 2006].

Cohen B. 2002. *Community Food Security Assessment Toolkit*. Washington, DC: Economic Research Service, U.S. Department of Agriculture. Report E-FAN-02-013. [Online]. Available: http://www.ers.usda.gov/publications/efan02013/efan02013.pdf [accessed June 8, 2004].

Cohen DA, Finch BK, Bower A, Sastry N. 2006. Collective efficacy and obesity: The potential influence of social factors on health. *Soc Sci Med* 62(3):769–778.

Cohen L, Larijani S, Aboelata M, Mikkelsen L. 2004. *Cultivating Common Ground: Linking Health and Sustainable Agriculture*. Oakland, CA: Prevention Institute. [Online]. Available: http://www.preventioninstitute.org/ pdf/Cultivating_Common_Ground_112204.pdf [accessed May 10, 2006].

Cradock AL, Kawachi I, Colditz GA, Hannon C, Melly SJ, Wiecha JL, Gortmaker SL. 2005. Playground safety and access in Boston neighborhoods. *Am J Prev Med* 28(4):357–363.

Crawford PB, Gosliner W, Strode P, Samuels SE, Burnett C, Craypo L, Yancey AK. 2004. Walking the talk: Fit WIC wellness programs improve self-efficacy in pediatric obesity prevention counseling. *Am J Public Health* 94(9):1480–1485.

Craypo L, Schwarte L, Samuels S. 2006 (April 3). *Evaluating Youth Engagement and Leadership in a Multi-Site Initiative to Change Community Food and Physical Activity Environments*. Abstract 526.3. Experimental Biology, San Francisco, CA, April 1–5, 2006.

CSREES (Cooperative State Research, Education, and Extension Service). 2006. *Cooperative State Research, Education, and Extension Service*. [Online]. Available: www.csrees.usda.gov [accessed May 10, 2006].

Dannenberg AL, Bhatia R, Cole BL, Dora C, Fielding JE, Kraft K, McClymont-Peace D, Mindell J, Onyekere C, Roberts JA, Ross CL, Rutt CD, Scott-Samuel A, Tilson H. 2006. Growing the field of health impact assessment in the United States: An agenda for research and practice. *Am J Pub Health* 92(2):262–270.

DeVault N, Watson S. 2005. (October 6). *Healthy Kids Partnerships*. Presentation at the Institute of Medicine Regional Symposium Progress in Preventing Childhood Obesity: Focus on Communities, Atlanta, Georgia. Institute of Medicine Committee on Progress in Preventing Childhood Obesity.

DHHS (U.S. Department of Health and Human Services). 2006. *Steps to a Healthier U.S. Initiative: Community Fact Sheets*. [Online]. Available: http://www.healthierus.gov/steps/grantees.html [accessed May 3, 2006].

Emery J, Crump C, Bors P. 2003. Reliability and validity of two instruments designed to assess the walking and bicycling suitability of sidewalks and roads. *Am J Health Promot* 18(1):38–46.

Fawcett SB, Francisco VT, Paine-Andrews A, Schultz JA. 2000. A model memorandum of collaboration: A proposal. *Public Health Rep* 115(2-3):174–179.

Fawcett SB, Carson V, Lloyd J, Collie-Akers VL, Schultz JA. 2005. *Promoting Healthy Living and Preventing Chronic Disease: An Action Planning Guide for Communities*. Lawrence, KS: University of Kansas. [Online]. Available: www.communityhealth.ku.edu [accessed May 15, 2006].

FHWA, DoT (Federal Highway Administration, U.S. Department of Transportation). 2006. *Safe Routes to School*. [Online]. Available: http://safety.fhwa.dot.gov/saferoutes/ [accessed May 2, 2006].

Fit City Madison. 2006. *Welcome to Fit City Madison!* [Online]. Available: http://www.fitcitymadison.com/ [accessed July 26, 2006].

Flournoy R, Treuhaft S. 2005. *Healthy Food, Healthy Communities: Improving Access and Opportunities Through Food Retailing*. Oakland, CA: PolicyLink and The California Endowment. [Online]. Available: http://www.policylink.org/pdfs/HealthyFoodHealthyCommunities.pdf [accessed August 1, 2006].

Food Trust. 2006. *Fresh Food Financing Initiative*. [Online]. Available: http://www.thefoodtrust.org/php/programs/super.market.campaign.php#1 [accessed July 26, 2006].

Frable PJ, Dart L, Bradley PJ. 2004. The Healthy Weigh/El Camino Saludable: A community campus partnership to prevent obesity. *J Interprof Care* 18(4):447–449.

Frank E, Breyan J, Elon L. 2000. Physician disclosure of healthy personal behaviors improves credibility and ability to motivate. *Arch Fam Med* 9(3):287–290.

Franks AL, Brownson RC, Bryant C, McCormack Brown K, Hooker SP, Pluto DM, Shepart DM, Pate RR, Baker EA, Gillespie KN, Leet TL, O'Neall MA, Simoes EJ. 2005. Prevention Research Centers: Contributions to updating the public health workforce through training. *Prev Chronic Dis* [Online]. Available: http://www.cdc.gov/Pcd/issues/2005/apr/04_0139.htm [accessed July 23, 2006].

Frieden TR. 2004. Asleep at the switch: Local public health and chronic disease. *Am J Public Health* 94(12):2059–2061.

Garden Mosaics. 2006. *TRUCE Carrie McCracken Community Garden*. New York, NY: Garden Mosaics. [Online]. Available: http://www.gardenmosaics.cornell.edu/pgs/data/inventoryread.aspx?garden=84 [accessed June 3, 2006].

Girl Scout Research Institute. 2006. *The New Normal? What Girls Say About Healthy Living*. [Online]. Available: http://www.girlscouts.org/research/publications/original/healthy_living.asp [accessed April 13, 2006].

Girl Scouts. 2006. *Health and Wellness*. [Online]. Available: http://www.girl scouts.org/program/program_opportunities/health_wellness/ [accessed May 12, 2006].

Girls on the Run. 2006. *Girls on the Run*. [Online]. Available: http://www.girlsontherun.org/ [accessed July 26, 2006].

Glanz K, Sallis JF, Saelens BE, Frank LD. 2005. Healthy nutrition environments: Concepts and measures. *Am J Health Promot* 19(5):330–333.

Glasgow RE, Vogt TM, Boles SM. 1999. Evaluating the public health impact of health promotion interventions: The RE-AIM framework. *Am J Public Health* 89(9):1322–1327.

Gordon-Larsen P, Nelson MC, Page P, Popkin BM. 2006. Inequality in the built environment underlies key health disparities in physical activity and obesity. *Pediatrics* 117(2): 417–424.

Green LA. 2005. Prescription for health: Round 1 initial results. *Ann Fam Med* 3(Suppl 2): S2–S3.

Greenberg JS, Howard D, Desmond D. 2003. A community-campus partnership for health: The Seat-Pleasant-University of Maryland Health Partnership. *Health Promot Pract* 4(4):393–401.

Hamilton N. 2002. Putting a face on our food: How state and local food policies can promote the new agriculture. *Drake J Agric Law* 7:408–443. [Online]. Available: http://www.statefoodpolicy.org/faceon.pdf [accessed May 8, 2006].

Handy S, Boarnet MG, Ewing R, Killingsworth RE. 2002. How the built environment affects physical activity: Views from urban planning. *Am J Prev Med* 23(2S):64–73.

Hannon C, Cradock A, Gortmaker SL, Wiecha J, El Ayadi A, Keefe L, Harris A. 2006. Play Across Boston: A community initiative to reduce disparities in access to after-school physical activity programs for inner-city youths. *Prev Chronic Dis* [Online]. Available: http://www.cdc.gov/Pcd/issues/2006/jul/ 05_0125.htm [accessed August 31, 2006].

Hardy D. 2005 (October 6). *Washington Wilkes County/Medical College of Georgia Partnership*. Presentation at the IOM Regional Symposium Progress in Preventing Childhood Obesity: Focus on Communities, Atlanta, GA. Institute of Medicine Committee on Progress in Preventing Childhood Obesity.

Health and Wellness Coalition of Wichita. 2005. *Community Comparisons and Common Language*. [Online]. Available: http://www.hwcwichita.org/images/Health%20Wellness%20Rprt.pdf [accessed May 12, 2006].

Health Collaborative. 2003. *2002 Community Health Assessment and Health Profiles*. San Antonio, TX: Health Collaborative. [Online]. Available: http://www.healthcollaborative.net/Assessment/AssessmentHome.html [accessed May 10, 2006].

Health Collaborative. 2006. *The Health Collaborative*. [Online]. Available: http://www. healthcollaborative.net/ [accessed July 26, 2006].

Hopson R. 2003. *Overview of Multicultural and Culturally Competent Program Evaluation. Oakland, CA: Social Policy Research Associates*. [Online]. Available: http://www. calendow.org/reference/publications/pdf/evaluations/TCE0509-2004_Overview_of_Mu. pdf [accessed April 18, 2006].

IHS (Indian Health Service). National Diabetes Program, U.S. Department of Health and Human Services. 2004. *Interim Report to Congress: Special Diabetes Program for Indians*. Washington, DC: Indian Health Service.

IOM (Institute of Medicine). 2003. *The Future of the Public's Health in the 21st Century*. Washington, DC: The National Academies Press.

IOM. 2005. *Preventing Childhood Obesity. Health in the Balance*. Washington, DC: The National Academies Press.

Israel BA, Schulz AJ, Parker EA, Becker AB. 1998. Review of community-based research: Assessing partnership approaches to improve public health. *Annu Rev Public Health* 19(1):173–202.

Jump Up and Go! 2006. *About Jump Up and Go!* [Online]. Available: http://jumpupand go.com/about.htm [accessed July 26, 2006].

Kahn EB, Ramsey LT, Brownson RC, Heath GW, Howze EH, Powell KE, Stone EJ, Rajab MW, Corso P. 2002. The effectiveness of interventions to increase physical activity. A systematic review. *Am J Prev Med* 22(4 Suppl 1):73–107.

Kaiser Permanente. 2004. *Kaiser Permanente Farmers' Market Resource Guide*. [Online]. Available: http://www.noharm.org/details.cfm?ID= 1112&type=document [accessed July 31. 2006].

Kaiser Permanente. 2006. *Kaiser Permanente's Comprehensive Approach to the Obesity Epidemic*. [Online]. Available: http://www.calwic.org/docs/ kaiserbroch_feb06.pdf [accessed July 31. 2006].

Kertesz L. 2006a. Weighing in on obesity. *AHIP Coverage* January/February Pp. 16–20.

Kertesz L. 2006b. Reaching out on obesity. *AHIP Coverage* March/April.

Kreuter MW, Lezin NA, Young LA. 2000. Evaluating community-based collaborative mechanisms: Implications for practitioners. *Health Promot Pract* 1(1):49–63.

Kreuter MW, Lukwago SN, Bucholtz RD, Clark EM, Sanders-Thompson V. 2003. Achieving cultural appropriateness in health promotion programs: Targeted and tailored approaches. *Health Educ Behav* 30(2):133–146.

Larsen L, Mandleco B, Williams M, Tiedeman M. 2006. Childhood obesity: Prevention practices of nurse practitioners. *J Am Acad Nurse Pract* 18(2):70–79.

Lasker RD, Weiss ES, Miller R. 2001. Partnership synergy: A practical framework for studying and strengthening the collaborative advantage. *Milbank Q* 79(2):179–205.

Latino New Urbanism. 2006. *Latino New Urbanism*. [Online]. Available: http://www.latino newurbanism.org/ [accessed May 16, 2006].

Leslie E, Coffee N, Frank L, Owen N, Bauman A, Hugo G. 2005. Walkability of local communities: Using geographic information systems to objectively assess relevant environmental attributes. *Health Place*. Dec. 29 Epub. [Online]. Available: www.elsevier. com/locate/healthplace [accessed May 16, 2006].

Lewis CE, Wells KB, Ware J. 1986. A model for predicting the counseling practices of physicians. *J Gen Intern Med* 1(1):14–19.

Librett JJ, Yore MM, Schmid TL. 2003. Local ordinances that promote physical activity: A survey of municipal policies. *Am J Public Health* 93(9):1399–1403.

Lumeng JC, Appugliese D, Cabral HJ. Bradley RH, Zuckerman B. 2006. Neighborhood safety and overweight status in children. *Arch Pediatr Adolesc Med* 160(1):25–31.

MacQueen KM, McLellan E, Metzger DS, Kegeles S, Strauss RP, Scotti R, Blanchard L, Trotter RT II. 2001. What is community? An evidence-based definition for participatory public health. *Am J Public Health* 91(12):1929–1937.

Mair JS, Pierce MW, Teret SP. 2005a. *The City Planner's Guide to the Obesity Epidemic: Zoning and Fast Food*. [Online]. Available: http://www.publichealthlaw.net/Zoning%20City%20Planners%20Guide.pdf [accessed May 11, 2006].

Mair JS, Pierce MW, Teret SP. 2005b. *The Use of Zoning to Restrict Fast Food Outlets: A Potential Strategy to Combat Obesity*. [Online]. Available: http://www.publichealthlaw.net/Zoning%20Fast%20Food%20Outlets.pdf [accessed May 11, 2006].

Mapping A Vision. 2006. *Mapping A Shared Vision of Hope*. [Online]. Available: http://mappingavision.unm.edu/ [accessed June 9, 2006].

Martin SL, Heath GW. 2006. A six-step model for evaluation of community-based physical activity programs. *Prev Chronic Dis* [Online]. Available: www.cdc.gov/pcd/issues/2006/jan/05_0111.htm [accessed May 2, 2006].

McCullum C, Desjardins E, Kraak VI, Lapido P, Costello H. 2005. Evidence-based strategies to build community food security. *J Am Diet Assoc* 105(2):278–283.

Meister JS, de Zapien JG. 2005. Bringing health policy issues front and center in the community: Expanding the role of community health coalitions. *Prev Chronic Dis* [Online]. Available: http://www.cdc.gov/Pcd/issues/2005/jan/04_0080.htm [accessed August 4, 2006].

Moore LV, Diez Roux AV. 2006. Associations of neighborhood characteristics with the location and type of food stores. *Am J Public Health* 96(2):325–331.

Moudon AV, Lee C. 2003. Walking and bicycling: An evaluation of environmental audit instruments. *Am J Health Promot* 18(1):21–37.

NACCHO (National Association of County and City Health Officials). 2004. *Achieving Healthier Communities Through MAPP. A User's Handbook*. [Online]. Available: http://mapp.naccho.org/MAPP_Handbook.pdf [accessed May 11, 2006].

National Community Youth Mapping. 2006. *National Community Youth Mapping*. [Online]. Available: http://www.communityyouthmapping.org/ Youth/ [accessed June 9, 2006].

National Research Center, Inc. 2004a. *Community Food Project Evaluation Handbook*. Venice, CA: Community Food Security Coalition. [Online]. Available: http://www.foodsecurity.org/Handbook2005JAN.pdf [accessed May 11, 2006].

National Research Center, Inc. 2004b. *Community Food Project Evaluation Toolkit*. Venice, CA: Community Food Security Coalition. [Online]. Available: http://www.foodsecurity.org/CFPTOOLKIT030805.pdf [accessed May 11, 2006].

NBGH (National Business Group on Health). 2006. *An Employer Toolkit: Reducing Child & Adolescent Obesity — Addressing Healthy Weight for Employees and Their Children*. [Online]. Available: http://www.wbgh.org/prevention/et_childobesity.cfm [accessed May 1, 2006].

New Urbanism. 2006. *New Urbanism: Creating Livable Sustainable Communities*. [Online]. Available: http://www.newurbanism.org/ [accessed June 2, 2006].

NICHQ (National Initiative for Children's Healthcare Quality). 2006. *Accelerating Improvement in Childhood Obesity*. [Online]. Available: http://www.nichq.org/NICHQ/Programs/ConferencesAndTraining/2006ObesityCongressSummit.htm?TabId=8 [accessed April 28, 2006].

NIHCM Foundation. 2006. *Prevention Corner*. [Online]. Available: http://www.nihcm.org/finalweb/pg_prevention.htm [accessed July 26, 2006].

Nike. 2006. *NikeGo*. [Online]. Available: http://www.nike.com/nikebiz/nikego/index.jsp [accessed July 26, 2006].

Norris T, Pittman M. 2000. The Healthy Communities Movement and the Coalition for Healthier Cities and Communities. *Public Health Rep* 115(2-3):118–124.

Northridge ME, Sclar ED, Biswas P. 2003. Sorting out the connections between the built environment and health: A conceptual framework for navigating pathways and planning healthy cities. *J Urban Health* 80(4):556–568.

O'Neall MA, Brownson RC. 2005. Teaching evidence-based public health to public health practitioners. *Ann Epidemiol* 15(7):540–544.

Partnership for a Healthy West Virginia. 2006. *Walkable Communities Workshop*. [Online]. Available: http://www.healthywv.com/community/ walkable_communities.aspx [accessed June 20, 2006].

PATH Foundation. 2006. *About the PATH Foundation*. [Online]. Available: http://www. pathfoundation.org/about/index.cfm [accessed June 3, 2006].

PBH (Produce for Better Health Foundation). 2006. *National 5 a Day Partnership Structure*. [Online]. Available: http://www.5aday.org/html/background/partners.php [accessed July 23, 2006].

PedNet Coalition. 2006. *PedNet*. [Online]. Available: http://www.pednet.org/ [accessed April 28, 2006].

Perrin EM, Flower KB, Ammerman AS. 2005. Pediatricians' own weight: Self-perception, misclassification, and ease of counseling. *Obes Res* 13(2):326–332.

Policy Leadership for Active Youth. 2005. *Addressing Overweight: Interventions Tailored to the Rural South*. Atlanta, GA: Georgia State University. [Online] Available: http:// publichealth.gsu.edu/pdf/PLAY%20Policy%20Brief%20II%20Community%20-%20 Readers%20Layout%206-6-05.pdf [accessed May 8, 2006].

Porter DE, Kirtland KA, Neet MJ, Williams JE, Ainsworth BE. 2004. Considerations for using a geographic information system to assess environmental supports for physical activity. *Prev Chronic Dis* [Online]. Available: http://www.cdc.gov/pcd/issues/2004/oct/ 04_0047.htm [accessed April 28, 2006].

Pothukuchi K, Joseph H, Burton H, Fisher A. 2002. *What's Cooking in Your Food System? A Guide to Community Food Assessment*. Venice, CA: Community Food Security Coalition.

Promoting Active Communities. 2006. *Welcome to the Promoting Active Communities Award Website*. [Online]. Available: http://www.mihealthtools.org/communities [accessed July 27, 2006].

Public Health Informatics Institute. 2005. *Charting the Information and Systems Needed to Support Effective Response to Childhood Obesity*. [Online]. Available: http://www. phii.org/Obesity.html [accessed February 21, 2006].

Resnicow K, Jackson A, Blissett D, Wang T, McCarty F, Rahotep S, Periasamy S. 2005. Results of the healthy body healthy spirit trial. *Health Psychol* 24(4):339–348.

Robinson TN, Killen JD, Kraemer HC, Wilson DM, Matheson DM, Haskell WL, Pruitt LA, Powell TM, Owens AS, Thompson NS, Flint-Moore NM, Davis GJ, Emig KA, Brown RT, Rochon J, Green S, Varady A. 2003. Dance and reducing television viewing to prevent weight gain in African-American girls: The Stanford GEMS pilot study. *Ethn Dis* 13(1 Suppl 1):S65–S77.

Roussos ST, Fawcett SB. 2000. A review of collaborative partnerships as a strategy for improving community health. *Annu Rev Public Health* 21:369–402.

RWJF (Robert Wood Johnson Foundation). 2006. *Healthy Eating Research: Building Evidence to Prevent Childhood Obesity*. [Online]. Available: http://www.healthyeating research.org/ [accessed May 16, 2006].

Saarlas KN, Hinman AR, Ross DA, Watson WC Jr, Wild EL, Hastings TM, Richmond PA. 2004. All Kids Count 1991–2004: Developing information systems to improve child health and the delivery of immunizations and preventive services. *J Public Health Manag Pract* (Suppl):S3–S15.

Sallis J, Glanz K. 2006. The role of built environments in physical activity, eating, and obesity in childhood. In: Paxon C, ed. *Future Child* 16(1):89–108.

San Antonio Metropolitan Health Department. 2006. *Overview of MAPP Process in San Antonio and Bexar County.* [Online]. Available: http://www.sanantonio.gov/health/MAPP/progress.asp?res=1024&ver=true [accessed June 2, 2006].

Schmid TL, Pratt M, Witmer L. 2006. A framework for physical activity policy research. *J Physical Activity Health* 3(Suppl 1):S20–S29.

Shortell SM. 2000. Community health improvement approaches: Accounting for the relative lack of impact. *Health Serv Res* 35(3):555–560.

Sisson SB, Lee SM, Burns EK, Tudor-Locke C. 2006. Suitability of commuting by bicycle to Arizona elementary schools. *Am J Health Promot* 20(3):210–213.

Smart Growth Network. 2003. *Getting to Smart Growth II: 100 More Policies for Implementation.* [Online]. Available: http://www.smartgrowth.org/library/articles.asp?art=870&res=1024 [accessed June 2, 2006].

Sonoma County. 2006. *Family Activity and Nutrition Task Force.* [Online]. Available: http://www.sonoma-county.org/health/prev/fantf.htm [accessed July 26, 2006].

Sparke A, Walters C, Byram M. 2005 (June 27). *Kansas Teen Leadership for Physically Active Lifestyles.* Presentation at the IOM Regional Symposium Progress in Preventing Childhood Obesity: Focus on Schools, Wichita, Kansas. Institute of Medicine Committee on Progress in Preventing Childhood Obesity.

Spokane and Kootenai Counties. 2005. *Spokane and Kootenai Regional Travel Survey.* [Online]. Available: http://www.srtc.org/HTCS%20final%20report.pdf [accessed June 20, 2006].

Story M, Orleans CT. 2006. Building evidence for environmental and policy solutions to prevent childhood obesity: The healthy eating research program. *Am J Prev Med* 30(1): 96–97.

Story M, Sherwood NE, Himes JH, Davis M, Jacobs DR Jr, Cartwright Y, Smyth M, Rochon J. 2003. An after-school obesity prevention program for African-American girls: The Minnesota GEMS pilot study. *Ethn Dis* 13(1 Suppl 1):S54–S64.

TFAH (Trust for America's Health). 2005. *F as in Fat: How Obesity Policies are Failing America 2005.* Washington, DC: The Trust for America's Health. [Online]. Available: http://healthyamericans.org/reports/obesity2005/Obesity2005Report.pdf [accessed July 23, 2006].

Thompson LS, Grey M. 2002. Fighting childhood obesity with university-community partnerships. *Nurs Leadership Forum* 7(1):20–24.

Thompson PD, Buchner D, Pina IL, Balady GJ, Williams MA, Marcus BH, Berra K, Blair SN, Costa F, Franklin B, Fletcher GF, Gordon NF, Pate RR, Rodriguez BL, Yancey AK, Wenger NK. 2003. Exercise and physical activity in the prevention and treatment of atherosclerotic cardiovascular disease. A statement from the Council on Clinical Cardiology (Subcommittee on Exercise, Rehabilitation, and Prevention) and the Council on Nutrition, Physical Activity, and Metabolism (Subcommittee on Physical Activity) of the American Heart Association. *Circulation* 107:3109–3116 and *Arterioscler Thromb Vasc Biol* 23(8):E42–E49.

TRB (Transportation Research Board) and IOM. 2005. *Does the Built Environment Influence Physical Activity? Examining the Evidence.* TRB Special Report 282. Washington, DC: The National Academies Press. [Online]. Available: http://books.nap.edu/html/SR282/SR282.pdf [accessed December 29, 2005].

Turnock BJ. 2001. *Public Health: What It Is and How It Works,* 2nd ed. Gaithersburg, MD: Aspen Publishers.

University of Kansas. 2006. *Community Tool Box.* [Online]. Available: http://ctb.ku.edu [accessed July 27, 2006].

U.S. Bureau of the Census. 2006. County, municipal, and township governments by population size: 2002, Table 417. In: *Statistical Abstract of the United States, 2006*. Washington, DC: U.S. Bureau of the Census.

USDA (U.S. Department of Agriculture). 2005. *Fit WIC: Programs to Prevent Childhood Overweight in Your Community*. Special Nutrition Program Report Series, No. WIC-05-FW. Alexandria, VA: Office of Analysis, Nutrition, and Evaluation, Food and Nutrition Service, USDA. [Online]. Available: http://www.fns.usda.gov/oane/MENU/Published/WIC/FILES/fitwic.pdf [accessed July 23, 2006].

Washington State Department of Health. 2006. *Healthy Communities Tool Kit*. [Online]. Available: http://www.doh.wa.gov/cfh/NutritionPA/healthy_communities_tool_kit.htm [accessed June 2, 2006].

Webb KL, Pelletier D, Maretzki AN, Wilkins J. 1998. Local food policy coalitions: Evaluation issues as seen by academics, project organizers, and funders. *Agric Human Values* 15(1):65–75.

WHO (World Health Organization). 2002. *A Physically Active Life through Everyday Transport*. [Online]. Available: http://www.euro.who.int/document/e75662.pdf [accessed June 20, 2006].

Williams JE, Evans M, Kirtland KA, Cavnar MM, Sharpe PA, Neet MJ, Cook A. 2005. Development and use of a tool for assessing sidewalk maintenance as an environmental support of a physical activity. *Health Promot Pract* 6(1):81–88.

Winnebago Tribe. 2006. *Ho-Chunk Community Development Corporation (HCCDC)*. [Online]. Available: http://www.hochunkcdc.org/aboutus.html [accessed July 26, 2006].

WNBA (Women's National Basketball Association). 2005. *WNBA Launches New Fitness Initiative*. [Online]. Available: http://www.wnba.com/community/fitnesseventtour release_050517.html [accessed May 12, 2006].

Wyatt HR, Peters, JC, Reed GW, Grunwald GK, Barry M, Thompson H, Jones J, Hill JO. 2004. Using electronic step counters to increase lifestyle physical activity: Colorado on the Move™. *J Physical Activity Health* 1:178–188.

YMCA. 2006. *YMCA Activate America*. [Online]. Available: http://www.ymca.net/activate america/ [accessed June 19, 2006].

Zimring C, Joseph A, Nicoll GL, Tsepas S. 2005. Influences of building design and site design on physical activity: Research and intervention opportunities. *Am J Prev Med* 28(2 Suppl 2):186–193.

7

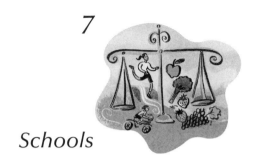

Schools

hildhood obesity prevention efforts have primarily focused on the
school environment because nearly all children, ages 5 years and
older, spend a large part of their days in school for 9 to 10 months
out of the year. Schools are an important setting to enhance students'
dietary intake and physical activity opportunities and to provide relevant
education and behavioral change programs. Policies and programs have the
potential to influence the behaviors of all the students in a classroom,
school, or school district. However, because the nation's estimated 66,000
public elementary schools, 12,000 middle schools, and 14,000 high schools
are often governed at the local school board, town, or district level, it is
difficult to systematically evaluate prevention strategies or to disseminate
promising strategies, policies, and programs (NCES, 2005). Further, more
attention needs to be paid to the provision of low-calorie and high-nutrient
foods and beverages that contribute to a healthful diet and opportunities
for physical activity in the child-care, after-school, and preschool environments regarding the.

The *Health in the Balance* report provided a range of recommendations
for schools (Box 7-1) with the goals of creating and maintaining a consistent environment that supports healthful eating behaviors and regular physical activity. The report also emphasized the need to help students understand the benefits of healthy lifestyles and the relationship between calorie
intake and energy expenditure to achieve energy balance at a healthy weight
(IOM, 2005).

BOX 7-1
Recommendations for Schools from the 2005 IOM report
Preventing Childhood Obesity: Health in the Balance

Schools should provide a consistent environment that is conducive to healthful eating behaviors and regular physical activity.

To implement this recommendation:

USDA, state and local authorities, and schools should
- Develop and implement nutritional standards for all competitive foods and beverages sold or served in schools.
- Ensure that all school meals meet the Dietary Guidelines for Americans.
- Develop, implement, and evaluate pilot programs to extend school meal funding in schools with a large percentage of children at high risk of obesity.

State and local education authorities and schools should
- Ensure that all children and youth participate in a minimum of 30 minutes of moderate to vigorous physical activity during the school day.
- Expand opportunities for physical activity through: physical education classes; intramural and interscholastic sports programs and other physical activity clubs, programs, and lessons; after-school use of school facilities; use of schools as community centers; and walking- and biking-to-school programs.
- Enhance health curricula to devote adequate attention to nutrition, physical activity, reducing sedentary behaviors, and energy balance, and to include a behavioral skills focus.
- Develop, implement, and enforce school policies to create schools that are advertising-free to the greatest possible extent.
- Involve school health services in obesity prevention efforts.
- Conduct annual assessments of each student's weight, height, and gender- and age-specific BMI percentile and make this information available to parents.
- Perform periodic assessments of each school's policies and practices related to nutrition, physical activity, and obesity prevention.

Federal and state departments of education and health and professional organizations should
- Develop, implement, and evaluate pilot programs to explore innovative approaches to both staffing and teaching about wellness, healthful choices, nutrition, physical activity, and reducing sedentary behaviors. Innovative approaches to recruiting and training appropriate teachers are also needed.

SOURCE: IOM (2005).

In June 2005, the committee sponsored the symposium Progress in Preventing Childhood Obesity: Focus on Schools in collaboration with the Kansas Health Foundation and sponsored by the Robert Wood Johnson Foundation (Appendix F). The symposium was held in Wichita, Kansas and provided the committee with the opportunity to interact with a range of stakeholders—teachers, students, principals, health educators, dietitians, after-school personnel, food service providers, industry representatives, state government and community leaders, and researchers—and learn about innovative interventions, challenges in implementing and evaluating school-based and after-school programs, and opportunities for evaluating policies and initiatives. In addition to the symposium, the committee draws from reports, scientific literature, and the media to provide examples of obesity prevention activities in schools for this chapter.

The obesity prevention effort in schools is an active area for change, and the committee recognizes that it can capture only a small proportion of the obesity prevention-, physical activity-, and nutrition-related policies and programs being implemented. This chapter focuses on assessing progress and ensuring that evaluations are conducted so that the most promising approaches can be identified and disseminated. As noted in the *Health in the Balance* report (IOM, 2005), there is a relative paucity of scientific data on obesity prevention efforts in schools. Teachers, schools, school districts, states, and the nation are in the midst of many exploratory efforts and new interventions, which provide opportunities to build the evidence base in order for promising efforts to be replicated and scaled up. Additionally, it is important that efforts found to be ineffective are either revised or discontinued, so they do not use resources that can be more effectively used for other efforts.

The multitude of actions revolving around nutrition and physical education in schools is a positive step forward. However, as detailed in a recent report examining state and regional obesity prevention-related policies, much remains to be done to provide a consistent healthy school environment that promotes energy balance for children and youth (TFAH, 2005). Although many states are addressing nutrition-related issues, these efforts are not being implemented in all states, and limited attention is focused on concurrently increasing physical activity levels and reducing sedentary behaviors.

Highlights from the 2005 Trust for America's Health (TFAH) report indicate that, as of the time of publication of the report:

- Six states (Arkansas, Kentucky, South Carolina, South Dakota, Tennessee, and Texas) have mandated nutritional standards for school meals and snacks that are stricter than current USDA requirements.
- Eleven states (Arizona, California, Hawaii, Kentucky, Maryland, New Mexico, Oklahoma, South Carolina, Tennessee, Texas, and West Virginia) have established nutritional standards for competitive foods sold in schools. Many of these changes had occurred recently with six states setting requirements for competitive foods since 2004.
- All states except South Dakota have physical education require-

ments for students; however Illinois is the only state that requires physical education for every grade in schools on a daily basis.

• Four states (Arkansas, Illinois, Tennessee, and West Virginia) have passed legislation that allows schools to measure students' body mass index (BMI) levels as part of health examinations or physical education activities.

OPPORTUNITIES AND CHALLENGES

One of the greatest challenges for school-based obesity prevention efforts may also be an opportunity to rapidly advance progress. As noted above, because schools are primarily controlled and administered at the local level, there are challenges in disseminating effective prevention interventions and for schools to learn about what has been effective or ineffective in other schools or school districts. However, this same lack of coordination between educational institutions may also provide the opportunity for a broad array of highly innovative approaches to emerge or for similar approaches to be implemented within many different settings. If evaluation efforts can be applied to these various approaches, there is an opportunity to rapidly expand the evidence base. In the absence of evaluation, this multiplication of efforts and approaches has less opportunity to support effective policies, programs, and initiatives or ensure the efficient use of resources.

Time and financial resources were two key barriers to the implementation of obesity prevention interventions identified by teachers and school administrators at the committee's regional symposium (Appendix F). The school year and school day are finite, and teachers report competing demands on their time. In particular, the school day is filled with nationally and state-mandated academic subjects, and there has been an increased emphasis in recent years on teaching to meet academic testing requirements. Teachers and school officials also reported that the effort to comply with the academic requirements set forth in the No Child Left Behind Act that was signed into law in 2002 (DoEd, 2006a) and similar state or local mandates often results in a de-emphasis on physical education and nutrition education programs.

Financial resources are also limited and are spread across many different competing priorities. Unless an individual school or school district has established health promotion as a high priority, financial resources will be insufficient to hire and train highly qualified physical education teachers, after-school program personnel, health educators, and school health professionals (e.g., school nutritionists and school nurses) and equip them with the space, equipment and supplies, and curricula that they require for creating a healthy school environment. Even when health promotion and obesity prevention have been identified as high priorities, school funding may still be insufficient to effectively implement and evaluate relevant policies, programs, and initiatives.

As with other sectors that affect the health and wellness of children and youth, schools are only one setting where young people spend part of their day and their year. Therefore, an important challenge is to promote and achieve collaborations between many stakeholders that provide healthful messages and opportunities. These collaboration should involve parents; after-school and child-care programs; media; sports organizations; non-profit organizations that sponsor after-school, evening, and summer activities (e.g., Girl Scouts, Boy Scouts, and Boys and Girls Clubs); and industry. Nevertheless, although schools are attractive partners and settings for collaborative initiatives, they are also asked to address many other health and social issues (e.g., violence prevention, sexual health education, and substance abuse prevention). Extra demands may create more competition for the time that children and adolescents spend in school and the human and financial resources needed to implement nutrition and physical activity programs.

Assessing progress in childhood obesity prevention in the school setting is assisted by many surveillance systems, surveys, and self-assessment tools— some of which have been actively used for 10 to 15 years. The discussions in this chapter frequently refer to the major surveillance systems or tools that are being used to assess progress in obesity prevention in the school setting (Table 7-1; Chapter 4; Appendixes C and D). However, as noted later in the chapter, most surveys do not comprehensively cover all school grades and local-level data are limited.

EXAMPLES OF PROGRESS IN PREVENTING CHILDHOOD OBESITY

With the myriad of obesity prevention initiatives occurring across the nation, the committee can provide only selected examples of innovative practices. This section examines the progress toward meeting the recommendations presented in the *Health in the Balance* report (IOM, 2005), provides examples of relevant efforts to fulfill the recommendations, and, where available, discusses the tools and strategies being used to evaluate and assess that progress.

Creating an Environment Conducive to Healthy Lifestyles

School wellness plans and councils are the focus of current efforts to address the comprehensive issues of creating and sustaining schools throughout the nation that promote healthy lifestyles. The Child Nutrition and

TABLE 7-1 Overview of Surveillance and Monitoring Systems

Surveillance System	Description
School Health Policies and Programs Study (SHPPS)	SHPPS has been conducted every six years by the Centers for Disease Control and Prevention (CDC) since 1994. SHPPS provides state, school district, school, and classroom information that is aggregated at the national and state levels. Of greatest relevance to childhood obesity prevention are the sets of questions about health education, physical education and activity, food service, and school policy and the school environment.
School Health Profiles (SHP)	SHP is a biennial survey, which CDC has conducted since 1994, of a representative sample of middle and senior high schools in a state or school district. Principals and health education teachers are asked to respond to surveys that encompass a range of school health issues.
Youth Risk Behavior Surveillance System (YRBSS)	YRBSS collects self-reported data on the risk behaviors primarily of 9th- to 12th-grade students, and has been conducted every two years since 1991. CDC provides technical assistance to states and municipalities that conduct the Youth Risk Behavior Survey (YRBS) at state or local levels concurrent to CDC conducting the YRBS at the national level. In 2005, weighted results (requiring a 60 percent or higher response rate) were collected for 40 states and 21 school districts (Eaton et al., 2006).
School Nutrition Dietary Assessment Study (SNDA)	SNDA has been conducted by the U.S. Department of Agriculture (USDA) in the 1991–1992 and 1998–1999 school years and data for SNDAS III were collected in the 2005 school year. The study examines calorie content, fat content, pricing, student participation, and other elements of school food sales for a nationally representative sample of elementary, middle, and high schools.
School Health Index (SHI)	The School Health Index (SHI), developed and promoted by CDC, is an eight-module assessment tool aimed at assisting individual schools examine and evaluate their comprehensive school health and safety policies. Two sets of SHI modules— one for elementary schools and the other for middle and high schools—have been developed.

WIC Reauthorization Act (Public Law 108-265) was initiated and passed by Congress in 2004 and requires school districts participating in the National School Lunch Program (NSLP) or School Breakfast Program (SBP) to establish local school wellness policies by the beginning of the 2006–2007 school year (CNWICRA, 2004). Local school wellness policies address a range of health-related issues, including nutrition and physical activity. The Act includes a plan for assessing the implementation of local school wellness policies supported by $4 million in appropriated funds (Chapter 4).

A number of organizations have developed model wellness policies and components of those policies. For example, the National Alliance for Nutrition and Activity has developed model nutrition and physical education policies that states and school districts can use and customize to local situations (NANA, 2006). The National Association of State Boards of Education in collaboration with the National School Boards Association has developed the resource Fit, Healthy, and Ready to Learn, which provides sample policies that reflect promising practices (NASBE, 2006). USDA has assembled reference materials in its online Team Nutrition: Local Wellness Policy database (USDA, 2006b). Action for Healthy Kids, in partnership with the Centers for Disease Control and Prevention (CDC) has developed the Wellness Policy Tool, which complements the Team Nutrition website and which assists school districts in identifying appropriate policy options (Action for Healthy Kids, 2006). Both websites also include evaluation resources. Additional resources include the wellness policy evaluation checklists developed by state agencies in Pennsylvania and Texas (Pennsylvania School Boards Association, 2006; Texas Department of Agriculture, 2006).

Most evaluations conducted to date have focused on outcome measures related to developing and implementing policy changes at the school or school district level (e.g., structural, institutional, and systemic outcomes). Future evaluations should examine the effect of these changes on students' cognitive, dietary, and physical activity behaviors, as well as health outcomes. It is unclear at this point whether most schools will have the resources required to conduct further evaluations that focus on behavioral and health outcomes.

A presentation at the committee's symposium in Wichita, Kansas highlighted the joint efforts of the Kansas Department of Education and the Kansas Department of Health and Environment. The two departments are collaborating to develop model wellness policies for school districts throughout the state (Appendix F). Additionally, tools are being developed that individual school districts can use to evaluate the implementation of their wellness policy and a state-level database will be used to track the implementation of these policies in each district. Technical assistance will be provided to the school districts, and efforts are under way to sustain local changes through school health advisory councils. In the next few years, as school wellness policies are adopted and promoted, it will be important to systematically evaluate the implementation of the wellness policies and to focus on sustainability issues.

The development and implementation of coordinated school health programs are the emphases of the funding and technical assistance available through CDC's Division of Adolescent and School Health (Kolbe et al., 2004). Currently 23 states receive funding focused on the coordinated school health program model, which has eight components, including nutrition, physical education, creating a healthy school environment, and health promotion for staff.

Many states and cities are currently enacting legislation that focuses on multiple aspects of enhancing a healthy school environment. For example, in June 2005 South Carolina's legislature and governor approved legislation that focused on school nutrition, physical activity, and health education particularly in elementary schools (Box 7-2). Arkansas took an early lead in this effort with a focus on assessing BMI levels, implementing changes in school foods, and promoting physical activity (Ryan et al., 2006).

Additionally, a number of organizations, foundations, government agencies, corporations, and others are partnering with schools on efforts that affect multiple aspects of the school environment. Examples of these

---

BOX 7-2
South Carolina's Students' Health and Fitness Act of 2005

Beginning in the 2006–2007 school year:

- Students in kindergarten through fifth grade must be provided 150 minutes a week of physical education and physical activity. A minimum of 60 minutes per week must be for physical education, with plans to increase it to 90 minutes per week.
- The fitness status of individual students, as determined during fifth and eighth grades and during high school physical education classes, must be reported to the student's parent(s) or guardian.
- All schools must administer the South Carolina Physical Education Assessment. The assessment of students in the second, fifth, eighth grade, and in high school are used to evaluate the effectiveness of the school's physical education program and its adherence to the South Carolina Education Curriculum Standards. Effectiveness scores will be developed and reported through the school district and school report cards.
- The State Board of Education will establish requirements for elementary school food service meals and competitive foods.
- The State Department of Education will make available to each school district a coordinated school health model. An assessment of district and school health education programs will be conducted.
- Each school district will establish a coordinated school health advisory council.

SOURCE: South Carolina General Assembly (2006).

broad-based initiatives include Action for Healthy Kids (a public-private partnership with state-based coalitions) and the Healthy Schools Program sponsored by the Alliance for a Healthier Generation (a joint effort of the American Heart Association and the William J. Clinton Foundation with support from the Robert Wood Johnson Foundation) (Chapters 2 and 5).

Improving School Food and Beverage Nutrition

The food and beverages sold or available in schools through the federal meal programs, as competitive (à la carte) items in the school cafeteria, in vending machines, in school stores, or in the classroom have been the focus of obesity prevention efforts in many localities (CSPI, 2006; Story et al., 2006). Policies related to the types of foods and beverages available in elementary, middle, and high schools generally differ, with more restrictive policies implemented for the lower grades. Many states are developing and implementing state nutrition standards for the foods and beverages served and sold in schools (see for example, Andersen et al., 2004; Connecticut State Department of Education, 2006). Certain cities and localities, such as Chicago and Philadelphia (Box 7-3) are enacting requirements stricter than those mandated by state law.

In 2004, the School Health Profiles (SHP) survey found that carbonated soft drinks, sports drinks, or fruit drinks were offered for sale in vending machines in 95.4 percent of the schools in the 27 states for which weighted data were available. Similarly, bottled water was offered by 94.3

BOX 7-3
Overview of Nutrition Standards of the
School District of Philadelphia

- Soft drinks will not be sold or served in school.
- Juice beverages must contain at least 25 percent real fruit juice.
- The total fat content of snack foods must be less than or equal to 7 grams per serving.
- The saturated fat content of snack foods must be less than or equal to 2 grams per serving.
- The sodium content of snack foods must be less than or equal to 360 milligrams per serving.
- The sugar content of snack foods must be less than or equal to 15 grams per serving.
- Candy will not be served or sold during the school day.

SOURCE: Philadelphia Comprehensive School Nutrition Policy Task Force (2002).

percent of the schools (Kann et al., 2005). In future SHP surveys, it will be important to track trends in the type of foods and beverages available for purchase by students.

Despite all the attention being paid to improving the nutritional quality of the foods and beverages provided in schools, however, the committee heard at the Wichita symposium that food service managers face ongoing challenges in improving school nutrition. These include insufficient funding, the use of sole-source contracts, open campuses where students can choose to leave schools to eat, a lack of nutrition education, short meal periods, and competition with vending machine options (Appendix F). Other barriers that food service managers face include preferences for fast foods, carbonated soft drinks, and salty snacks; the mixed messages sent by school personnel; and school food preparation and serving space limitations (Gross and Cinelli, 2004).

At the more local level, individual schools and school districts have made innovative changes to their menus, food sales, and beverage choices (Box 7-4) (Kojima et al., 2002). One of the challenges, however, has been in disseminating that information. The Produce for Better Health Foundation, in conjunction with 5 a Day and Fresh from Florida, has compiled promo-

---

BOX 7-4
Key Considerations in Improving School Foods and Beverages from the Minneapolis Public Schools Food Service Presentation at the IOM Symposium on Schools

- Ensure that Minneapolis Public School students have access to nutritious meals and ensure that nutritional and cultural needs of the diverse community are met.
- Meet or exceed USDA standards for nutrition requirements, food safety, and food security (offering more fresh fruits and vegetables, more whole grains). For example, a free "fixin's bar" that provides fresh vegetables and salsa can be added outside the serving area so students can help themselves.
- Broaden community involvement by establishing and maintaining Nutrition Advisory Councils, conducting student and parent annual surveys, and providing school meal and nutrition information on the school's website.
- Establish nutrition standards for à la carte items, considering portion size, and sugar and fat content.
- Form partnerships with local universities and technical colleges, local extension agencies, and state and county health departments.
- Evaluations can include tracking what students are selecting and consuming; conducting annual student/parents/staff surveys; and using input from partnerships.

SOURCE: Dederichs (2005).

tional ideas and implementation models to help food service managers increase students' fruit and vegetable consumption (PBH, 2005a,b). A recent CDC and USDA publication, *Making It Happen: School Nutrition Success Stories*, documents some of those changes. Examples include efforts made in Ennis, Montana, where students were involved from the initial planning in 2002–2003 in restocking vending machines and removing brand logos from vending machine signage. The vending services for the Oceanside, California school district were placed under the auspices of the food services program; and the results included healthier options and increased revenue from vending sales for the high school. In McComb, Mississippi, school policies were changed so that fundraising through the sale of candy or other less nutritious food items is not permitted in kindergarten through the eighth grade (USDA, DHHS, and DoE, 2005).

Federal, state, and community programs are increasingly focused on improving the nutritional quality of school foods and beverages—those offered as part of the NSLP and SBP, as well as those sold competitively. As discussed in Chapter 4, USDA's Team Nutrition program provides technical assistance to school food service personnel and child-care professionals, including Fruit and Vegetables Galore, a tool to assist schools in promoting fruit and vegetable consumption (USDA, 2006c). Additionally, innovative approaches to increase fruit and vegetable availability and consumption are being implemented by students, teachers, food service personnel, and the community through farm-to-school programs and school gardens (Graham and Zidenberg-Cherr, 2005; USDA, 2005). The U.S. Department of Defense (DoD), in partnership with USDA, conducts the DoD Fresh program, which in the 2005–2006 school year distributed produce to school food-service programs in 46 states and more than 100 American Indian reservations (Chapter 4) (David Leggett, USDA, personal communication, July 13, 2006; USDA, 2006a).

Fresh fruits, dried fruits, and fresh vegetables are also being made available to students outside the regular school meal periods through USDA's Fresh Fruit and Vegetable Program (FFVP). Established as a pilot program in the 2002–2003 school year, the program aims to increase student consumption of fruits and vegetables by increasing the availability of these foods in the school environment (Chapter 4). In 2004, the Child Nutrition and WIC Reauthorization Act (Public Law 108-265) established FFVP as a permanent program and expanded the program from four to eight states and added additional American Indian reservations (UFFVA, 2006); subsequent appropriations legislation in 2006 expanded the program to 14 states, and additional funding for a nationwide program is being sought. FFVP has undergone a preliminary evaluation, and further evaluation efforts are under way (Buzby et al., 2003) (Appendix D). For example, an evaluation of 25 schools in Mississippi that participated in the

FFVP suggests that the distribution of free fruit to middle school students might be effective as a component of a more comprehensive approach to improve dietary behaviors (Schneider et al., 2006). The committee encourages increased funding for implementing and evaluating innovative programs such as the FFVP.

A major focus of recent obesity prevention analyses and efforts has been the competitive foods and beverages—those foods and beverages offered at schools other than those available through the school meals programs (e.g., NSLP, SBP) often through school vending machines (Bachman et al., 2006; California Endowment, 2005; CSPI, 2006; Forshee et al., 2005; Westcott, 2005). In many parts of the country, school districts, localities, and states have set standards for foods and beverages that can be sold, have enacted restrictions on when vending machines are available to students, and in some cases, have removed vending machines from school grounds. Recently, major beverage companies announced an alliance to restrict the sales of some beverages in schools, particularly in elementary and middle schools (Alliance for a Healthier Generation, 2006) (Chapters 2 and 5).

In a recently published study of competitive foods in schools (Greves and Rivara, 2006) investigators interviewed school district representatives with the largest student enrollment in each state and Washington, DC, and compared the policies with the recommendations in the *Health in the Balance* report (IOM, 2005). Nineteen of the 51 districts evaluated had policies with requirements that went beyond state or federal requirements, with most having criteria for food and beverage content. Fewer school districts had policies related to portion size, advertising, or fund-raising. Interview questions regarding district policies also indicated that changes in product lines have been made and that snack food and beverage vendors have developed and offer new products (Greves and Rivara, 2006).

IOM is currently conducting a study, sponsored by CDC, to develop recommendations on appropriate nutrition standards for foods that are available, sold, and consumed at school, with attention given to competitive foods and beverages (IOM, 2006a). The committee recommends that Congress, USDA, and the U.S. Department of Health and Human Services (DHHS) provide leadership in establishing nutrition standards for competitive foods in schools by marshalling the political will needed to develop, implement, and evaluate appropriate standards that are consistent with the Dietary Guidelines for Americans 2005.

Evaluating Progress in Improving School Foods and Beverages

National surveys, particularly SHPPS, ask extensive questions about the school food environment. These questions examine the nutritional content of school meal programs and competitive foods, in addition to infor-

---

BOX 7-5
Examples of Survey Questions Related to the
Availability of Foods and Beverages Offered in Schools

2006 SHPPS School Questionnaire (CDC, 2006b)
- Are faculty and staff at this school prohibited from using food or food coupons as a reward for good behavior or good academic performance?
- Has this school adopted a policy stating that, if food is served at student parties, fruits or vegetables will be among the foods offered?
- During the past 12 months, have the school food service staff worked on school food service or nutrition activities with health education staff from this school?

SHP 2006 School Principal Questionnaire (CDC, 2006g)
- How long do students usually have to eat lunch once they are seated?
- Can students purchase each snack food or beverage [list of 12 foods or beverages] from vending machines or at the school store, canteen, or snack bar?

SHI for Middle and High Schools (CDC, 2005):
- Does the school food service offer low-fat milk and skim milk every day?
- Do school meals include at least one appealing, low-fat fruit, vegetable, and dairy product every day?

---

mation about the foods and beverages sold through other school venues (Box 7-5). For example, the segment of the 2006 SHPPS questionnaire related to food services included 55 questions at the state level, 78 questions at the school-district level, and 88 questions for individual schools,[1] with additional questions focused on the foods and beverages sold in vending machines and other school venues (CDC, 2006b). The results of the 2006 survey and future surveys will provide extensive data that can be used to examine trends in the school food environment since 2000. The most recent School Nutrition Dietary Assessment Study, SNDA III, is in the process of collecting and analyzing data (Mathematica Policy Research, 2005). When these results become available, they can be compared with the data from the 1991–1992 and 1998–1999 SNDA studies to examine the level of progress made toward improving the nutritional quality of available foods, dietary intake of students, and student participation rates in the federal school meals programs. The focus of the SNDA study is on the federally funded school meal programs with fewer data collected on competitive foods or on vending machine usage.

---

[1] SHPPS questions cover a wide range of food service issues including personnel, training, and food safety issues.

Individual surveys of school nutrition policies and program implementation are also useful tools for assessing and encouraging progress in preventing childhood obesity. A survey of school food service directors at a sample of high schools in Pennsylvania found that à la carte sales provided an estimated $700 a day to each school food service program, with 85 percent of those programs not receiving financial support from their school districts (Probart et al., 2005). Ninety-four percent of respondents indicated that vending machines are accessible to students, with bottled water being the most commonly offered item (71.5 percent). A survey of vending machine-related policies and practices in Delaware school districts provides similar baseline data against which future progress can be assessed (Gemmill and Cotugna, 2005). Given the number of changes in school foods and beverages, a baseline assessment of nutritional content and sales data against which data from later follow-up assessments can be compared is a useful evaluation tool.

Evaluations of farm-to-school programs to enhance the fruit and vegetable consumption of children and youth have been conducted. For example, Feenstra and Ohmart (2004, 2005, 2006) evaluated farm-to-school salad bar programs in Yolo County, California using a variety of methods: school food expenditures and distributor documentation; interviews and focus groups with students, farmers, school garden coordinators, and food service personnel; a plate wastage study; and digital photographs of student meals. Results showed that the salad bars raised the fruit and vegetable consumption of students. It also found that choice and variety are two important dimensions of school meals; when multiple varieties of fruits and vegetables were provided, children selected them.

Initiatives such as the Team Nutrition program are developing evaluation resources that can be provided to schools, and often include sample data collection instruments. The Team Nutrition school-based evaluation instruments are currently undergoing pilot testing (Murimi et al., 2006).

Other researchers are exploring the factors associated with student purchase of competitive foods, including the timing of school meals, open campus policies, the number of vending machines accessible to students during and after school, and policies regarding the type of food and beverages sold (see, for example, Neumark-Sztainer et al., 2005; Probart et al., 2006).

Increasing Physical Activity

Schools offer the opportunity for children and youth to be engaged in physical activity and to establish the foundation for lifelong habits of incorporating physical activity into their daily lives. However, physical activity is often not a priority consideration in school, child-care, and after-school policies and practices. Schools, school districts, preschools, and after-school and child-care programs may vary widely in the extent to which they are engaged in promoting regular physical activity. The results of the YRBSS show that the percentage of students in grades 9 to 12 who attended physical education classes on a daily basis decreased between 1991 and 1995 (from 41.6 percent to 25.4 percent) but has since remained relatively constant at approximately one-third of students (25.4 percent to 33 percent from 1995 to 2005) (Eaton et al., 2006). Among the 40 states that participated in this most recent YRBSS, there was a substantial variation in students who attended physical education classes daily (from 6.7 percent to 60.7 percent).

Although, many changes in school policies and practices in improving the nutritional content of the foods and beverages offered to students are occurring, there appears to be less progress in making changes in physical education requirements, enforcing state standards where they do exist, or expanding intramural and other physical activity opportunities.

The state policy assessment conducted by TFAH found that in 2004–2005, 17 states passed legislation, resolutions, or policies aimed at improving their physical education programs (TFAH, 2005). A large proportion of the legislation created task forces to examine and revamp state physical education policies. Further, some states have not yet been able to pass legislation that implements changes in physical education requirements. For example, in Georgia, legislation requiring 150 minutes per week of physical education in kindergarten through the fifth grade and plans for 225 minutes of physical education per week for sixth to eighth graders was defeated upon adjournment of the 2006 legislative session (NetScan, 2006). The National Conference of State Legislatures (NCSL) also found that few states have physical education requirements that specify the duration and frequency of physical education (Figure 7-1) (NCSL, 2006).

The National Association for Sport and Physical Education (NASPE), in partnership with the American Heart Association (AHA), recently released the *Shape of the Nation Report* on physical education in U.S. schools (NASPE and AHA, 2006). Although physical education is mandated in most states (e.g., 36 states mandate physical education for elementary-school students, 33 states mandate physical education for middle-school students, and 42 states mandate physical education for high-school students), far fewer states specify the number of minutes of physical education per week. Two states (Louisiana and New Jersey) mandate the recommended 150 or more minutes of weekly physical education for students (NASPE and AHA, 2006). Only 15 states require student assessment in physical education (NASPE and AHA, 2006). Health-related physical edu-

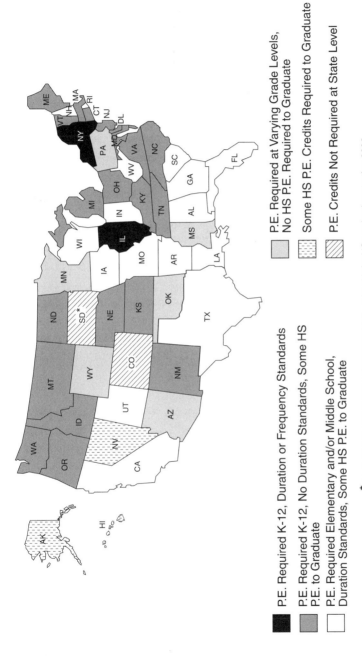

FIGURE 7-1 State physical education (PE) requirements, 2005. Reprinted, with permission, from the National Conference of State Legislatures (NCSL), 2006. SOURCE: NCSL (2006).

Legend:

■ P.E. Required K-12, Duration or Frequency Standards

▨ P.E. Required K-12, No Duration Standards, Some HS P.E. to Graduate

☐ P.E. Required Elementary and/or Middle School, Duration Standards, Some HS P.E. to Graduate

▨ P.E. Required at Varying Grade Levels, No HS P.E. Required to Graduate

▨ Some HS P.E. Credits Required to Graduate

▨ P.E. Credits Not Required at State Level

*South Dakota will require 1/2 credit of P.E. or health for HS graduation starting 2006

cation is the focus in some school districts with an emphasis on developing the skills and interest in lifelong physical activity (Pate et al., 2006).

Recess provides another opportunity in the school day for promoting physical activity among children and youth. In a recent U.S. Department of Education survey of 1,198 public elementary schools, 83 to 88 percent reported providing daily recess for students with the average number of minutes ranging from 27.8 minutes in first grade to 23.8 minutes in sixth grades; among these schools, the rates at which physical education classes were provided on a daily basis ranged from 17 to 22 percent across the elementary grades (Parsad and Lewis, 2006).

Although several organizations monitor state physical education policies, including the Trust for America's Health and the National Council of State Legislatures (Chapter 2), enforcement of state physical education standards and requirements is more difficult to monitor.

A variety of perceived barriers to increasing physical activity opportunities were shared by stakeholders at the committee's symposium in Wichita, Kansas (Appendix F). These include a lack of time throughout the school day due to the efforts that schools must make to meet the requirements for standardized testing and a lack of resources to develop or supplement intramural or other physical activity programs. A survey of physical education teachers in Texas working with the Coordinated Approach To Child Health (CATCH) program similarly reported that one of the greatest barriers to providing quality physical education is the low priority it is given relative to the priority given to other academic subjects (Barroso et al., 2005). Large class sizes and inadequate financial resources were also concerns.

Incorporating physical activity into the standard curriculum is a subject of study and exploration. Several programs, including Take 10!®, encourage teachers to allow students to be physically active as they answer questions, cite mathematics facts, or engage in other learning activities (Cardon et al., 2004; Donnelly, 2005; Lloyd et al., 2005; Stewart et al., 2004) (Chapter 3). The effects of implementing school-based and community-based physical activity programs is being examined through various research efforts, such as the National Institutes of Health (NIH)-funded Trial of Activity for Adolescent Girls, a randomized multicenter study involving girls in 36 middle schools across the country (Gittelsohn et al., 2006).

Many opportunities exist to promote physical activity in school and child-care settings. States, school districts, schools, preschools, and after-school and child-care programs should expand opportunities for physical activity. The federal government and state governments have responsibilities in increasing the capacity, standards, and resources needed to implement regular physical activity in schools. The U.S. Department of Education's Carol M. White Physical Education Program awarded more than

$73 million in grants to schools and communities in 2005, with each of the awards ranging from $75,000 to $650,000 to support physical education programs, including after-school programs, for students in kindergarten through 12th grade (DoEd, 2006b) (Appendix D). These efforts, in addition to those of the CDC and the President's Council on Physical Fitness and Sports (DHHS, 2006), should be strengthened, coordinated, sustained, and evaluated.

Intramural and Interscholastic Sports and Physical Activity Programs

Limited data are available to assess the extent to which intramural sports programs in schools are changing or the number of schools that are moving beyond competitive extramural athletics to expand opportunities for more students to participate in physical activity clubs. The 2005 Youth Sports National Report Card noted a strong concern about early sports specialization and a highly competitive atmosphere that is more focused on winning than encouraging children and youth to have fun, increase their fitness, or develop important skills (CTSA, 2006).

Awareness of the value of nontraditional physical activity programs as a component of school programs appears to be growing. Activities such as dance classes may attract students who have not shown an interest in other types of physical activity (Chapter 3). For example, West Virginia is incorporating a video-based dance game, Dance Dance Revolution®, into its physical education curriculum for public schools, in partnership with the game's producer, Konami Digital Entertainment. An evaluation of this effort is being conducted by a consortium that includes West Virginia University, the West Virginia Department of Education, Mountain State Blue Cross Blue Shield, and Konami (Konami Digital Entertainment, 2006).

Efforts to document innovative physical activity policies, programs, and success stories in schools are needed, similar to the efforts by CDC and USDA in documenting examples of changes to school food programs through publications such as *Making It Happen: School Nutrition Success Stories* (USDA, DHHS, and DoEd, 2005). Further, national surveillance systems should include a more extensive focus on intramural and other physical activity programs so that progress can be tracked on the nature and extent of these efforts.

Walking and Biking-to-School Programs

The level of progress made in increasing the number of students who walk or bike to and from school is difficult to assess. Comparisons of the 2006 SHPPS and SHP surveys with prior results may indicate the extent to which schools are more or less actively engaged in walking and biking programs, than they were in prior years. As discussed in Chapter 6, specific programs that have focused on improving sidewalks and crosswalks, or in providing supervision for active transport to school, have resulted in greater student participation. For example, in Marin County, California, the Safe Routes to School (SRTS) program included mapping efforts, promotional activities and contests, classroom education, and organized "walking school buses" and bike trains. Comparisons of the rates of walking and biking among students between fall 2000 and spring 2002 found a 64 percent increase in the number of students who walked to and from school and a 114 percent increase in the number of students cycling to school among students in the participating schools (Staunton et al., 2003). Community-school partnerships and other efforts to enhance programs that promote active transport to and from school are greatly needed.

Research efforts continue to explore the community, safety, built environment (e.g., intersection design, crosswalks), and other factors that relate to the success of active transport programs and initiatives (Boarnet et al., 2005; Carver et al., 2005; Sisson et al., 2006; Timperio et al., 2006). Efforts to evaluate these programs are under way in many areas (FHWA/DOT, 2006) (Chapter 2). The distances to school and traffic-related danger have been the most commonly reported barriers to children walking to and from school (Martin and Carlson, 2005). The National SRTS Clearinghouse promises to be a useful resource in disseminating information on evaluations of these programs (SRTS, 2006).

After-School Programs

After-school programs are increasingly being recognized as opportunities for increasing physical activity and providing fruits, vegetables, and other low-calorie and high-nutrient foods and beverages to children and youth. In addition to a number of informal programs in individual schools and community centers, several research-based approaches are being evaluated. For example, the CATCH program—which involves multiple modifications related to school food service, physical activity, and classroom curricula—piloted a CATCH Kids Club as an after-school program for elementary school students. The program underwent pilot testing in 16 after-school programs in Texas (Kelder et al., 2005) and involved an education component, in addition to snack and physical activity segments.

Similar research-based programs examining after-school opportunities include the Georgia FitKid Project, which involves third graders in an after-school program (Yin et al., 2005a,b); the Sports, Play, and Active Recreation for Kids (SPARK) After-School program (SPARK, 2006), and the Students and Parents Actively Involved in Being Fit After-School program, which works with African-American students and parents at urban middle schools in Michigan (Engels et al., 2005). As discussed in Chapter 6, the Girls Health Enrichment Multisite Studies (GEMS) funded by the National Heart, Lung, and Blood Institute (NHLBI) have examined pilot studies of after-school obesity prevention programs targeting African-American girls (Klesges et al., 2004, Robinson et al., 2003; Story et al., 2003) (Chapter 3), and subsequent full-scale trials are underway in Memphis, Tennessee, and Oakland, California.

As noted in the *Health in the Balance* report (IOM, 2005), after-school programs can be either school- or community-based and may vary widely in their content. Although the infrastructure for after-school programs is limited nationwide, organizations such as the Afterschool Alliance and the National Network of Statewide Afterschool Networks are focused on obesity prevention in children and youth and are working to include nutrition and physical activity guidelines for after-school programs into school wellness policies (Afterschool Alliance, 2006).

Use of Schools as Community Centers

A recent statewide survey of West Virginia schools found that 80.7 percent of schools permitted public access to outdoor physical activity facilities and 42.3 percent provided student and community access to indoor facilities beyond the usual school hours (O'Hara Tompkins et al., 2004). Similarly, a survey of schools in specific regions of four states (Maryland, Minneapolis, Mississippi, and North Carolina) found that of the 313 schools with outdoor physical activity facilities, 240 (77 percent) allowed some public use of the facilities. Among the 210 schools with indoor facilities, 134 (64 percent) permitted some public use (Evenson and McGinn, 2004). The reasons for not opening the school facilities to the public included supervision and personnel requirements, safety concerns, and insurance and liability issues. The benefits of permitting the public use of school facilities included positive publicity for the school and keeping children physically active.

Beyond individual surveys, surveillance of the extent of community use of school physical activity facilities is conducted through the SHP and the SHPPS surveys. Efforts in some communities to combine school and community needs often include a focus on the use of school athletic facilities and other space for sports, for activity classes, and as recreation centers (Box 7-6).

Evaluating Progress to Increase Physical Activity in Schools

As discussed earlier, several national surveillance systems examine the nature and the extent of physical activity opportunities in schools (Box 7-7).

BOX 7-6
Schools as Community Centers

Los Angeles County is examining the potential to use state school construction funds to create incentives for urban school districts and municipalities to jointly build mixed-use projects that co-locate schools with parks, libraries, health facilities, and other parts of the public infrastructure. Mixed-use concepts aim to meet both school and community needs such as having gymnasiums and play fields double as community parks and recreation centers. By utilizing school property after regular class hours and incorporating centralized libraries, health clinics and other community services, community access and engagement is increased. The state health department is also supporting these joint-use efforts, for example, by funding university research on legislative policies that the state might adopt to provide limited liability protection for the individuals and the organizations that provide space and facilities for physical activity opportunities.

SOURCE: NSBN (2002).

Several of these surveys (e.g., SHPPS, SHP) are collecting data in 2006 that will provide informative comparisons with data from prior years (Table 7-1). The 2006 SHPPS survey has a broad range of questions to assess students' physical activity at the state, district, school, and classroom levels. The resulting data are aggregated at the national and state levels and state report cards are categorized by whether the state requires or recommends various aspects of physical education (CDC, 2006d). Furthermore, the SHP study examines several aspects of physical activity with a focus on physical education requirements. SHP results are available in a format that compares individual states and cities with other participating states and cities (CDC, 2006e).

State- and district-level surveys are also valuable for the assessment of the progress that has been made. For example, West Virginia adapted some of the 2000 SHPPS survey questions for a statewide survey of opportunities for physical activity. Questions were also added to assess community recreation opportunities and walking safety (O'Hara Tompkins et al., 2004). Individual schools can track their progress in developing opportunities for physical activity through self-assessment tools such as the School Health Index. Possible enhancements of the SHI could include a greater emphasis on intramural physical activity opportunities. Tools such as CDC's Physical Education Curriculum Analysis Tool provide valuable technical assistance in evaluating physical activity-related curricula (CDC, 2006c).

Tracking the physical fitness progress of individual students is also an important evaluation measure. The tracking tools that schools use include

---

BOX 7-7
Examples of Survey Questions on
Increasing Physical Activity Levels in Schools

2006 SHPPS School District Questionnaire (CDC, 2006h)
- Does your district require or recommend that elementary schools provide students with regularly scheduled recess?
- How many minutes per day of recess are required or recommended for elementary school students?
- Has your district adopted a policy that prohibits elementary schools from excluding students from all or part of recess as punishment for bad behavior?

2005 YRBSS (CDC, 2006f)
- In an average week when you are in school, how many days do you go to physical education classes?
- During an average physical education class, how many minutes do you spend actually exercising or playing sports?
- During the past 12 months, on how many sports teams (school and community) did you play?

SHP 2006 School Principal Questionnaire (CDC, 2006g)
- Does this school offer opportunities for students to participate in intramural activities or physical activity clubs?
- Does your school promote walking or biking to and from school?
- How many required physical education courses do students take in grades 6 through 12 in this school?
- Can students be exempted from taking a required physical education course for one grading period or longer for any of the following reasons [list of reasons follows in the questionnaire]?

SHI for Middle and High Schools (CDC, 2005)
- Do all students in each grade receive physical education for at least 225 minutes per week throughout the school year?
- Are students moderately to vigorously active for at least 50 percent of the class time?

---

the Fitnessgram/Activitygram® and the President's Challenge (President's Challenge, 2006). Both of these tools compare a student's performance on a set of physical fitness tests with fitness standards specific to the student's age and gender. The President's Challenge also offers a health fitness test, an active lifestyle program, and the Presidential Champion's program. As discussed below, there is wide variation in the extent and the manner in which schools report the student's physical fitness results to parents and caregivers.

A number of states have awards programs for students, school personnel, schools, and school districts that have demonstrated progress in increasing physical fitness or physical activity levels. For example, in Michigan the Governor's Council on Physical Fitness, Health, and Sports and the Michigan Fitness Foundation recognize school districts and teachers that provide high-quality physical education (Michigan Governor's Council on Physical Fitness, Health, and Sports, 2006). The Virginia Department of Education (2006) offers a physical activity award program to school personnel (Virginia Department of Education, 2006), and Indiana offers the Governor's Physical Fitness Award to students at all levels (Indiana Governor's Council for Physical Activity and Sports, 2006).

Behavioral Nutrition and Physical Activity Curricula

Curricula aimed at improving nutrition and physical activity behaviors have been developed in research settings and are available for dissemination to schools. These curricula focus on skill-building activities and provide students with the opportunity to set goals, engage in the desired behaviors, self-monitor their efforts, and receive feedback, as well as provide incentives and reinforcement of positive lifestyle changes. Examples include curricula for reducing leisure screen time for third and fourth graders (Robinson, 1999; Stanford SMART, 2006) and improving nutrition and physical activity among middle school students (Bauer et al., 2006; Gortmaker et al., 1999).

Some indicators of progress in offering health education related to physical activity and nutrition are available by comparing the 2002 and 2004 results of the SHP survey, which found an increase across states in the percentage of schools that required health education courses included information on choosing a variety of fruits and vegetables daily (from 84.6 to 89.8 percent), preparing healthy meals and snacks (from 74.0 to 82.7 percent), and aiming for a healthy weight (from 86.3 to 93.5 percent), although decreases in providing information about choosing a variety of grains daily were seen (91.5 to 86.4 percent) (Grunbaum et al., 2005). Information is limited on which to assess whether or not these courses have a behavioral skills focus instead of an educational or informational focus. The 2006 SHPPS survey may help provide data on this aspect of health curricula, as it includes questions about goal setting, decision making, self-monitoring, and other behavioral skills. Greater attention should be focused on implementing and evaluating the outcomes of behaviorally focused curricula.

School Health and Student Assessments

School health services are the focus of attention in programs such as CDC's comprehensive school health programs. However, it is difficult to assess whether progress in involving school health services in obesity prevention efforts is being made. The committee did not find a systematic assessment of obesity prevention efforts in school health services, which indicates a need for a comprehensive evaluation. SHPPS has a section devoted to school health services with relevant questions focused on school screening for height, weight, or BMI. The upcoming results from the 2006 SHPPS may provide insight into current screening efforts.

Assessments of the weight, height, and BMI of each student are implemented in some states as an additional form of health screening, similar to screening for vision or hearing problems (Scheier, 2004). Concerns regarding BMI screening have focused on protecting the privacy of students and ensuring that, along with the screening results, information is provided to assist students and parents in determining next steps and reducing the potential negative impact of the results on students' mental health.

Arkansas was one of the first states to actively explore and implement assessments of the weight, height, and BMI of each student in which the results are reported to parents and guardians (Ryan et al., 2006). In addition to other provisions regarding childhood obesity prevention, the Arkansas Act 1220 (enacted in 2003) mandated that parents be provided with an annual measure of their child's BMI, along with an explanation of BMI and the health effects associated with childhood obesity. The recently completed year 2 evaluation of Arkansas Act 1220 was conducted through surveys of school principals, school district superintendents, and licensed Arkansas pediatricians, as well as telephone interviews with a randomly selected sample of families (e.g., parents and adolescents were interviewed if consent was obtained), site visits to assess the presence and content of school vending machines, and interviews with key officials (University of Arkansas for Medical Sciences, 2006). The evaluation found that parents and adolescents were generally accepting of BMI measurements and comfortable with the confidentiality provisions. Parents had increased their awareness of the health consequences of obesity, and increased numbers of families reported changes in planning and preparation of healthier meals. Potential negative outcomes or consequences—such as teasing, use of diet pills, or skipping meals—have not detectably increased with the distribution of BMI measurements compared with those at the baseline assessments. School principals and superintendents reported that some parents expressed concerns regarding the assessments; however, approximately one-third (34 percent) of the superintendents reported that no parent had contacted them about the BMI reporting issues and 75 percent had been contacted by less than 10 parents.

Other states are also assessing student BMI levels or are planning similar assessments. Illinois requires schools to measure BMIs in their first-, fifth-, and ninth-grade students, and California schools measure BMI levels in the fifth, seventh, and ninth grade (NASPE and AHA, 2006). In September 2005, the Pennsylvania Department of Health began a growth screening program that required BMIs to be determined during annual screenings in kindergarten through the fourth grade; in the 2006–2007 school year this will extend up to the eighth grade, and in 2007–2008 it will encompass all students (PANA, 2006).

Evidence gathered from the studies conducted by Arkansas and evaluations of BMI assessment programs in other states will be valuable in clarifying the impact of BMI reporting. Similar issues are being evaluated in school systems that provide the results of physical fitness testing to students and parents.

Advertising in Schools

A recent IOM report focused on food marketing to children and youth examined issues related to commercial activities in schools including product sales, direct and indirect advertising, and conducting marketing research on students (IOM, 2006b). The *Health in the Balance* report recommended that state and local education authorities and schools should develop, implement, and enforce school policies to create schools that are advertising-free to the greatest possible extent (IOM, 2005). The San Francisco Unified School District Board of Education was an early leader on this issue. In 1999, the board passed the Commercial-Free Schools Act that prohibited food and tobacco advertising in educational settings (Wynns and Chin, 1999). More recent attention on this issue includes the efforts by the National Association of Secondary School Principals in developing guidelines for partnerships between schools and beverage companies that address the use of logos and signage on school grounds and the visibility of company logos (NASSP, 2004). A recent survey of 20 California high schools found that nearly 65 percent of vending machine advertisements were for sweetened beverages and that 60 percent of the posters for products were for foods or beverages that were high in fat, sugar, or sodium or low in nutrients (Craypo et al., 2006). Advertising by soft drink companies is examined by the SHPPS survey. Research and evaluations are needed to assess the ongoing trends in advertising and other commercial activities in schools and to examine whether changes in the school environment with regard to advertising can be linked to improved dietary and physical activity behaviors and health outcomes of children and youth.

Evaluation of School Programs and Policies

With the numerous programs, interventions, and policy changes being implemented in schools, it is important that they be evaluated and that those found to be effective be disseminated to other schools.

As noted earlier, the SHI is a self-assessment and planning tool designed to provide schools with a systematic means of assessing progress and planning for changes. Several elementary schools in Rhode Island used the SHI to assess their physical activity and nutrition environments and to evaluate the outcomes of a school-based intervention. The outcome measures included changes in the SHI module scores from the baseline point (October 2002) to the end of the school year (June 2003) and changes in the number of relevant policies that had been developed and implemented (Pearlman et al., 2005). A study of the use of the SHI in schools in Arizona with a high predominance of Hispanic/Latino students from low-income families found that external factors were often associated with changing policies and implementing recommendations (Austin et al., 2006; Staten et al., 2005). Both studies found similar perceived barriers to implementing nutrition and physical activity changes, including pressures to focus on reading and math test scores, low staff morale, budgetary concerns, and inconsistent support from the school administrators (Pearlman et al., 2005).

A recent study by Brener and colleagues (2006) matched school and classroom-level data from the SHPPS 2000 with comparable questions in the SHI to examine the percentage of schools meeting the SHI recommendations in four areas: school health and safety policies and environment; health education; physical education and other physical activity programs; and nutrition services. The study found that most schools are addressing school health issues to some extent, but few schools are providing a comprehensive approach. For example, the analysis of elementary school responses in SHPPS found that 38.2 percent had credentialed physical education teachers, 20.2 percent had a teacher-student ratio for physical education comparable to the ratio for classroom instruction, and only 8.0 percent met the SHI levels of 150 minutes of physical education per week (Brener et al., 2006). Data set linkages of this sort are useful in providing progress assessments.

It will be important for research and evaluation efforts to assess whether process and policy outcomes, such as those included in the School Health Index, lead to associated improvements in dietary and physical activity outcomes. A 2006 initiative of CDC, in partnership with the American School Health Association and corporate sponsors, will provide small grants to schools to support physical activity- or nutrition-related activities that are part of action plans developed through the use of the SHI (CDC, 2006a).

APPLYING THE EVALUATION FRAMEWORK TO SCHOOLS

What Constitutes Progress for Schools?

Progress resulting from changes in school-based programs and policies can be assessed through the evaluation of a range of intermediate-term and long-term outcomes. The evaluation framework introduced in Chapter 2 can be used to consider issues in evaluating school policies, programs, and other interventions. Two examples are provided: one focuses on efforts to implement after-school extracurricular physical activity opportunities and the other focuses on evaluating efforts to increase the use of schools as community centers (Figures 7-2 and 7-3). Intermediate outcomes (e.g., revising and enforcing school policies, coordinating schedules, and enhancing facilities) are important in both of these examples, as these changes are needed in order to improve access to and availability of facilities and opportunities for families and children to engage in physical activity.

Structural and systemic outcomes include the legislative and policy changes, often made by the state legislature or local school district, that pave the way for positive changes to the school environment. Examples include the implementation of school wellness policies, policies regarding comprehensive school health programs, legislative or regulatory adoption or changes in school nutrition standards, and legislative or administrative changes in physical activity requirements.

Changes in the school environment to promote more healthful behaviors are intermediate outcomes that denote increased opportunities for physical activity and healthful eating. These include increased availability of fruits and vegetables through food service choices, self-serve salad bars, or vending machines; reduced availability of high-calorie, high-sugar, and/ or high-fat foods and beverages available as à la carte items or in vending machines; increased duration, quality, and variety of physical activity classes; increased opportunities for physical activity through intramural sports and other avenues; an increased emphasis on nutrition- and physical activity-related topics in health education and other classroom curricula; and the support and promotion of walking- and biking-to-school programs.

Individual- and population-level outcomes include individual student and school population consumption of fruits, vegetables, and other low-calorie and high nutrient foods and beverages and improved physical activity testing levels and reduced sedentary behaviors. Health outcomes include reduced BMI levels in the population, reduced obesity prevalence and related morbidity, and improved child and adolescent health.

As noted throughout the report, evaluation does not need to be a complex process. Policy-monitoring efforts can report on specific state- or local-level legislative or policy changes. For individual schools and child-

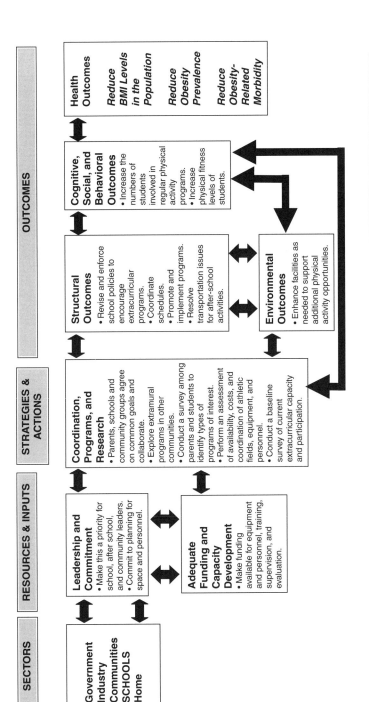

FIGURE 7-2 Evaluating school efforts to increase extracurricular opportunities for children and youth to engage in regular physical activity.

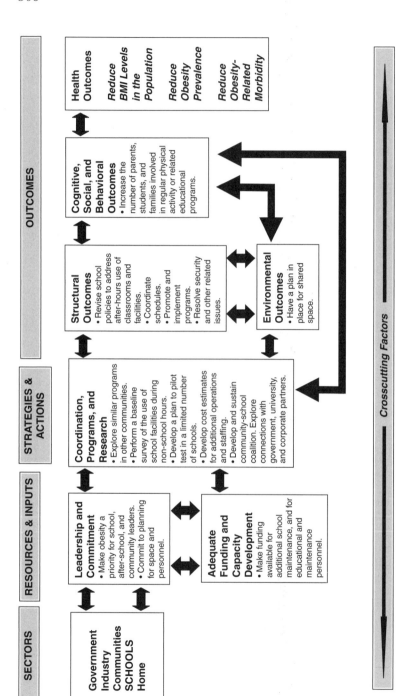

FIGURE 7-3 Evaluating school efforts to increase the use of schools as community centers.

care programs, outcomes could be as basic as developing and implementing a local school wellness policy; completing the needed capital improvements on sidewalks and street crossings in a community that allows children to walk and bicycle to school; increasing student awareness about the importance of healthful diets and physical activity; enhancing student knowledge about energy balance at a healthy weight; increasing the number of students who walk or bicycle to school; increasing the number of students participating in intramural programs over time; and improving the physical fitness levels of students. Specific interventions, such as a spring intramural track program, could base its evaluation on participation but could also collect baseline data on a measure of physical fitness (e.g., the time that it takes each student to run a mile) and at the end of the season assess each student's progress. Additionally, schools can assess their overall progress toward achieving a healthy school environment by using self-assessment tools such as the SHI. Initial evaluation efforts often focus on process evaluation and then move toward linking changes in process or programs with behavioral and health outcomes (Box 7-8). The collection of baseline data is always an important first step.

NEEDS AND NEXT STEPS IN ASSESSING PROGRESS

In the midst of the numerous changes that have been made in schools to promote healthy lifestyles, the committee was encouraged by the number of resources that are currently available to monitor progress in schools at the national and the state levels. However, few of the data sets provide details at the local level. Furthermore, linkages between surveillance systems could provide needed insights into how environmental changes in schools are

---

BOX 7-8
Examples of Outcome Measures for Schools, Preschools,
and Child-Care and After-School Programs

- Changes in the amount of time that students spend being active.
- Proportion of physical education time spent being physically active.
- Changes in before- and after-school physical activity opportunities.
- Meal participation rates for school breakfast and lunch.
- Performance on student fitness tests.
- Number of schools that provide self-serve salad bars.
- Extent of student consumption of fruits and vegetables.
- Frequency of using food and other non-food incentives as rewards for behaviors.

SOURCES: Boyle et al. (2004); Connecticut State Department of Education (2006).

affecting food and beverage choices, physical activity levels, or other relevant behavioral changes. Evaluating a range of outcomes of school-based programs and interventions appears to be occurring only on a limited basis, at least in part because of the lack of emphasis on evaluation and limited time and resources.

Although the committee could explore only a small subset of the ongoing efforts by states, localities, school districts, and schools in implementing and evaluating obesity prevention policies and interventions, it is apparent that throughout the country there are wide differences in the resources available, the level of evaluation activity, and the extent of commitment to improving the school environment to promote healthy lifestyles. Some schools have implemented extensive changes, with wellness policies in place and improvements occurring in the foods and beverages they offer, the relevant curricula that they present, and the opportunities for physical activity that they provide. Other schools have not yet made changes or are focused on only one aspect of the school environment. Often, the first area of change is in the food and beverage choices made available to students.

The committee urges continued efforts to promote a healthy school environment that encompasses a breadth of changes relevant to nutrition and physical activity and extensive evaluation, as suggested in the *Health in the Balance* report (IOM, 2005). Additionally, emphasis must be placed on evaluating nutrition and physical activity in child-care, after-school, and preschool settings.

Each of the committee's four recommendations is directly relevant to improving the efforts to evaluate school-based interventions, policies, and initiatives. The following section highlights the specific implementation actions needed.

Promote Leadership and Collaboration

Given the multiple competing priorities that schools are asked to address—priorities that cover an array of academic, social, and health concerns—there has been a tendency until recently to pay less attention to efforts related to nutrition and physical activity. Leadership is needed at the federal, state, school district, and school levels to:

- recognize childhood obesity as a serious health concern;
- implement and prioritize the changes needed to improve nutrition and increase physical activity;
- establish the expectation and the tracking mechanisms to ensure that standards are followed; and
- foster creativity and student and parent involvement in developing,

refining, implementing, and evaluating policies, programs, and other interventions relevant to childhood obesity prevention.

Federal and state leadership is needed in providing adequate and sustained resources to implement changes relevant to obesity prevention in the school environment. Not only are political will and leadership needed to improve school nutrition and physical activity opportunities, but it is critically important that adequate and sustained funding be provided to reinforce these priorities so that attention to this issue does not result in unfunded mandates.

Develop, Sustain, and Support Evaluation Capacity and Implementation

Evaluation is vital to schools, school districts, localities, and states in determining if their initiatives are producing an impact and are effectively using the limited available resources. Currently, the evidence base on the effectiveness of school-based policy change and interventions is quite slim (Katz et al., 2005). Despite its central importance, however, limited resources to date have been devoted to evaluation efforts. As the committee heard at its Wichita symposium (Appendix F), many schools and school officials acknowledge the need for evaluations but often report that they do not have the skills, expertise, time, personnel, or financial resources to implement evaluation efforts.

One of the critical areas needing technical support and focused attention is evaluation of the effectiveness of individual programs and interventions. Individual teachers, schools, school districts, preschools, and afterschool and child care programs are implementing innovative changes that need to be assessed. It is also desirable to evaluate the obesity prevention-related policies, programs, and practices of individual schools. These evaluation efforts will need to range from rigorous randomized controlled trials to determine the specific outcomes of specific interventions for specific populations to observational assessments of the associations between outcomes at all levels and the policies and practices in single classrooms, single schools, or groups of schools.

In order to initiate evaluation efforts, the committee recommends that funding be made available through CDC, USDA, and other federal agencies to provide technical assistance support through the development and dissemination of evaluation materials; the expansion of opportunities for evaluation-related training; and increases in the numbers of technical assistance personnel who are available to assist with evaluation efforts in states, localities, and school districts. Furthermore, the evaluation of obesity-prevention efforts should be made a priority and a necessary component of school-based interventions. Partnerships between schools and school districts and their neighboring universities, colleges, public health departments, foundations and other public and private agencies and entities that have the requisite experience and skills in developing and conducting evaluations need to be developed and encouraged.

Enhance Surveillance, Monitoring, and Research

Expand and Fully Utilize Current Surveillance Systems and Tools

One of the strengths for assessing progress in obesity prevention in the school setting is the range of surveillance and assessment tools that have been developed and implemented in recent years. Because of the interest in collecting data from and about the school setting, it may be easier to assess progress in the school setting than for most, if not all, of the other relevant settings. However, despite the availability of data, gaps remain in the age groups surveyed, the depth and nature of the questions asked and the information collected, the size and representativeness of the samples surveyed, and the ability to retrieve data on a specific state or city. Furthermore, it is difficult to link changes in individual behaviors with changes in the school environment and the availability of data does not guarantee that appropriate feedback will be communicated to policy makers, schools and individuals or that the changes that result are guided by the evidence. Enhancements to current surveillance systems are needed to increase the utility of the information to policy makers and decision makers, and those who work with the students on a daily basis. A number of improvements are under way or should be implemented.

CDC is developing and testing a new component of the YRBSS that will focus on physical activity and nutrition and plans to administer it in 2010. The committee supports this effort to collect more extensive information on students' dietary and physical activity behaviors and hopes that this survey will be conducted by a number of states at the middle school and perhaps upper elementary school levels.

Innovations in monitoring changes in the school foodservice environment also deserve additional emphasis. The third School Nutrition Dietary Assessment Study (SNDA) is currently being conducted and analyzed by USDA. Previous SNDA studies were conducted in the 1991–1992 and 1998–1999 school years and provide comparative data. Efforts are needed by USDA and other agencies and organizations to further monitor and assess changes in food and beverage purchases and consumption. Innovative evaluation strategies should be explored. Marketing data and some limited data on the foods and beverages that students consume in schools are available. Strategies and mechanisms need to be in place to allow local-level monitoring of the outcomes related to changes in the foods and beverages made available to students on sales and consumption.

SHPPS is conducted only every six years so short-term incremental changes in policies and practices are difficult to detect. Even every 6 years, however, the fact that this survey is repeated periodically with consistency in its methods and content makes it one of the most promising sources for assessing progress over time. The committee feels that the SHPPS data appear to have been underutilized. Increased analysis and dissemination of the SHPPS results and trends are needed. Given the numerous changes implemented by states and school districts, SHPPS is a vital resource for tracking progress and identifying areas needing refined interventions. Ideally, SHPPS (or separate modules of SHPPS) could be administered and the data could be aggregated at a more local level to allow progress to be tracked in schools in large metropolitan areas (as is done for the School Health Profiles study) or in other school districts that could potentially help fund the data collection and analysis. The timeliness of the 2006 SHPPS data collection, given the recent interest in improving the school environment, will provide an opportunity for analyses of the accomplishments that have been made and of the ongoing gaps and needs for further improvement.

Implement a National Survey Focused on Physical Activity

School-based efforts often focus on changing food and beverage availability, but less attention is devoted to physical activity. More needs to be learned about progress in increasing the physical activity levels and fitness of the nation's students. The last comprehensive evaluation of this issue was in the late 1980s through the first National Children and Youth Fitness Study (NCYFS I) (1984), the President's Council on Physical Fitness and Sports School Population Fitness Survey (1985), and a second NCYFS (1987) (Brandt and McGinnis, 1985; Pate and Ross, 1987). An ongoing survey of physical activity levels and physical fitness—spanning from children and youth, preschool through adolescence—should be explored and should be conducted, either as a stand-alone survey or as a component of a current national surveillance system such as NHANES that has sustained long-term funding to track the progress of a representative sample of children and youth.

Support Research

Current measures for measuring the physical activity levels of children and youth are often cumbersome or intrusive. Pilot studies for the expanded YRBSS focused on physical activity and nutrition could provide opportunities for exploring various approaches to measurement. Similarly, research on more accurate methods of measuring the dietary intake of children and youth is needed (IOM, 2006b). Measures, such as 24-hour food intake logs, are subject to the inconsistencies and other challenges of self-reported data, and other measures, such as assessing plate waste, are difficult and time consuming to obtain.

Expand and Adapt Self-Assessment Tools for Schools, Preschools, Child-Care, and After-School Programs

The SHI is a potentially useful tool that could serve as a model for similar types of self-assessment tools for preschools, after-school programs, or child-care programs. Although these settings are often independent and frequently decentralized in the manner in which they are administered, it would be valuable to develop a health index for each of these settings and encourage the dissemination of the self-assessment tools through relevant professional associations and organizations. It will also be important to assess whether performance on these tools predicts subsequent improvements in nutrition and physical activity behaviors and health outcomes.

Link Data Sets

Opportunities for linking data sets also need to be explored to allow geographic and school-level matching of policy and program outcomes with behavioral and health outcomes. The linking of these data sets has the potential to allow tracking of these associations over time. If the systematic use of the SHI could be linked with assessments of the school environment and student health behaviors and health status, such as through the YRBSS, schools could obtain substantial guidance on implementing the most promising policy-related strategies for the prevention of obesity.

Disseminate and Use Evaluation Results

The added value of an emphasis on surveillance, monitoring, and evaluation is in the lessons learned and the evidence gained from assessments of whether specific interventions and policies have a positive impact on improving nutrition, increasing physical activity, and reducing childhood obesity. As discussed in Chapter 2, there is much to be learned from those efforts that are both effective and ineffective in achieving the desired intermediate and long-term outcomes. Successful efforts need to be replicated, scaled up, and evaluated to be further refined. Unsuccessful efforts should be substantially changed and reevaluated or discontinued. In either case, the dissemination of evaluation results is crucial.

The lessons learned need to be disseminated through the traditional mechanisms, such as through presentations at professional meetings and the publication of findings in professional journals. They also, however, need to be disseminated through innovative mechanisms that can provide teachers, principals, school administrators, and food service personnel with examples of specific interventions that can be implemented. Sharing the innovative changes through publications with concrete examples and details, such as the recent compilation by CDC and USDA of innovations in school food and beverages, *Making It Happen: School Nutrition Success Stories*, should be continued. Such publications should provide as much detail on the intervention and on the results of its evaluation as possible.

Mechanisms to incentivize evaluation and disseminate promising practices include the provision of awards or recognition for schools or school districts that implement and evaluate relevant programs and policies and that are able to demonstrate positive changes on the path to obesity prevention. For example, the Keystone Healthy Zone Schools program in Pennsylvania provides schools with technical assistance in improving the school wellness environment and offers competitive minigrant funding to make improvements. The program also assists schools with collecting benchmark measures of progress and actively disseminates school success stories through its website (Keystone Healthy Zone, 2006). Another example is the Utah Gold Medal Schools program, which was begun just before the 2002 Olympic Games. With the support of the Utah Department of Health, Intermountain Healthcare and other organizations, the program offers incentives for schools that implement policies and programs focused on increasing physical activity, improving nutrition, and reducing tobacco use (Utah Department of Health, 2006). In addition to bronze, silver, and gold awards, schools can work toward the platinum award, which in addition to other nutrition- and physical activity-related stipulations, requires the involvement of families and the community in health-related efforts; a policy of selling only food and beverage choices that contribute to healthful diets at school events, in vending machines, and at school stores; policies that ensure that meal periods are of the appropriate length or policies that schedule recess before lunch; and the implementation of a faculty wellness program (Utah Department of Health, 2006).

SUMMARY AND RECOMMENDATIONS

Current childhood obesity prevention efforts are largely focused on changes in the school environment, with much of the attention on improving the nutritional quality and the portion sizes of the foods and beverages made available in schools. Momentum related to promoting increased opportunities for physical activity seems to be growing; however, the limited time available in the school day and the many competing demands on school time are presenting obstacles to these efforts.

Similar to community obesity prevention efforts, wide variations in the extent of resources and the amount of effort devoted to increasing physical activity and making changes in the school nutrition environment are seen across states, school districts, and individual schools. Wide variations in other areas, such as improving the school curriculum on energy balance, discouraging branded marketing in schools, and assessing and communicating student BMI and fitness levels, as well as the collaborative efforts between schools and communities to use schools as community centers, are also found. Less attention appears to be being paid to improving nutrition and increasing the levels of physical activity in the preschool, child-care, and after-school environments, although again, some locations are quite focused on this issue, whereas others are not yet engaged.

Throughout the nation there appears to be only limited efforts to evaluate the many policies and programs being implemented in states, local school districts, individual schools, and classrooms. Each of the report's four recommendations (Chapter 2) is directly relevant to promoting leadership and collaboration and improving the evaluation of school-based childhood obesity prevention efforts. The following provides the report's recommendations and summarizes the specific implementation actions (detailed in the preceding sections) that are needed to improve childhood obesity prevention efforts in schools.

Recommendation 1: Government, industry, communities, schools, and families should demonstrate leadership and commitment by mobilizing the resources required to identify, implement, evaluate, and disseminate effective policies and interventions that support childhood obesity prevention goals.

Implementation Actions for Schools
School boards, administrators, and staff should elevate the priority that is placed on creating and sustaining a healthy school environment and advance school policies and programs that support this priority.

To accomplish this:
- Relevant federal and state agencies and departments, local school districts, individual schools and preschools, and child-care and after-school programs should prioritize opportunities for physical activity and expand the availability and access in schools to fruits, vegetables, and other low-calorie and high nutrient foods and beverages that contribute to healthful diets.

Increased resources are needed to develop, implement, and evaluate policies and programs. State and local school-based nutrition and physical activity standards need to be implemented, and the relevant educational entities should be held accountable for promoting and adhering to these standards.

Recommendation 2: Policy makers, program planners, program implementers, and other interested stakeholders—within and across relevant sectors—should evaluate all childhood obesity prevention efforts, strengthen the evaluation capacity, and develop quality interventions that take into account diverse perspectives, that use culturally relevant approaches, and that meet the needs of diverse populations and contexts.

Implementation Actions for Schools
Schools and school districts should strengthen evaluation efforts by partnering with state and federal agencies, foundations, and academic institutions to develop, implement, and support evaluations of all relevant school-based programs.

To accomplish this:
Federal agencies (e.g., CDC, USDA, Department of Education), state departments of education and health, foundations, academic institutions, school districts, and local schools should
- Increase the resources devoted to technical assistance for evaluating school-based childhood obesity prevention policies, programs, and interventions and
- Develop partnerships to fund, develop, and implement childhood obesity prevention evaluations.

Recommendation 3: Government, industry, communities, and schools should expand or develop relevant surveillance and monitoring systems and, as applicable, should engage in research to examine the impact of childhood obesity prevention policies, interventions, and actions on relevant outcomes, paying particular attention to the unique needs of diverse groups and high-risk populations. Additionally, parents and caregivers should monitor changes in their family's food, beverage, and physical activity choices and their progress toward healthier lifestyles.

Implementation Actions for Schools
Schools and school districts should conduct self-assessments to enhance and sustain a healthy school environment, and mechanisms

for examining links between changes in the school environment and behavioral and health outcomes should be explored.

To accomplish this:
Relevant federal agencies (e.g., CDC, NIH, USDA, and the Department of Education), state education departments, school districts, and local schools should

- Expand and fully use current surveillance systems related to children's dietary and physical activities, obesity-related health indicators, and relevant school policies and programs;
- Implement a national survey focused on the physical activity behaviors of all children and youth;
- Support research on means to improve the monitoring of diet and physical activity;
- Establish mechanisms to link health, educational, economic, and sociological data sources across a variety of areas related to childhood obesity prevention; and
- Expand and adapt self-assessment tools for schools, preschools, child-care, and after-school programs and evaluate their validity for predicting changes in children's levels of physical activity, dietary intakes, and weight.

Recommendation 4: Government, industry, communities, schools, and families should foster information-sharing activities and disseminate evaluation and research findings through diverse communication channels and media to actively promote the use and scaling up of effective childhood obesity prevention policies and interventions.

Implementation Actions for Schools
Schools should partner with government, professional associations, academic institutions, parent-teacher organizations, foundations, communities, and the media to publish and widely disseminate the evaluation results of school-based childhood obesity prevention efforts and related materials and methods.

To accomplish this:
- Schools, preschools, child-care and after-school programs, and relevant stakeholders should broadly disseminate the evaluation results using diverse communication channels and media and develop incentives to encourage the use of promising practices.

REFERENCES

Action for Healthy Kids. 2006. *Wellness Policy Development Tool.* [Online]. Available: http://actionforhealthykids.org/wellnesstool/index.html [accessed July 6, 2006].

Afterschool Alliance. 2006. *After School and Children's Health.* [Online]. Available: http://www.afterschoolalliance.org/active_hours_ob_kit.cfm [accessed May 16, 2006].

Alliance for a Healthier Generation. 2006. *Alliance for a Healthier Generation and Industry Leaders Set Healthy School Beverage Guidelines for U.S. Schools.* [Online]. Available: http://www.healthiergeneration.org/docs/ afhg_nr_school_beverage_5-3-06.pdf [accessed July 7, 2006].

Andersen K, Caldwell D, Dunn C, Hoggard L, Thaxton S, Thomas C. 2004. *Eat Smart: NC's Recommended Standards for All Foods Available in School.* Raleigh, NC: North Carolina Division of Public Health.

Austin SB, Fung T, Bearak AC, Wardle K, Cheung LWY. 2006. Facilitating change in school health: A qualitative study of schools' experiences using the School Health Index. *Prev Chronic Dis* [Online]. Available: http://www.cdc.gov/Pcd/issues/2006/apr/05_0116.htm [accessed July 23, 2006].

Bachman CM, Baranowski T, Nicklas T. 2006. Is there an association between sweetened beverages and adiposity? *Nutr Rev* 64(4):153–174.

Barroso CS, McCullum-Gomez C, Hoelscher DM, Kelder SH, Murray NG. 2005. Self-reported barriers to quality physical education by physical education specialists in Texas. *J School Health* 75(8):313–319.

Bauer KW, Patel A, Prokop LA, Austin SB. 2006. Swimming upstream: Faculty and staff members from urban middle schools in low-income communities describe their experience implementing nutrition and physical activity initiatives. *Prev Chronic Dis* [Online]. Available: http://www.cdc.gov/Pcd/issues/2006/apr/05_0113.htm [accessed July 23, 2006].

Boarnet MG, Anderson CL, Day K, McMillan T, Alfonzo M. 2005. Evaluation of the California Safe Routes to School legislation: Urban form changes and children's active transportation to school. *Am J Prev Med* 28(2 Suppl 2):134–140.

Boyle M, Purciel M, Craypo L, Stone-Francisco S, Samuels S. 2004. *National Evaluation & Measurement Meeting on School Nutrition and Physical Activity Policies.* Conducted by Samuels & Associates. Commissioned by The Robert Wood Johnson Foundation and The California Endowment.

Brandt EN Jr, McGinnis JM.1985. National Children and Youth Fitness Study: Its contribution to our national objectives. *Public Health Rep* 100(1):1–3.

Brener ND, Pejavara A, Barrios LC, Crossett L, Lee SM, McKenna M, Michael S, Wechsler H. 2006. Applying the school health index to a nationally representative sample of schools. *J School Health* 76(2):57–66.

Buzby JC, Guthrie JF, Kantor LS. 2003. *Evaluation of the USDA Fruit and Vegetable Pilot Program: Report to Congress.* E-FAN-03-006. Washington, DC: USDA. [Online]. Available: http://www.fns.usda.gov/cnd/Research/FV030063.pdf [accessed May 8, 2006].

California Endowment. 2006. *Beverage Vending Machines in California High Schools.* [Online]. Available: http://www.calendow.org/reference/publications/pdf/disparities/Beverage%20Vending%20Brief.pdf [accessed July 14, 2006].

Cardon G, De Clercq D, De Bourdeaudhuij I, Breithecker D. 2004. Sitting habits in elementary schoolchildren: A traditional versus a "moving school." *Patient Educ Couns* 54(2): 133–142.

Carver A, Salmon J, Campbell K, Baur L, Garnett S, Crawford D. 2005. How do perceptions of local neighborhood relate to adolescents' walking and cycling? *Am J Health Promot* 20(2):139–147.

CDC (Centers for Disease Control and Prevention). 2005. *School Health Index: A Self-Assessment and Planning Guide, Middle School, High School.* [Online]. Available: http://apps.nccd.cdc.gov/shi [accessed August 1, 2006].

CDC. 2006a. *School Health Index (SHI): Mini-Grants for Physical Activity and Nutrition Improvements.* [Online]. Available: http://www.cdc.gov/HealthyYouth/SHI/grants.htm [accessed February 14, 2006].

CDC. 2006b. *SHPPS 2006 Questionnaires.* [Online]. Available: http://www.cdc.gov/healthy youth/shpps/2006/questionnaires.htm [accessed May 17, 2006].

CDC. 2006c. *Physical Education Curriculum Analysis Tool.* [Online]. Available: http://www.cdc.gov/healthyyouth/PECAT/index.htm [accessed May 24, 2006].

CDC. 2006d. *SHPPS 2000, State Health Report Cards.* [Online]. Available: http://www.cdc.gov/HealthyYouth/shpps/report_cards/index.htm [accessed May 25, 2006].

CDC. 2006e. *School Health Profiles, State and District Fact Sheets.* [Online]. Available: http://www.cdc.gov/healthyyouth/profiles/facts.htm [accessed May 25, 2006].

CDC. 2006f. *2005 State and Local Youth Risk Behavior Survey.* [Online]. Available: http://www.cdc.gov/HealthyYouth/yrbs/pdfs/2005highschoolquestionnaire.pdf [accessed May 25, 2006].

CDC. 2006g. *2006 School Health Profile School Principal Questionnaire.* [Online]. Available: http://www.cdc.gov/Healthyyouth/profiles/2006/QuestionnaireP.pdf [accessed July 12, 2006].

CDC. 2006h. *SHPPS 2006, Physical Education District Questionnaire.* [Online]. Available: http://www.cdc.gov/HealthyYouth/SHPPS/2006/pdf/pe-district.txt [accessed May 26, 2006].

CNWICRA (Child Nutrition and WIC Reauthorization Act). 2004. *Child Nutrition and WIC Reauthorization Act of 2004.* PL 108-265. 108th Congress. June 30, 2004. [Online]. Available: http://www.fns.usda.gov/cnd/Governance/Legislation/PL_108-265.pdf [accessed March 22, 2006].

Connecticut State Department of Education. 2006. *Action Guide for School Nutrition and Physical Activity Policies.* Hartford: Connecticut State Department of Education.

Craypo L, Francisco SS, Boyle M, Samuels S. 2006. *Food and Beverage Marketing on California High School Campuses Study.* Conducted by Samuels & Associates. Commissioned by the Public Health Institute.

CSPI (Center for Science in the Public Interest). 2006. *School Foods Report Card.* [Online]. Available: http://www.cspinet.org/nutritionpolicy/sf_reportcard.pdf [accessed July 17, 2006].

CTSA (Citizenship Through Sports Alliance). 2006. *2005 Youth Sports National Report Card.* [Online]. Available: http://www.sportsmanship.org/News/1105%20Report%20Card-Fgrade.pdf [accessed May 26, 2006].

Dederichs R. 2005 (June 27). *School District Food Service Policies.* Presentation at the IOM Symposium on Progress in Preventing Childhood Obesity: Focus on Schools, Wichita, Kansas. Institute of Medicine Committee on Progress in Preventing Childhood Obesity. [Online]. Available: http://www.iom.edu/Object.File/Master/28/217/RDederichs.2005.pdf [accessed July 9, 2006].

DHHS (U.S. Department of Health and Human Services). 2006. *President's Challenge.* [Online]. Available: http://www.fitness.gov/home_pres_chall.htm [accessed May 16, 2006].

DoEd (U.S. Department of Education). 2006a. *No Child Left Behind.* [Online]. Available: http://www.ed.gov/nclb/landing.jhtml [accessed July 30, 2006].

DoEd. 2006b. *Carol M. White Physical Education Program.* [Online]. Available: http://www.ed.gov/programs/whitephysed/index.html [accessed March 6, 2006].

Donnelly JE. 2005 (June 27). *Physical Activity Across the Curriculum/Take 10!* Presentation at the Institute of Medicine Symposium Progress in Preventing Childhood Obesity: Focus on Schools, Wichita, Kansas. Institute of Medicine Committee on Progress in Preventing Childhood Obesity.

Eaton DK, Kann L, Kinchen S, Ross J, Hawkins J, Harris WA, Lowry R, McManus T, Chyen D, Shanklin S, Lim C, Grunbaum JA, Wechsler H. 2006. Youth risk behavior surveillance—United States, 2005. *MMWR* 55(5):1–108.

Engels HJ, Gretebeck RJ, Gretebeck KA, Jimenez L. 2005. Promoting healthful diets and exercise: Efficacy of a 12-week after-school program in urban African-Americans. *J Am Diet Assoc* 105(3):455–459.

Evenson KR, McGinn AP. 2004. Availability of school physical activity facilities to the public in four U.S. communities. *Am J Health Promot* 18(3):243–250.

Feenstra G, Ohmart J. 2004. *"Plate Tectonics": Do Farm-to-School Programs Shift Students' Diets?* University of California Sustainable Agriculture Research and Education Program. [Online]. Available: http://www.sarep.ucdavis.edu/newsltr/v16n3/sa-1.htm [accessed August 1, 2006].

Feenstra G, Ohmart J. 2005. *Yolo County Farm-to-School Project Evaluation. Year Two Annual Report, 2004–2005.* Kellogg Foundation Project. University of California Sustainable Agriculture Research and Education Program.

Feenstra G, Ohmart J. 2006. *Yolo County Farm-to-School Project Evaluation. Year Four Annual Report, Fall/Winter 2005–2006.* Kellogg Foundation Project. University of California Sustainable Agriculture Research and Education Program.

FHWA/DoT (Federal Highway Administration/Department of Transportation). 2006. *Safe Routes to Schools.* [Online]. Available: http://safety.fhwa.dot.gov/saferoutes/ [accessed June 10, 2006].

Forshee RA, Storey ML, Ginevan ME. 2005. A risk analysis model of the relationship between beverage consumption from school vending machines and risk of adolescent overweight. *Risk Analysis* 25(5):1121–1135.

Gemmill E, Cotugna N. 2005. Vending machine policies and practices in Delaware. *J School Nurs* 21(2):94–99.

Gittelsohn J, Steckler A, Johnson CC, Pratt C, Grieser M, Pickrel J, Stone EJ, Conway T, Coombs D, Staten LK. 2006. Formative research in school and community-based health programs and studies: "State of the art" and the TAAG approach. *Health Educ Behav* 33(1):25–39.

Gortmaker SL, Peterson K, Wiecha J, Sobol AM, Dixit S, Fox MK, Laird N. 1999. Reducing obesity via a school-based interdisciplinary intervention among youth: Planet Health. *Arch Pediatr Adolesc Med* 153(4):409–418.

Graham, H, Zidenberg-Cherr, S. 2005. California teachers perceive school gardens as an effective nutritional tool to promote healthful eating habits. *J Am Diet Assoc* 105(11):1797–1800.

Greves HM, Rivara FP. 2006. Report card on school snack food policies among the United States' largest school districts in 2004–2005: Room for improvement. *Int J Behav Nutr Phys Act* 3:1.

Gross SM, Cinelli B. 2004. Coordinated school health program and dietetics professionals: Partners in promoting healthful eating. *J Am Diet Assoc* 106(5):793–798

Grunbaum JA, Di Pietra J, McManus T. Hawkins J, Kann L. 2005. *School Health Profiles: Characteristics of Health Programs Among Secondary Schools (Profiles 2004).* Atlanta, GA: CDC. [Online]. Available: http://www.cdc.gov/HealthyYouth/profiles/2004/report.pdf [accessed July 20, 2006].

Indiana Governor's Council for Physical Activity and Sports. 2006. *Governor's Fitness Award*. [Online]. Available: http://www.in.gov/isdh/programs/GovernorsCouncil/award.htm [accessed May 26, 2006].

IOM (Institute of Medicine). 2005. *Preventing Childhood Obesity: Health in the Balance*. Washington, DC: The National Academies Press.

IOM. 2006a. *Nutrition Standards for Foods in Schools*. [Online]. Available: http://www.iom.edu/project.asp?id=30181 [accessed May 15, 2006].

IOM. 2006b. *Food Marketing to Children and Youth: Threat or Opportunity?* Washington, DC: The National Academies Press.

Kann L, Grunbaum J, McKenna ML, Wechsler H, Galuska DA. 2005. Competitive foods and beverages available for purchase in secondary schools—Selected sites, United States, 2004. *J School Health* 75(10):370–374.

Katz DL, O'Connell M, Yeh M-C, Nawaz H, Njike V, Anderson LM, Cory S, Dietz W. 2005. Public health strategies for preventing and controlling overweight and obesity in school and worksite settings: A report on recommendations of the Task Force on Community Preventive Services. *MMWR* 54(RR10):1–12.

Kelder S, Hoelscher DM, Barroso CS, Walker JL, Cribb P, Hu S. 2005. The CATCH Kids Club: A pilot after-school study for improving elementary students' nutrition and physical activity. *Public Health Nutr* 8(2):133–140.

Keystone Healthy Zone. 2006. *Keystone Healthy Zone Schools*. [Online]. Available: http://www.panaonline.org/programs/khz/ [accessed June 3, 2006].

Klesges LM, Baranowski T, Beech B, Cullen K, Murray DM, Rochon J, Pratt C. 2004. Social desirability bias in self-reported dietary, physical activity and weight concerns measures in 8- to 10-year-old African-American girls: Results from the Girls Health Enrichment Multisite Studies (GEMS). *Prev Med* 38(Suppl):S78–S87.

Kojima D, Teare C, Dill L, Boyle M. 2002. *Improving Meal Quality in California's Schools: A Best Practices Guide for Health School Food Service*. California Food Policy Advocates. [Online]. Available: http://www.cfpa.net/obesity/MealQualityReport_May2003.pdf [accessed August 6, 2006].

Kolbe L, Kann L, Patterson B, Wechsler H, Osorio J, Collins J. 2004. Enabling the nation's schools to help prevent heart disease, stroke, cancer, COPD, diabetes, and other serious health problems. *Public Health Rep* 119(3):286–302.

Konami Digital Entertainment. 2006. *Konami Digital Entertainment and West Virginia Schools Develop Ground-Breaking Partnership*. [Online]. Available: http://www.konami.com/gs/newsarticle.php?id=726 [accessed May 26, 2006].

Lloyd LK, Cook CL, Kohl HW III. 2005. A pilot study of teachers' acceptance of a classroom-based physical activity curriculum too: TAKE 10! *TAHPERD Journal* Spring: 8–11.

Martin S, Carlson S. 2005. Barriers to children walking to or from school—United States, 2004. *J Am Med Assoc* 294(17):2160–2162.

Mathematica Policy Research. 2005. *National School Meals Study*. [Online]. Available: http://www.mathematica-mpr.com/nutrition/schoolmeals study.asp [accessed July 13, 2006].

Michigan Governor's Council on Physical Fitness, Health, and Sports. 2006. *Governor's Council on Physical Fitness, Health and Sports Exemplary Physical Education Awards*. [Online]. Available: http://www.michiganfitness.org/awardsprogram/exemplarypeawards.htm [accessed May 26, 2006].

Murimi M, Colvin J, Liner K, Guin J. 2006. *Methodology to Evaluate the Outcomes of the Team Nutrition Initiative in Schools*. USDA Contractor and Cooperator Report No. 20, Economic Research Service. [Online]. Available: http://www.ers.usda.gov/publications/ccr20/ccr20.pdf [accessed July 14, 2006].

NANA (National Alliance for Nutrition and Activity). 2006. *Model School Wellness Policies.* [Online]. Available: http://www.schoolwellnesspolicies.org [accessed May 12, 2006].

NASBE (National Association of State Boards of Education). 2006. *Fit, Healthy, and Ready to Learn: A School Health Policy Guide.* [Online]. Available: http://www.nasbe.org/HealthySchools/fithealthy.html [accessed May 12, 2006].

NASPE (National Association for Sport and Physical Education) and AHA (American Heart Association). 2006. *2006 Shape of the Nation Report.* [Online]. Available: http://www.aahperd.org/naspe/ShapeOfTheNation/ [accessed June 7, 2006].

NASSP (National Association of Secondary School Principals). 2006. *NASSP Guidelines for Beverage-Provider Business Agreements.* [Online]. Available: http://www.principals.org/s_nasspsec.asp?TrackID=&SID=1&DID=47375&CID=63&VID=2&RTID=0&CIDQS=&Taxonomy=False&specialSearch=False [accessed July 31, 2006].

NCES (National Center for Education Statistics). 2005. *Digest of Education Statistics, 2004* (NCES 2006-2005), Chapter 2.

NCSL (National Conference of State Legislatures). 2006. *Physical Education and Physical Activity for Children.* [Online]. Available: http://www.ncsl.org/programs/health/pe requirement.htm [accessed July 13, 2006].

NetScan. 2006. *State Actions to Promote Nutrition, Increase Physical Activity, and Prevent Obesity: A 2006 First Quarter Legislative Overview.* [Online]. Available: http://www.rwjf.org/files/research/NCSL%20FinalApril%202006%20Report.pdf [accessed June 3, 2006].

Neumark-Sztainer D, French SA, Hannan PJ, Story M, Fulkerson JA. 2005. School lunch and snacking patterns among high school students: Associations with school food environment and policies. *Int J Behav Nutr Phys Act* 2(1):14.

NSBN (New Schools, Better Neighborhoods). 2002. *A New Strategy for Building Better Neighborhoods.* [Online]. Available: http://www.nsbn.org/publications/cra/cra-new strategy.pdf [accessed July 13, 2006].

O'Hara Tompkins N, Zizzi S, Zedosky L, Wright J, Vitullo E. 2004. School-based opportunities for physical activity in West Virginia public schools. *Prev Med* 39(4):834–840.

PANA (Pennsylvania Advocates for Nutrition and Activity). 2006. *Growth Screening.* [Online]. Available: http://www.panaonline.org/programs/ khz/screening/index.php [accessed May 26, 2006].

Parsad B, Lewis L. 2006. *Calories In, Calories Out: Food and Exercise in Public Elementary Schools, 2005.* Washington, DC: National Center for Education Statistics. NCES 2006–057.

Pate RR, Ross JG. 1987. Factors associated with health-related fitness. *J Phys Educ Rec Dance* November–December:93–95.

Pate RR, Davis MG, Robinson TN, Stone EJ, McKenzie TL, Young JC. 2006. Promoting physical activity in children and youth. A leadership role for schools. *Circulation* 114(11): 1214–1224.

PBH (Produce for Better Health Foundation). 2005a. *School Foodservice Guide: Successful Implementation Models for Increased Fruit and Vegetable Consumption.* Wilmington, DE: PBH.

PBH. 2005b. *School Foodservice Guide: Promotions, Activities, and Resources to Increase Fruit and Vegetable Consumption.* Wilmington, DE: PBH.

Pearlman DN, Dowling E, Bayuk C, Cullinen K, Thacher AK. 2005. From concept to practice: Using the School Health Index to create healthy school environments in Rhode Island elementary schools. *Prev Chronic Dis* [Online]. Available: http://www.cdc.gov/PCD/issues/2005/nov/05_0070.htm [accessed July 23, 2006].

Pennsylvania School Boards Association. 2006. *Local Wellness Policy Checklist* [Online]. Available: http://www.psba.org/policy/localwellnesspolicychecklist.pdf [accessed June 16, 2006].

Philadelphia Comprehensive School Nutrition Policy Task Force. 2002. *Comprehensive School Nutrition Policy* [Online]. Available: http://www.thefoodtrust.org/pdf/snpolicy.pdf [accessed May 16, 2006].

President's Challenge. 2006. *President's Challenge, Educators.* [Online]. Available: http://www.presidentschallenge.org/educators/program_details. aspx [accessed May 26, 2006].

Probart C, McDonnell E, Weirich JE, Hartman T, Bailey-Davis L, Prabhakher V. 2005. Competitive foods available in Pennsylvania public high schools. *J Am Diet Assoc* 105(8):1243–1249.

Probart C, McDonnell E, Hartman T, Weirich JE, Bailey-Davis L. 2006. Factors associated with the offering and sale of competitive foods and school lunch participation. *J Am Diet Assoc* 106(2):242–247.

Robinson TN. 1999. Reducing children's television viewing to prevent obesity: A randomized controlled trial. *J Am Med Assoc* 282(16):1561–1567.

Robinson TN, Killen JD, Kraemer HC, Wilson DM, Matheson DM, Haskell WL, Pruitt LA, Powell TM, Owens AS, Thompson NS, Flint-Moore NM, Davis GJ, Emig KA, Brown RT, Rochon J, Green S, Varady A. 2003. Dance and reducing television viewing to prevent weight gain in African-American girls: The Stanford GEMS pilot study. *Ethn Dis* 13(1 Suppl 1):S65–S77.

Ryan KW, Card-Higginson P, McCarthy SG, Justus MB, Thompson JW. 2006. Arkansas fights fat: Translating research into policy to combat childhood and adolescent obesity. *Health Aff* 25(4):992–1004.

Scheier LM. 2004. School health report cards attempt to address the obesity epidemic. *J Am Diet Assoc* 104(3):341–344.

Schneider DJ, Carithers T, Coyle K, Endahl J, Robin L, McKenna M, Debrot K, Seymour J. 2006. Evaluation of a fruit and vegetable distribution program—Mississippi, 2004–05 school year. *MMWR* 55(35):957–961.

Sisson SB, Lee SM, Burns EK, Tudor-Locke C. 2006. Suitability of commuting by bicycle to Arizona elementary schools. *Am J Health Promot* 20(3):210–213.

South Carolina General Assembly. 2006. *Students Health and Fitness Act of 2005.* Act No. 102. [Online]. Available: http://www.scstatehouse.net/sess116_2005-2006/bills/3499.htm [accessed June 9, 2006].

SPARK (Sports, Play, and Active Recreation for Kids Program). 2006. *The SPARK After School Program.* [Online]. Available: www.sparkpe.org/programAfterSchool.jsp [accessed May 24, 2006].

SRTS (Safe Routes to School). 2006. *National Safe Routes to School Clearinghouse.* [Online]. Available: http://www.saferoutesinfo.org/ [accessed June 9, 2006].

Stanford SMART (Student Media Awareness to Reduce Television). 2006. *Examining the Negative Effects of Excessive Television.* [Online]. Available: http://notv.stanford.edu/ [accessed June 9, 2006].

Staten LK, Teufel-Shone NI, Steinfelt VE, Ortega N, Halverson K, Flores C, Lebowitz MD. 2005. The School Health Index as an impetus for change. *Prev Chronic Dis* [Online]. Available: http://www.cdc.gov/PCD/issues/2005/jan/04_0076.htm [accessed July 23, 1976].

Staunton CE, Hubsmith D, Kallins W. 2003. Promoting safe walking and biking to school: The Marin County success story. *Am J Public Health* 93(9):1431–1434.

Stewart JA, Dennison DA, Kohl HW III, Doyle JA. 2004. Exercise level and energy expenditure in the TAKE 10! in-class physical activity program. *J School Health* 74(10):397–400.

Story M, Sherwood NE, Himes JH, Davis M, Jacobs DR Jr, Cartwright Y, Smyth M, Rochon J. 2003. An after-school obesity prevention program for African-American girls: The Minnesota GEMS pilot study. *Ethn Dis* 13(1 Suppl 1):S54–S64.

Story M, Kaphingst KM, French S. 2006. The role of schools in obesity prevention. In: Paxon C, ed. *The Future of Children* 16(1):109–142.

Texas Department of Agriculture. 2006. *Local Wellness Policy Checklist*. [Online]. Available: http://www.psba.org/policy/localwellnesspolicy checklist.pdf [accessed June 16, 2006].

TFAH (Trust for America's Health). 2005. *F As in Fat: How Obesity Policies Are Failing in America 2005*. Washington, DC: Trust for America's Health. [Online]. Available: http://healthyamericans.org/reports/obesity2005/Obesity2005Report.pdf [accessed December 22, 2005].

Timperio A, Ball K, Salmon J, Roberts R, Giles-Corti B, Simmons D, Baur LA, Crawford D. 2006. Personal, family, social, and environmental correlates of active commuting to school. *Am J Prev Med* 30(1):45–51.

UFFVA (United Fresh Fruit and Vegetable Association). 2006. *Fruit and Vegetable Snack Program Resource Center*. [Online]. Available: http://www.uffva.org/fvpilotprogram.htm [accessed May 10, 2006].

University of Arkansas for Medical Sciences. 2006. *Year Two Evaluation: Arkansas Act 1220 of 2003 to Combat Childhood Obesity*. Little Rock, AR: University of Arkansas. [Online]. Available: http://www.uams.edu/coph/ reports/Act1220Eval.pdf [accessed May 16, 2006].

USDA (U.S. Department of Agriculture), Food and Nutrition Service. 2005. *Eat Smart— Farm Fresh: A Guide to Buying and Serving Locally-Grown Produce in School Meals*. [Online]. Available: http://www.fns.usda.gov/cnd/Guidance/Farm-to-School-Guidance_ 12-19-2005. pdf [accessed June 16, 2006].

USDA. 2006a. *Department of Defense Fresh Fruit and Vegetable Program*. [Online]. Available: http://www.fns.usda.gov/FDD/programs/dod/default.htm [accessed July 13, 2006].

USDA. 2006b. *Local Wellness Policy*. [Online]. Available: http://www.fns.usda.gov/tn/ Healthy/wellnesspolicy.html [accessed June 8, 2006].

USDA. 2006c. *Team Nutrition*. [Online]. Available: http://www.fns.usda.gov/tn/ [accessed May 17, 2006].

USDA, DHHS, and DoEd. 2005. *Making It Happen! School Nutrition Success Stories*. [Online]. Available: http://www.cdc.gov/healthyyouth/nutrition/Making-It-Happen/index. htm [accessed June 13, 2006].

Utah Department of Health. 2006. *Gold Medal Schools*. [Online]. Available: http://www. hearthighway.org/gms.html [accessed July 18, 2006].

Virginia Department of Education. 2006. *Health Education, Physical Education, and Driver Education*. [Online]. Available: http://www.pen.k12.va.us/VDOE/Instruction/PE/ [accessed May 26, 2006].

Westcott RF. 2005. *Measuring the Purchases of Soft Drinks by Students in U.S. Schools: An Analysis for the American Beverage Association*. Washington, DC: American Beverage Association. [Online]. Available: http://www.ameribev.org/pressroom/measuring%20the %20purchases%20of%20soft%20drinks%20by%20students%20in%20u.s.%20 schools.pdf [accessed July 17, 2006].

Wynns J, Chin EY. 1999. *Healthy Food and Physical Activity in the San Francisco Unified School District*. Resolution No. 95-25A6.

Yin Z, Hanes J Jr, Moore JB, Humbles P, Barbeau P, Gutin B. 2005a. An after-school physical activity program for obesity prevention in children. *Eval Health Prof* 28(1): 67–89.

8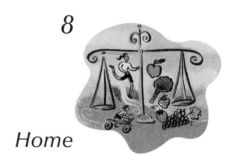

Home

Families can play an essential role in preventing childhood obesity. The Institute of Medicine (IOM) *Health in the Balance* report proposed a set of recommended actions for families and the home environment (Box 8-1) (IOM, 2005). The central recommendation is that parents should promote healthful eating behaviors and regular physical activity for their children. In addition, as noted throughout that report, actions need to be taken by government, industry, communities, and schools that will provide an environment that supports and reinforces the healthy behaviors promoted at home.

Parents and other household caregivers are influential role models, policy makers, and change agents in the home. They can control the home environment, monitor their children's and adolescents' behaviors, set goals for the family or household, reward successful behavioral changes, address problems to overcome barriers to change, and apply their parenting skills to maintain in their households attitudes and actions that are consistent with healthy behaviors (Dietz and Robinson, 2005). For example, if toddlers and young children are given multiple opportunities to try new foods without being coerced to eat them, many of the foods, including fruits and vegetables, will become a part of their diet even if they initially reject them (Birch and Marlin, 1982; Wardle et al., 2003).

Because parents and other caregivers are often strong influences in their children's lives, many of the policies and programs implemented in other settings (e.g., schools, communities, and the marketplace) target behaviors that manifest in the family and home context. Thus, the home environment

---

BOX 8-1
Recommendations for the Home from
Preventing Childhood Obesity: Health in the Balance

Parents should promote healthful eating behaviors and regular physical activity for their children.

To implement this recommendation parents can

- Choose exclusive breastfeeding as the method for feeding infants for the first 4 to 6 months of life.
- Provide healthful food and beverage choices for children by carefully considering nutrient quality and energy density.
- Assist and educate children in making healthful decisions regarding types of foods and beverages to consume, how often, and in what portion size.
- Encourage and support physical activity.
- Limit children's television viewing and other recreational screen time to less than two hours per day.
- Discuss weight status with their child's health care provider and monitor age- and gender-specific body mass index (BMI).
- Serve as positive role models for their children regarding eating and physical activity behaviors.

SOURCE: IOM (2005).

---

represents a setting that is particularly relevant to the prevention of childhood obesity. Parents and families can respond to policy changes and initiatives implemented in other settings. For example, if communities develop safe walkways and bikeways or initiate neighborhood farmers markets, parents can encourage family involvement in physical activity or purchasing fresh produce in these settings. If industry creates healthier calorie-controlled packaged foods and beverages, then adults and adolescents can purchase these products and work to ensure that nutrition is a priority when they plan meals for their families.

Parents can serve as advocates to promote changes that encourage and support healthy choices in their children's schools and communities as well as in their homes. Parents' Action for Children, a nonprofit organization dedicated to advancing the interests of families and children, suggests that parents get involved in their children's school wellness programs (Mansukhani, 2005).

Other useful resources that provide guidance to parents are the Parents as Teachers National Center (2005), which works to expand parents' knowledge of early childhood development and to improve parenting practices, as well as the resources and support provided by the national Parent

Teacher Association to promote health and wellness and prevent obesity (PTA, 2006). Parents can make the school environment healthier by advocating for the greater availability of low-calorie and nutrient-dense food and beverage products in vending machines and expanding opportunities for their children to be physically active throughout the school day. The Child Nutrition and WIC (Special Supplemental Nutrition Program for Women, Infants, and Children) Reauthorization Act of 2004 (Public Law 108-265) required school districts to involve parents in the process of establishing a local school wellness policy by the 2006–2007 school year (CNWICRA, 2004) (Chapters 4 and 7).

State-level efforts are also actively engaging parents. Recent legislation proposed or passed in many states requires parental representation on state and school advisory committees or task forces established to prevent childhood obesity (CDC, 2005; NCSL, 2006). For example, elementary, middle, and junior high schools in Texas are required to adopt by 2007 a state-approved coordinated school health program that includes a strong parental involvement component (Texas Department of State Health Services, 2006). Additionally, Oklahoma enacted legislation that requires each public school to establish a Healthy and Fit School Advisory Committee comprised of teachers, administrators, parents, health care professionals, and business community representatives to examine and make recommendations to the school principal regarding health education, physical education and physical activity, and nutrition and health services (NCSL, 2006).

OPPORTUNITIES AND CHALLENGES

Families in the United States face many potential opportunities and challenges that influence the efforts of household members to engage in healthy behaviors. The challenges include the stresses and pressures of daily living, along with economic and time constraints that make healthful eating and daily physical activity difficult for many families to achieve (Devine et al., 2003). The *Health in the Balance* report acknowledged that since the early 1970s expanded job opportunities as well as economic necessities have led to the entry of more women into the work force (IOM, 2005). In an estimated 62.4 percent of two-parent households, both parents are working; and in single-parent households, more than three-quarters of mothers (77.1 percent) and fathers (88.7 percent) are working (Fields, 2003). In 2004, both parents of 59 percent of children under 6 years of age were in the labor force and neither parent of 10 percent of children under 6 years of age was in the work force (Annie E. Casey Foundation, 2006). In addition to long work and commute hours, many families have busy schedules, with both parents and their children participating in activities outside the home, all of which can lead to reduced time for free play or for families to engage in physical activity together. Family meals may also be more irregular, and family members with busy schedules may rely more on take-out meals and fast food (Devine et al., 2003).

McIntosh and colleagues (2006) conducted an analysis of more than 300 household telephone interviews and self-administered questionnaires and examined the effects of parental work experiences on selected aspects of children's diet and health. Children's and youths' percentage of total calories from fat and saturated fat were examined in relation to their waist circumference and body mass index (BMI). The findings showed that household income, the quality and amount of parental time spent with their children, and parents' work experiences are associated with the total calorie and fat intake and obesity-related outcomes for children and youth ages 9 to 15 years. Mothers' behaviors tended to be more closely associated with their children's dietary intake than fathers' behaviors. Additionally, the characteristics and behaviors of both parents were strongly related to the behaviors of younger children ages 9 to 11 years than youth ages 13 to 15 years (McIntosh et al., 2006).

Family meals may have an important role in promoting positive dietary intakes in adolescents. Teens who consume meals with their families more frequently or who assist with the preparation of dinner for their families report higher intakes of fruits, vegetables, grains, and essential nutrients and lower intakes of low-nutrient foods, such as sweetened soft drinks and dietary fat, and are at lower risk for developing eating disorders (Larson et al., 2006; Neumark-Sztainer, 2006; Neumark-Sztainer et al., 2003). Adolescents living in families that prioritize eating meals together, provide structure around meals, and maintain an enjoyable meal-time atmosphere are less likely to engage in less healthful dietary practices and dieting behaviors. However, it has been suggested that a challenge for families, given current work and other life pressures, is the establishment of broader social networks to support healthful family meals (Neumark-Sztainer, 2006).

Another formidable challenge that parents face is the conflicted relationship that they have with television in their families. Although some parents have guidelines for the content of what their children view, especially in entertainment media, few parents appear to have rules restricting the amount of time that their children spend watching television (Hersey and Jordan, 2006). Moreover, the vast majority of families have multiple televisions in their homes, with children and teens often having televisions in their bedrooms (Rideout, 2004; Roberts et al., 2005).

Parents have identified several barriers to reducing television viewing to two hours or less per day, as recommended by the *Health in the Balance* report (IOM, 2005), the American Academy of Pediatrics (AAP, 2001), and *Healthy People 2010* (DHHS, 2000). These barriers include their own heavy television viewing habits, the use of television as a safe and affordable distraction for their children, the central role that television plays in family routines (e.g., relaxing, eating, and falling asleep), and the perspective that children should choose how to spend their leisure time (Hersey and Jordan, 2006; Rideout and Hamel, 2006). Parents often use electronic media such as television to manage busy family schedules, maintain peace in the household, facilitate family routines with their children, and teach their children things that parents do not have the time to teach themselves (Rideout and Hamel, 2006).

Several promising strategies can facilitate bringing about reductions in children's television viewing time, although they have not yet been fully evaluated. These strategies include encouraging parents to refrain from placing a television in their child's bedroom, establishing family rules about television viewing when children are young and consistently enforcing the rules, limiting the amount of time that children can watch television and use other electronic media on school days, not placing a television in household eating areas, disconnecting television viewing with eating meals or snacks, being attentive to how much time children spend with electronic media during their leisure time, and role modeling by limiting parental television viewing (Hersey and Jordan, 2006). School-based curricula promoting some of these behaviors have proven effective in reducing the sedentary television viewing habits of children (Robinson, 1999), adolescents (Gortmaker et al., 1999), and other family members (Robinson and Borzekowski, 2006).

Life experiences and opportunities are associated with the knowledge and behaviors of parents and caregivers. Demographic factors and personal perceptions about obesity are associated with parents' readiness to help their children who are obese or who are at risk for obesity to lose weight (Rhee et al., 2005). A review of barriers and facilitating factors for healthful eating among 11- to 16-year-olds found that family support, the broad availability of foods and beverages that contribute to a healthful diet, and a desire to take care of one's appearance were important factors in promoting healthy choices (Shepherd et al., 2006). Other barriers to changing adolescents' behaviors include adolescents' perceptions of low levels of caring by their parents, the difficulty that adolescents have with talking to their parents about problems, and the fact that adolescents value their friends' opinions over their parents' opinions for serious decisions. The feelings accompanying these barriers were associated with body dissatisfaction, depression, and low self-esteem (Ackard et al., 2006). If parents are unwilling or unable to change family behaviors, then interventions to promote positive lifestyle behaviors for the family are unlikely to be effective.

An additional challenge is a belief held by some that obesity is primarily an issue of personal or family responsibility and that government should not intervene in the home environment. This perspective makes it difficult to directly influence family behaviors and leads to a situation in difficult to directly influence family behaviors and leads to a situation in which parents face even greater obstacles to providing a healthy home environment.

Parents and caregivers are often unaware that their child is obese or at risk for obesity. A study conducted by the Centers for Disease Control and Prevention (CDC) showed that one-third of mothers of obese 2- to 11-year-old children thought that their child's weight was in the normal range (Maynard et al., 2003). In another study, parents involved in the Fit WIC pilot program of the U.S. Department of Agriculture (USDA), which was designed to evaluate social and environmental approaches to the prevention of obesity, showed that many parents of obese preschoolers neither viewed their children as being obese, nor were they concerned about their children's weight (USDA, 2005b). Thus, it is important for health care providers to discuss with parents and caregivers their child's weight and BMI, and the important roles of nutrition and physical activity in the promotion of normal growth and development and a healthy weight in their child.

Health care providers face several challenges when they address childhood obesity (Chapter 6). They report that they are often reluctant to discuss obesity with families because of the associated stigma, concern that parents will feel blamed, and apprehension that a discussion of weight may lead to unintended consequences, such as further stigmatization or an eating disorder. A neutral, nonjudgmental approach to weight management and obesity prevention may help parents and caregivers take responsibility for helping their children and teens reach a healthy weight and also assess the family's readiness to change (Dietz and Robinson, 2005). Ongoing efforts are focused on assisting individual health care providers with becoming more informed and comfortable with counseling children and their parents about obesity. Professional health care organizations such as the American Academy of Family Physicians, the American Academy of Pediatrics (AAP), and the American Dietetic Association provide evidence-based position statements, online patient and provider tool kits, and websites to help them manage obesity in children and adolescents (AAFP, 2004; AAP, 2006b; Ritchie et al., 2006).

The use of a combination of family-based and school-based multicomponent programs may more likely be effective at preventing obesity in children and youth if they address both the physical environment (e.g., food availability and portion size or access to opportunities for physical activity) and the social environment (e.g., socioeconomic and sociocultural factors and the mealtime structure) (Patrick and Nicklas, 2005). It has been suggested that multifaceted interventions should include the promotion of physical activity, parent training and modeling, behavioral counseling, and nutrition education for children and youth (Ritchie et al., 2006). Additionally, an integrated approach that promotes both healthy eating and physical activity choices and the acceptance of diverse body shapes and sizes among children and youth may have a greater likelihood of preventing both obesity and eating disorders and the health consequences of these weight-related eating disorders (Neumark-Sztainer, 2005a).

Although childhood obesity treatment research has demonstrated the importance of involving parents in interventions to change obese children's and adolescents' dietary and physical activity behaviors (Epstein et al., 1990), the challenges identified have contributed to the modest efficacies of parent and family interventions in obesity prevention studies. Challenges that remain in the home setting are motivating parents and families to participate in obesity prevention programs (Perry et al., 1989) and designing and implementing evaluations to assess changes in the home environment. Even when the level of parent participation is high, family-based interventions that have been evaluated have generally only produced relatively modest short-term effects on behavioral outcomes with limited effects on children's BMI levels and other anthropometric and health outcomes (Hearn et al., 1992; Nader et al., 1983; Perry et al., 1987, 1989; Vega et al., 1988).

For example, in a study of a home correspondence intervention for families of third grade students in Minnesota and North Dakota, a parent participation rate of 86 percent was achieved and the home-only and home-plus-school curriculum groups reported significant improvements in targeted dietary behaviors compared with the improvements for the school-curriculum-only and untreated control groups. There were no significant changes in anthropometric measures, however, and the dietary behavior differences were not maintained at a one-year follow-up (Perry et al., 1989).

Similarly, the large National Heart, Lung, and Blood Institute's (NHLBI's) Child and Adolescent Trial for Cardiovascular Health found only modest added benefits of the family intervention when it was combined with a school intervention in a comparison with the school intervention alone (Luepker et al., 1996). Parent-child interventions implemented independently of school programs have also had limited effects. A 12-week culturally tailored obesity prevention program for African-American mothers and daughters in households of low socioeconomic status resulted in statistically significant improvements in mothers' self-reported diets; but only minimal behavioral changes were observed for their daughters, and there were no significant changes in the daughters' BMI levels (Stolley and Fitzgibbon, 1997).

To intervene earlier in childhood, parents and families of preschool-aged children have recently been targeted by prevention programs. For example, a 16-week controlled trial that involved 43 American-Indian mothers of preschool-aged children used peer educators to deliver a home-based childhood obesity prevention program that included encouraging parental role modeling of healthy eating behaviors and establishing household rules about food and beverage choices. The trial produced nonstatistically significant differences between groups, although there was a trend toward lower weight for height and lower calorie intakes for children in the intervention group compared with those for the group receiving standard home-based parenting sessions (Harvey-Berino and Rourke, 2003). No differences between groups in the percentage of preschool children who were obese or at risk for obesity or in the children's physical activity levels emerged. There also were no differences in the mothers' BMIs, dietary intakes, or activity levels.

In 1999, the USDA began funding Fit WIC, an initiative to support and evaluate social and environmental approaches to the prevention and reduction of the levels of obesity in preschool children ages 2 to 4 years. Four state WIC programs (California, Kentucky, Vermont, Virginia) and the Inter-Tribal Council of Arizona were funded for a 3-year period to identify ways in which WIC could respond to the childhood obesity epidemic for program participants (USDA, 2005b) (Chapter 4).

Evaluation results of the Fit WIC pilot program in Virginia compared participating parents' behaviors in the intervention WIC clinic with those of parents at a non-randomly selected control WIC site. Parents who participated in the program were encouraged to perform six behaviors that affect their children. These included increasing their physical activity, monitoring mealtime behaviors, limiting household television, offering water instead of sweetened beverages, consuming five fruits and vegetables per day, and increasing family activities to promote physical fitness. WIC staff was asked to model these behaviors for parents, and complementary educational materials were sent to community agencies serving WIC clients. After one year of the intervention, Fit WIC program participants reported that they more frequently offered water to their children and more frequently engaged in more active play with their children than the participants at the comparison site (McGarvey et al., 2004). However, in the evaluation, limited and differential follow-up response rates and ethnic differences between the intervention and control sites complicated the attribution of differences between the groups to the Fit WIC intervention.

A promising preschool intervention that has been evaluated is Hip-Hop to Health Jr., a two-year randomized controlled trial with 420 low-income, predominantly African-American children enrolled in the Head Start program at 12 sites (Fitzgibbon et al., 2005). A 14-week intervention included 20-minute healthy eating or physical activity educational lessons and 20 minutes of aerobic activity three times per week. Control group participants received general health education on a weekly basis. The parents of the children received newsletters and homework assignments on a weekly basis and a $5.00 gift certificate for each completed assignment. After the intervention there were no differences in BMI levels between the groups. After one year of follow-up, the change in BMI levels (adjusted for age and baseline BMI) was significantly less for the treatment group. Smaller but statistically significant effects were maintained after two years (Fitzgibbon et al., 2005).

A systematic evidence-based review of obesity interventions for children and youth showed that multicomponent family-based programs are the most likely to be effective for children ages 5 to 12 years. However, there is limited evidence regarding effective obesity interventions for adolescents ages 13 years and older (Ritchie et al., 2006). Although there is the potential for a range of childhood obesity prevention interventions that involve parents and families, much more remains to be learned about effective strategies and how these strategies can be widely disseminated across various contexts.

CURRENT EFFORTS

Many different ongoing efforts are focused on improving dietary patterns, increasing physical activity, and preventing childhood obesity in the home environment. However, evaluations of the interventions are generally not performed; therefore there is limited evidence of whether and how these efforts may assist families, whether they have effects on family lifestyles, or even whether they produce unintended adverse effects and outcomes. Federal, state, and local government programs, as well as industry, community, and school-based efforts, often focus on reaching parents and their children at home or include a family-based component.

We Can! (Ways to Enhance Children's Activity and Nutrition) is a collaborative effort of four institutes of the National Institutes of Health (NIH)[1] and is one of many government-funded obesity prevention interventions focused on families. We Can! is designed to prevent obesity in children and tweens (tweens refer to young people from the ages of 9 to 13 years) by providing practical advice, resources, and community-based programs to parents, caregivers, children, and youth to adopt healthy lifestyles. The handbook developed for parents focuses on three critical behaviors: improve food choices, increase physical activity, and reduce leisure screen time. An evaluation of this effort is in progress (NIH, 2005) (Appendix D).

USDA's Food and Nutrition Service developed Eat Smart. Play Hard. as a national nutrition education and promotion campaign to convey

---

[1]We Can! is a collaboration between the NHLBI; the National Institute of Diabetes & Digestive & Kidney Diseases; the National Institute of Child Health and Human Development; and the National Cancer Institute.

evidence-based, behavior-focused, and motivational messages about healthy eating and physical activity (USDA, 2005a). The campaign uses an animated cartoon character, the Power Panther™, to deliver messages to children and their caregivers. A formative evaluation of this campaign has been conducted (Appendix C). However, a long-term evaluation examining the campaign's influence on children's behavioral outcomes is needed.

Some food companies have developed programs and tools to assist families and parents in planning healthy meals or engaging in regular physical activity. For example, parents and a group of several food companies and food retailers, including Annie's Homegrown, Applegate Farms, Horizon Organic, Newman's Own, Newman's Own Organics, and Whole Foods Market, initiated the Eat Smart, Grow Strong™ campaign in 2005. The campaign is focused on encouraging families to consume more healthful foods and promoting healthy eating habits at home (Public Interest Media Group, 2005). The campaign's interactive website offers parents a range of ideas for healthy recipes and includes games to teach children about healthy eating habits.

In August 2002, Gerber Products Company launched the Start Healthy, Stay Healthy™ campaign that was designed to provide parents and consumers with educational materials on raising healthy infants and toddlers and preventing childhood obesity (Gerber Products Company, 2006). A recent addition to the campaign is the Start Healthy, Stay Healthy Promise, a program aimed at mobilizing parents across the country to pledge to give their children a healthy start. Parents who enroll in the program receive advice on healthy feeding practices (Gerber Products Company, 2005). In some states, such as Arkansas, Gerber has entered into a public-private partnership with Wal-Mart and state government agencies, under the leadership of Governor Michael Huckabee, to reach parents through state programs. The Arkansas program has established the goal of increasing the number of healthier preschoolers by 50 percent by 2010 (Gerber Products Company, 2005). The committee recommends comprehensive and independent evaluations of industry-supported programs to assess the programs and to examine the direct and indirect effects of industry sponsorship (Chapter 5).

As noted above, health care professionals and health care-related organizations have frequent interactions with families. These interactions provide opportunities for obesity prevention information to be conveyed to parents. A recent policy statement by AAP recommends that physicians regularly assess a child's weight, diet, and level of physical activity; work with families to identify possible barriers to healthy living; encourage parents to serve as role models for healthy living through their own diet and exercise regimens; and encourage parents to support their children's regular participation in sports and other physical activities (AAP, 2006a).

A number of ongoing school-based interventions include a family-based component that may involve activities or work sheets that families may complete together or logs of family meals, television viewing, and physical activity. For example, the Stanford SMART (Student Media Awareness to Reduce Television) classroom curriculum, which was intended to reduce third and fourth graders' leisure screen time, included periodic newsletters for parents to teach parenting skills about television use and distributed electronic television time managers to families to help children budget their television time in the home. The intervention statistically significantly slowed the gain in BMI, triceps skinfold thickness, waist circumference, and waist-to-hip ratio in children receiving the curriculum compared with the values for the controls (Robinson, 1999) and also significantly reduced the television viewing times of the mothers, fathers, older siblings, and other children in the household (Robinson and Borzekowski, 2006).

Many parents can improve their modeling of healthy behaviors for their children. It is clear that much progress is needed, given that two-thirds of the American adult population is either overweight or obese (Ogden et al., 2006), only 22.2 percent of adults regularly engage in leisure-time physical activity for at least 30 minutes per day five or more times per week, and less than a quarter (23.3 percent) of adults consume five or more fruits and vegetables per day (Reeves and Rafferty, 2005). Families have an important role to play in reinforcing positive behaviors as well as protecting their children from negative influences or unintended consequences. Parents can assist their children with engaging in more healthful eating and physical activity behaviors by modeling the behaviors themselves, providing a supportive environment that facilitates the selection of healthier choices by their children, emphasizing healthy lifestyles and behaviors rather than weight or BMI, and engaging in supportive communication with their children (Neumark-Sztainer, 2005b).

EVALUATING PROGRESS AND NEXT STEPS

Coordinated public health interventions may successfully shape parental behaviors in the home, and lessons can be learned from other public health efforts. A frequently cited example is the Back to Sleep campaign to reduce the risk of sudden infant death syndrome (SIDS). In 1994, AAP, in partnership with the National Institute of Child Health and Human Development, the SIDS Alliance (now First Candle/SIDS Alliance), the Association of SIDS and Infant Mortality Programs, and the Maternal and Child Health Bureau of the Health Resources and Services Administration, launched the Back to Sleep campaign to inform all parents, infant caregivers, and health care professionals about the importance of placing healthy infants on their backs instead of their stomachs when they go to sleep. This required behavioral changes among parents and caregivers. Since the Back to Sleep campaign was introduced, the percentage of infants placed on their backs has increased substantially, and the rates of SIDS have declined by more than 50 percent (NICHD, 2005). Through the examination of multiple sources of data, these changes have generally been attributed to the campaign (Moon et al., 2004).

Limited efficacy and effectiveness data hinder the development of best practices for childhood obesity prevention in the home environment. However, several promising practices have been published in the literature. The Stanford GEMS (Girls Health Enrichment Multisite Studies) pilot study confirmed the feasibility and efficacy of using after-school dance classes and a family-based intervention to decrease television viewing time and videogame use to reduce weight gain in African-American girls (Robinson et al., 2003). Reducing television viewing time and videogame use (Robinson, 1999), closely monitoring children's eating behaviors (Brann and Skinner, 2005), emphasizing regular breakfast consumption (Fiore et al., 2006), and substituting noncaloric beverages for sugar-sweetened beverages at home (Ebbeling et al., 2006) are all promising approaches to preventing childhood obesity. However, these interventions require continued evaluations and research to confirm the findings. A recent Cochrane systematic review of childhood obesity prevention interventions concluded that the appropriateness of the development, design, intensity, and duration of interventions must be considered along with the comprehensive reporting of the scope of the intervention and the process (Summerbell et al., 2006). It has also been confirmed that sufficient data from randomized clinical trials to support any particular obesity prevention strategy are currently lacking (Summerbell et al., 2006). Thus, an integrated approach to using the best available evidence is recommended and reinforced by a systematic evaluation of the interventions (IOM, 2005).

APPLYING THE EVALUATION FRAMEWORK TO THE HOME ENVIRONMENT

What Constitutes Progress for Families and at Home?

Progress in preventing childhood obesity through family- and home-based interventions can be categorized as progress in providing environments that facilitate obesity prevention; progress in changing parental, familial, and caregiver behaviors and practices; and progress in research, evaluation, and surveillance. As noted earlier in this chapter, numerous external stresses, pressures, and challenges make it difficult for parents and caregivers to provide guidance and care for their children. Changes in some of these external conditions may facilitate desirable parental behavior. For example, the more widespread availability of convenient and private rooms for pumping breastmilk at worksites could potentially facilitate mothers' continued breastfeeding of their infants for the recommended 4 to 6 months. Modifications to the built environment to reduce work-related travel time or to provide common outdoor play areas for children are other examples of changes that may facilitate parents' and caregivers' efforts to prevent childhood obesity.

The recommendations for parents and caregivers from the *Health in the Balance* report (Box 8-1), can be used as a guide for parents to assess their own progress. These recommendations were based on the IOM committee's consensus of the best available evidence for changing physical activity and eating behaviors to prevent childhood obesity and represent promising practices that require further and ongoing evaluation. The majority of the available evidence was derived from small-scale behavioral research and population-based surveys and, by extension, from research on other types of behaviors (IOM, 2005).

Many of the policies and programs implemented in other settings influence the behaviors of parents, caregivers, families, and households. Therefore, the present IOM committee's recommendations and next steps for assessing progress focus on actions for parents, caregivers, families, and households (detailed below) and also on the actions needed by industry, government, communities, and schools (Chapters 4, 5, 6, and 7).

One of the challenges in assessing progress and evaluating the childhood obesity prevention initiatives implemented by families is the difficulty in collecting data at the individual parent-caregiver or family-household level. Sampling to determine overall national-level estimates may be feasible, but doing so at a meaningful level for each local area and every state is likely to be costly in terms of human and financial resources. Therefore, evaluations may need to rely on a combination of national data sources, as well as many different types of state and local data sources (Appendix C). A range of evaluation designs and research on families is needed in order to build a sufficient evidence base of promising obesity prevention strategies that can be widely disseminated. Some of the most useful data for planners and policy makers will come from evaluations of local programs that can be translated and adapted to other communities and populations (Chapters 3 and 6).

Another challenge to evaluating progress is a lack of reliable and valid measures with demonstrated sensitivities to changes in many of the outcomes that should be measured and that are recommended in Chapter 2. New methods and measures will need to be developed to monitor progress in reaching a variety of outcomes in the home setting. Additionally, there is a need to account for the possibility that obesity prevention interventions may have adverse or unanticipated outcomes, such as the stigmatization of children or the development of eating disorders (Doak et al., 2006).

As is the case for government, industry, communities, and schools, the efforts of families and caregivers at home to prevent childhood obesity involve all aspects of the evaluation framework. For example, if promoting the consumption of healthful foods, beverages, and snacks at home is the desired outcome (Figure 8-1), the following events might be expected to occur. In terms of resources and inputs, parents commit to healthful eating at home, develop a plan to model and encourage healthful eating, and modify the household budget, as necessary. Relevant strategies and actions include educating parents about the nutritional value of foods and beverages; encouraging parents and families to establish household guidelines or rules limiting the availability and consumption of less healthful foods, beverages, meals, and snacks at home and limiting leisure screen time; and assisting parents and families with the development of weekly menus to ensure a balanced and diverse diet. Outcomes that could be examined include the increased availability of and access to healthful foods, beverages, meals, and snacks in the home; the use of weekly menu planning; and the extent to which family members adhere to healthful diets that are consistent with the Dietary Guidelines for Americans 2005. Figure 8-1 assesses efforts to promote the consumption of fruits, vegetables, and other low-calorie and high nutrient foods, beverages, meals, and snacks at home; and Figure 8-2 applies the framework to assess how parents may promote regular physical activity at home.

Box 8-2 provides a checklist that parents, families, and caregivers can use to assess their ongoing progress in adopting a healthy lifestyle for their families.

NEEDS AND NEXT STEPS IN ASSESSING PROGRESS

Promote Leadership, Commitment, and Collaboration

The *Health in the Balance* report emphasized that "a child's health and well-being are fostered by a home environment with engaged and skillful parenting that models, values, and encourages sensible eating habits and a physically active lifestyle. By promoting certain values and attitudes, by rewarding or reinforcing specific behaviors, and by serving as role models, parents can have a profound influence on their children" (IOM, 2005, p. 285). Parents should provide leadership in the home and act as positive role models for healthy lifestyles. They can also act as community change agents and advocates to create healthy communities for their families by getting involved in school and community wellness programs and other activities at their children's schools and in the community. Collaboration among all

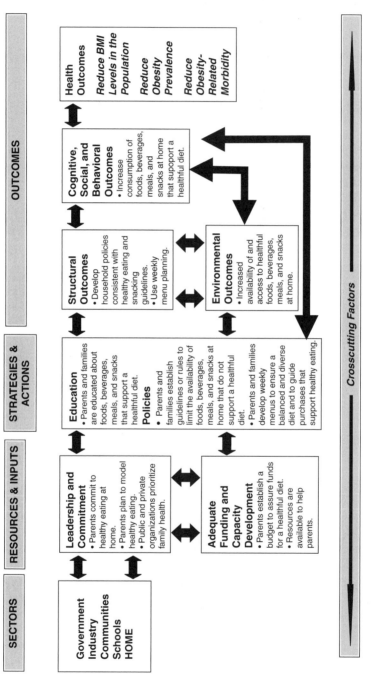

FIGURE 8-1 Evaluating family efforts to promote the consumption of fruits, vegetables, and other low-calorie and high nutrient foods, beverages, snacks, and meals in the home.

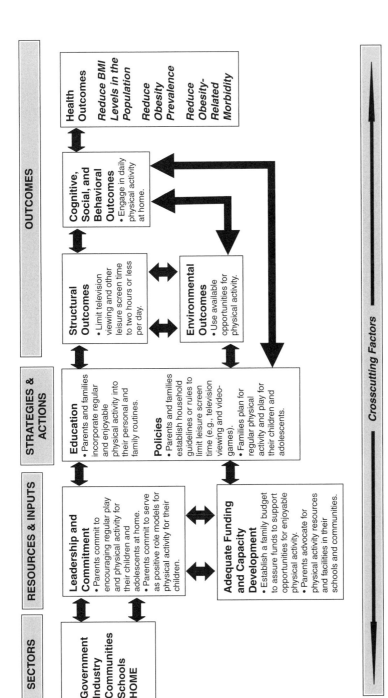

FIGURE 8-2 Evaluating family efforts to promote physical activity in the home.

BOX 8-2
Checklist for Parents, Families, and Caregivers

- Are you promoting healthful eating behaviors and regular physical activity to your children?

- Are you choosing exclusive breastfeeding as the method for feeding your infant for the first 4 to 6 months of life?

- Are you providing food and beverage choices for your children that reflect careful consideration of nutrient quality and energy density?

- Are you assisting and educating your children with making healthful food choice decisions and educating them about the types of foods and beverages that they should consume, how often they should consume them, and the correct portion size?

- Are you encouraging, supporting, and participating in physical activity among the members of your household?

- Are you limiting your children's television viewing and other leisure screen time to less than two hours per day?

- Are you discussing weight status with your child's health care provider and monitoring your child's age- and gender-specific BMI level?

- Are you serving as positive role models for your children regarding eating and physical activity behaviors?

SOURCE: Adapted from IOM (2005).

---

sectors is needed to create healthy environments for children both at home and away from home.

Develop, Sustain, and Support Evaluation Capacity and Implementation

Evaluation capacity refers to assisting families with developing or strengthening their ability to meet specific goals or objectives, as well as monitoring and evaluating their strategies and actions to promote healthier lifestyles in the home setting. Families need to recognize that even small incremental advances are valuable in improving dietary quality, decreasing sedentary time, and increasing physical activity.

Just as families may periodically evaluate their household budgets and financial well-being and their children's academic progress, it is important for parents, caregivers, children, and adolescents to periodically assess their health-related family practices and home environment. They can use such informal evaluation strategies as keeping regular food and physical activity diaries or use MyPyramid and MyPyramid for Kids, which have online tracking tools that can be used to monitor the lifestyle changes made in the home. Checklists of strategies for behavioral change can also be helpful (Box 8-2).

Enhance Surveillance, Monitoring, and Research

Further research on family interventions, as well as more family-targeted interventions, is needed to prevent childhood obesity (Jackson et al., 2005; Lindsay et al., 2006). Few rigorous evaluations on the effectiveness of these programs have been performed. However, current evidence suggests that parent interventions may work most effectively as a component of comprehensive interventions across a variety of settings, including schools, health care services, communities, and federal food and nutrition programs such as the WIC program.

Appendix C contains data sources and evaluation tools that can be used to measure obesity prevention-related outcomes, several of which are related to the home environment. Among these are the Behavioral Risk Factor Surveillance System, which assesses fruit and vegetable consumption and physical activity levels reported by parents and caregivers. The National Survey of Children's Health and the National Survey of Early Childhood Health collect information from families on a variety of relevant behaviors, including breastfeeding, family mealtime, physical activity, and family rules concerning television viewing. The Youth Risk Behavior Surveillance System assesses the physical activity levels, television viewing times, leisure-time computer use, and fruit and vegetable consumption of middle school and high school students.

Disseminate and Use Evaluation Results

Although families play a central role in childhood obesity prevention, parents and families have only a limited number of information sources on obesity prevention. These include television and other media; materials brought home from preschool, school, child-care, and after-school care; and interactions with teachers, health care professionals, social workers, and coaches. Innovative approaches are needed to provide families with relevant obesity prevention information, particularly information that is practical, that is easily implemented, and that does not judge or lecture parents, who are often overwhelmed with multiple health-related messages and competing priorities. The federal government, state governments, local governments, communities, and the media should find ways to disseminate promising interventions and initiatives such as Small Steps and Small Step Kids!; the Dietary Guidelines for Americans; MyPyramid and MyPyramid for Kids; the Eat Smart. Play Hard. campaign; the Food Stamp Nutrition Education Program; the WIC program; 5 a Day for Better Health; the Fresh Fruit and Vegetable Program; and We Can!. Consideration should be given to the development of channels that provide parents with information at multiple points through the child's development, from prenatal and baby care to adolescence.

SUMMARY AND RECOMMENDATIONS

Each of the committee's four recommendations is directly relevant to improving the implementation and evaluation of family-based interventions, policies, and initiatives.

Recommendation 1: **Government, industry, communities, schools, and families should demonstrate leadership and commitment by mobilizing the resources required to identify, implement, evaluate, and disseminate effective policies and interventions that support childhood obesity prevention goals.**

Implementation Actions for Home
Families, parents, and caregivers should commit to promoting healthful eating and regular physical activity to create a healthy home environment.

To accomplish this:
- Parents and caregivers should make physical activity and healthful eating priorities at home. They should provide food and beverage choices for their children that contribute to a healthful diet, encourage and support physical activity, limit children's television viewing and other leisure screen time, and serve as positive role models. Parents can also serve as advocates to promote changes that encourage and support healthy behaviors in their local schools and communities.

Recommendation 2: **Policy makers, program planners, program implementers, and other interested stakeholders—within and across relevant sectors—should evaluate all childhood obesity prevention efforts, strengthen the evaluation capacity, and develop quality interventions that take into account diverse perspectives, that use culturally relevant approaches, and that meet the needs of diverse populations and contexts.**

Implementation Actions for Home
Parents and caregivers, as the policy makers in the household, should assess their family's progress in achieving positive lifestyle changes.

To accomplish this,
- Families should regularly assess their progress in adopting and maintaining healthful behaviors at home and achieving positive lifestyle changes.

Recommendation 3: Government, industry, communities, and schools should expand or develop relevant surveillance and monitoring systems and, as applicable, should engage in research to examine the impact of childhood obesity prevention policies, interventions, and actions on relevant outcomes, paying particular attention to the unique needs of diverse groups and high-risk populations. Additionally, parents and caregivers should monitor changes in their family's food, beverage, and physical activity choices and their progress toward healthier lifestyles.

Implementation Actions for Home
Parents and caregivers should monitor their families' lifestyle changes; and government, foundations, and industry should support applied research that examines family interventions in real-world settings.

To accomplish this:
- Parents and caregivers should monitor their families' lifestyle changes on an ongoing basis, including their capabilities as role models, the family's dietary intake and levels of physical activity, and their children's weight status.
- Parents should work with their child's physician to track body mass indices and healthy growth.
- The federal government should create and make available simple tools for parents and families to track their children's dietary intake and physical activity behaviors.
- Relevant federal agencies (e.g., CDC, NIH, USDA, and U.S. Department of Education), foundations, and other organizations should fund and support applied research that examines family interventions focused on specific ways that families can improve diets, reduce sedentary behaviors, and increase levels of physical activity in the home setting.
- Relevant federal and state agencies, foundations, and academic institutions should develop and enhance surveillance systems

and other data sources and assessment tools to expand knowledge about the relationship between changes in the home environment and a variety of outcomes for children and youth.

Recommendation 4: Government, industry, communities, schools, and families should foster information-sharing activities and disseminate evaluation and research findings through diverse communication channels and media to actively promote the use and scaling up of effective childhood obesity prevention policies and interventions.

Implementation Actions for Home
Government (federal, state, and local), communities, families, and the media should disseminate and widely promote the evaluation results of effective family- and home-based childhood obesity prevention efforts.

To accomplish this:
- Government agencies (federal, state, and local), communities, and the media should promote the results of evaluations and specific practical guidance related to promising family-based obesity prevention interventions such as approaches for reducing children's television viewing, promoting leisure-time physical activity, and promoting healthier food and beverage choices at home.
- Parents, children, and youth should share information about promising obesity-prevention strategies and activities with other families through parenting groups and school meetings and in family, social, faith-based, and other venues.

REFERENCES

AAFP (American Academy of Family Physicians). 2004. *Obesity and Children: Helping Your Child Keep a Healthy Weight.* [Online]. Available: http://www.aafp.org/afp/20040215/928ph.html [accessed June 2, 2006].

AAP (American Academy of Pediatrics). 2001. Children, adolescents, and television. *Pediatrics* 107(2):423–426.

AAP. 2006a. Active healthy living: Prevention of childhood obesity through increased physical activity. *Pediatrics* 117(5):1834–1842.

AAP. 2006b. *Overweight and Obesity.* [Online]. Available: http://www.aap.org/healthtopics/overweight.cfm [accessed June 2, 2006].

Ackard DM, Neumark-Sztainer D, Story M, Perry C. 2006. Parent-child connectedness and behavioral and emotional health among adolescents. *Am J Prev Med* 30(1):59–66.

Annie E. Casey Foundation. 2006. *2006 Kids Count Data Book.* [Online]. Available: http://www.aecf.org/kidscount/sld/databook.jsp [accessed July 10, 2006].

Birch LL, Marlin DW. 1982. I don't like it; I never tried it: Effects of exposure on two-year-old children's food preferences. *Appetite* 3(4):353–360.

Brann LS, Skinner JD. 2005. More controlling child-feeding practices are found among parents of boys with an average body mass index compared with parents of boys with a high body mass index. *J Am Diet Assoc* 105(9):1411–1416.

CDC (Centers for Disease Control and Prevention). 2005. *State Legislative Information: Search for Bills.* [Online]. Available: http://apps.nccd.cdc.gov/ DNPALeg/ [accessed April 24, 2006].

CNWICRA (Child Nutrition and WIC Reauthorization Act). 2004. *Child Nutrition and WIC Reauthorization Act of 2004.* Public Law 108-265 108th Congress. June 30, 2004. [Online]. Available: http://www.fns.usda.gov/cnd/Governance/ Legislation/PL_108-265. pdf [accessed March 22, 2006].

Devine CM, Connors MM, Sobal J, Bisogni CA. 2003. Sandwiching it in: Spillover of work onto food choices and family roles in low- and moderate-income urban households. *Soc Sci Med* 56(3):617–630.

DHHS (U.S. Department of Health and Human Services). 2000. *Healthy People 2010: Understanding and Improving Health.* Washington, DC: DHHS. [Online]. Available: http:// www.healthypeople.gov/Document/ [accessed July 17, 2006].

Dietz WH, Robinson TN. 2005. Overweight children and adolescents. *N Engl J Med* 352(20): 2100–2109.

Doak CM, Visscher TL, Renders CM, Seidell JC. 2006. The prevention of overweight and obesity in children and adolescents: A review of interventions and programmes. *Obes Rev* 7(1):111–136.

Ebbeling CB, Feldman HA, Osganian SK, Chomitz VR, Ellenbogen SJ, Ludwig DS. 2006. Effects of decreasing sugar-sweetened beverage consumption on body weight in adolescents: A randomized, controlled pilot study. *Pediatrics* 117(3):673–680.

Epstein LH, Valoski A, Wing RR, McCurley J. 1990. Ten-year follow-up of behavioral, family-based treatment for obese children. *J Am Med Assoc* 264(19):2519–2523.

Fields J. 2003. *Children's Living Arrangements and Characteristics: March 2002. Current Population Reports.* Washington, DC: U.S. Bureau of the Census.

Fiore H, Travis S, Whalen A, Auinger P, Ryan S. 2006. Potentially protective factors associated with healthful body mass index in adolescents with obese and nonobese parents: A secondary data analysis of the third National Health and Nutrition Examination Survey, 1988–1994. *J Am Diet Assoc* 106(1):55–64.

Fitzgibbon ML, Stolley MR, Schiffer L, Van Horn L, KauferChristoffel K, Dyer A. 2005. Two-year follow-up results for Hip-Hop to Health Jr.: A randomized controlled trial for overweight prevention in preschool minority children. *J Pediatr* 146(5):618–625.

Gerber Products Company. 2005. *Gerber Aims to Increase Number of Healthier Preschoolers by 50 Percent by 2010.* News release. September 20. [Online]. Available: http://www. gerber.com/content/usa/bin/pdf/press/Arkansas_Start_ Healthy_Press_Event_20Sep05.pdf [accessed June 17, 2006].

Gerber Products Company. 2006. *Start Healthy, Stay Healthy™ Fact Sheet.* [Online]. Available: http://www.gerber.com/content/usa/bin/pdf/press/Start_Healthy_Fact_Sheet.pdf [accessed June 11, 2006].

Gortmaker SL, Peterson K, Wiecha J, Sobol AM, Dixit S, Fox MK, Laird N. 1999. Reducing obesity via a school-based interdisciplinary intervention among youth: Planet Health. *Arch Pediatr Adolesc Med* 153(4):409–418.

Harvey-Berino J, Rourke J. 2003. Obesity prevention in preschool Native-American children: A pilot study using home visiting. *Obes Res* 11(5):606–611.

Hearn MD, Bigelow C, Nader PR, Stone E, Johnson C, Parcel G, Perry CL, Luepker RV. 1992. Involving families in cardiovascular health promotion: The CATCH feasibility study. *J Health Educ* 23(1):22–31.

Hersey JC, Jordan A. 2006. *Reducing Children's TV Time to Reduce the Risk of Childhood Overweight: The Children's Media Use Study*. Final report. Prepared for the Centers for Disease Control and Prevention and The Association of Preventive Medicine Teaching and Research. Washington, DC: Research Triangle Institute International.

IOM (Institute of Medicine). 2005. *Preventing Childhood Obesity: Health in the Balance*. Washington, DC: The National Academies Press.

Jackson D, Mannix J, Faga P, McDonald G. 2005. Overweight and obese children: Mother's strategies. *J Adv Nurs* 52(1):6–13.

Larson NI, Story M, Eisenberg ME, Neumark-Sztainer D. 2006. Food preparation and purchasing roles among adolescents: Associations with sociodemographic characteristics and diet quality. *J Am Diet Assoc* 106(2):211–218.

Lindsay AC, Sussner KM, Kim J, Gortmaker S. 2006. The role of parents in preventing childhood obesity. In: Paxon C, ed. *Future Child* 16(1):169–186.

Luepker RV, Perry CL, McKinlay SM, Nader PR, Parcel GS, Stone EJ, Webber LS, Elder JP, Feldman HA, Johnson CC. 1996. Outcomes of a field trial to improve children's dietary patterns and physical activity. The Child and Adolescent Trial for Cardiovascular Health (CATCH). *J Am Med Assoc* 275(10):768–776.

Mansukhani R. 2005. *Why Are So Many Kids Today Overweight? What Every Parent Needs to Know*. [Online]. Available: http://www.parentsaction.org/news/parenting-info/nutrition/why-are-so-many-kids-today-overweight/ [accessed May 8, 2006].

Maynard LM, Galuska DA, Blanck HM, Serdula MK. 2003. Maternal perceptions of weight status of children. *Pediatrics* 111(5 Pt 2):1226–1231.

McGarvey E, Keller A, Forrester M, Williams E, Seward D, Suttle D. 2004. Feasibility and benefits of a parent-focused preschool child obesity intervention. *Am J Public Health* 94(9):1490–1495.

McIntosh A, Davis G, Nayga R Jr, Anding J, Torres C, Kubena K, Perusquia E, Yeley G, You W. 2006. *Parental Time, Role Strain, and Children's Fat Intake and Obesity-Related Outcomes*. Economic Research Service, U.S. Department of Agriculture. [Online]. Available: http://www.ers.usda.gov/Publications/CCR19/ccr19.pdf [accessed June 17, 2006].

Moon RY, Oden RP, Grady KC. 2004. Back to Sleep: An educational intervention with Women, Infants, and Children program clients. *Pediatrics* 113(3 Pt 1):542–547.

Nader PR, Baranowski T, Vanderpool NA, Dunn K, Dworkin R, Ray L. 1983. The family health project: Cardiovascular risk reduction education for children and parents. *J Dev Behav Pediatr* 4(1):3–10.

NCSL (National Conference of State Legislatures). 2006. *Childhood Obesity—2005 Update and Overview of Policy Options*. [Online]. Available: http://www.ncsl.org/programs/health/ChildhoodObesity-2005.htm [accessed July 17, 2006].

Neumark-Sztainer D. 2005a. Can we simultaneously work toward the prevention of obesity and eating disorders in children and adolescents? *Int J Eat Disord* 38(3):220–227.

Neumark-Sztainer D. 2005b. Preventing the broad spectrum of weight-related problems: Working with parents to help teens achieve a healthy weight and a positive body image. *J Nutr Educ Behav* 37(Suppl 2):S133–S140.

Neumark-Sztainer D. 2006. Eating among teens: Do family mealtimes make a difference for adolescents' nutrition? *New Dir Child Adolesc Dev* Spring(111):91–105.

Neumark-Sztainer D, Hannan PJ, Story M, Croll J, Perry C. 2003. Family meal patterns: Associations with sociodemographic characteristics and improved dietary intake among adolescents. *J Am Diet Assoc* 103(3):317–322.

NICHD (National Institute of Child Health and Human Development). 2005. *SIDS: "Back to Sleep" Campaign.* [Online]. Available: http://www.nichd.nih.gov/sids/sids.cfm [accessed May 9, 2006].

NIH (National Institutes of Health). 2005. *Welcome to We Can!* [Online]. Available: http://www.nhlbi.nih.gov/health/public/heart/obesity/wecan/index.htm [accessed May 9, 2006].

Ogden CL, Carroll MD, Curtin LR, McDowell MA, Tabak CJ, Flegal KM. 2006. Prevalence of overweight and obesity in the United States, 1999–2004. *J Am Med Assoc* 295(13): 1549–1555.

Parents as Teachers National Center. 2005. *Parents as Teachers.* [Online]. Available: http://www.parentsasteachers.org/site/pp.asp?c= ekIRLcMZJxE&b=272091 [accessed July 17, 2006].

Patrick H, Nicklas TA. 2005. A review of family and social determinants of children's eating patterns and diet quality. *J Am Coll Nutr* 24(2):83–92.

Perry CL, Crockett SJ, Pirie P. 1987. Influencing parental health behavior: Implications of community assessments. *Health Educ* 18(5):68–77.

Perry CL, Luepker RV, Murray DM, Hearn MD. 1989. Parent involvement with children's health promotion: A one-year follow-up of the Minnesota Home Team. *Health Educ Q* 16(2):171–180.

PTA (Parent Teacher Association). 2006. *Health and Wellness.* [Online]. Available: http://www.pta.org/pr_category_details_1117232379734.html [accessed July 17, 2006].

Public Interest Media Group. 2005. *Eat Smart, Grow Strong.* [Online]. Available: http://www.eatsmartgrowstrong.com/ [accessed May 9, 2006].

Reeves MJ, Rafferty AP. 2005. Healthy lifestyle characteristics among adults in the United States, 2000. *Arch Intern Med* 165(8):854–857.

Rhee KE, DeLago CW, Arscott-Mills T, Mehta SD, Davis RK. 2005. Factors associated with parental readiness to make changes for overweight children. *Pediatrics* 116(1):94–101.

Rideout V. 2004. *Parents, Media and Public Policy: A Kaiser Family Foundation Survey.* Menlo Park, CA: Henry J. Kaiser Family Foundation.

Rideout V, Hamel E. 2006. *The Media Family: Electronic Media in the Lives of Infants, Toddlers, Preschoolers and Their Parents.* Menlo Park, CA: Henry J. Kaiser Family Foundation.

Ritchie LD, Crawford PB, Hoelscher DM, Sothern MS. 2006. Position of the American Dietetic Association: Individual-, family-, school-, and community-based interventions for pediatric overweight. *J Am Diet Assoc* 106(6):925–945.

Roberts DF, Foehr UG, Rideout V. 2005. *Generation M: Media in the Lives of 8–18 Year Olds.* Menlo Park, CA: Henry J. Kaiser Family Foundation. [Online]. Available: http://www.kff.org/entmedia/upload/Generation-M-Media-in-the-Lives-of-8-18-Year-olds-Report.pdf [accessed July 22, 2006].

Robinson TN. 1999. Reducing children's television viewing to prevent obesity. A randomized controlled trial. *J Am Med Assoc* 282(16):1561–1567.

Robinson TN, Borzekowski DLG. 2006. Effects of the SMART classroom curriculum to reduce child and family screen time. *J Communic* 56(1):1–26.

Robinson TN, Killen JD, Kraemer HC, Wilson DM, Matheson DM, Haskell WL, Pruitt LA, Powell TM, Owens AS, Thompson NS, Flint-Moore NM, Davis GJ, Emig KA, Brown RT, Rochon J, Green S, Varady A. 2003. Dance and reducing television viewing to prevent weight gain in African-American girls: The Stanford GEMS pilot study. *Ethn Dis* 13(1 Suppl 1):S1.65–S1.77.

Shepherd J, Harden A, Rees R, Brunton G, Garcia J, Oliver S, Oakley A. 2006. Young people and healthy eating: A systematic review of research on barriers and facilitators. *Health Educ Res* 21(2):239–257.

Stolley MR, Fitzgibbon ML. 1997. Effects of an obesity prevention program on the eating behavior of African American mothers and daughters. *Health Educ Behav* 24(2):152–164.

Summerbell CD, Waters E, Edmunds LD, Kelly S, Brown T, Campbell KJ. 2006. *The Cochrane Database of Systematic Reviews. Interventions for Preventing Obesity in Children*. The Cochrane Collaboration. John Wiley & Sons, Ltd. [Online]. Available: http://www.cochrane.org/reviews/en/ab001871.html [accessed November 28, 2006].

Texas Department of State Health Services. 2006. *A Guide to School Health Advisory Councils (SHACs): A Basic Primer for Texas*. [Online]. Available: www.dshs.state.tx.us/schoolhealth/ [accessed June 2, 2006].

USDA (U.S. Department of Agriculture). 2005a. *Eat Smart. Play Hard.™ Campaign Overview*. [Online]. Available: http://www.fns.usda.gov/eatsmartplayhard/Original/default.htm [accessed August 19, 2006].

USDA. 2005b. *Fit WIC: Programs to Prevent Childhood Overweight in Your Community*. Special Nutrition Program Report Series, No. WIC-05-FW. Food and Nutrition Service, USDA. Alexandria, VA: Office of Analysis, Nutrition, and Evaluation. [Online]. Available: http://www.fns.usda.gov/oane/MENU/Published/WIC/FILES/fitwic.pdf [accessed February 28, 2006].

Vega WA, Sallis JF, Patterson TL, Rupp JW, Morris JA, Nader PR. 1988. Predictors of dietary change in Mexican-American families participating in a health behavior change program. *Am J Prev Med* 4(4):194–199.

Wardle J, Cooke LJ, Gibson EL, Sapochnik M, Sheiham A, Lawson M. 2003. Increasing children's acceptance of vegetables: A randomized trial of parent-led exposure. *Appetite* 40(2):155–162.

9

Assessing the Nation's Progress in Preventing Childhood Obesity

The nation's growing recognition of the obesity crisis as a major health concern for its children and youth has led to an array of diverse efforts aimed at increasing physical activity and promoting healthful eating. These efforts, however, generally remain fragmented and are implemented on a small-scale. Furthermore, there is a lack of systematic tracking and evaluation of childhood obesity prevention interventions. Compared with the strong commitment and heavy infusion of governmental and private-sector resources to other major public health concerns, such as an impending infectious disease outbreak or bioterrorism, there is a marked underinvestment in the prevention of childhood obesity and related chronic diseases.

Accelerating the pace of change toward healthier lifestyles will require leadership, political will, increased resources, and sustained commitment. Additionally, broader-based efforts are needed to scale up programs and interventions found to be effective.

It is time to think strategically about what is required to create and institutionalize changes now to reverse the childhood obesity epidemic over future decades. Which state will be the first to reverse its escalating obesity rate? How will industry contribute to the response, beyond its incremental expansion of food, beverage, and meal products to full and profitable healthful product lines? When will social norms shift toward embracing active lifestyles and foods and beverages that contribute to a healthful diet?

The Institute of Medicine (IOM) *Health in the Balance* report (IOM, 2005) emphasized the collective responsibility that all sectors share for shaping an adequate response to the childhood obesity epidemic. All stakeholders can be instrumental in making changes to social norms throughout the nation so that obesity will be acknowledged as an important and preventable health outcome and healthful eating and regular physical activity will be accepted and encouraged as the standard (IOM, 2005). What is needed is for the childhood obesity epidemic to reach a "tipping point" (Gladwell, 2000), where small collective changes within and across all sectors will produce a substantial effect so that the obesity epidemic will be acknowledged, environmental changes will take hold, communities will be mobilized, and individuals and families will aspire to pursue healthy behaviors and active lifestyles as the social norm.

This report has sought to provide an extension of the *Health in the Balance* report. It has emphasized the need for the evaluation of obesity prevention actions across all sectors so that effective evidence-based approaches can be identified, scaled up, adapted to diverse settings and contexts, and widely disseminated. The committee developed five broad conclusions (Box 9-1) based on its assessment of progress in preventing

---

BOX 9-1
Conclusions

1. The country is beginning to recognize that childhood obesity is a serious public health problem that increases morbidity and mortality and that has substantial economic and social costs. However, the current level of investment by the public and private sectors still does not match the extent of the problem.

2. Government, industry, communities, schools, and families are responding to the childhood obesity epidemic by implementing a variety of policies, programs, and other interventions. All of these stakeholders bring strong values and beliefs to obesity-related issues, but evidence-based approaches are needed to guide the nation's collective actions in the response.

3. Current data and evidence are inadequate for a comprehensive assessment of the progress that has been made in preventing childhood obesity across the United States. Although the best available evidence should be used to develop an immediate response to the childhood obesity epidemic, a more robust evidence base that identifies promising practices must be developed so that these interventions can be scaled-up and supported in diverse settings.

4. Evaluation serves to foster collective learning, accountability, responsibility, and cost-effectiveness to guide improvements in childhood obesity prevention policies and programs. Multiple sectors and stakeholders should commit adequate resources to conduct these evaluations. Surveillance, monitoring, and research are fundamental components of childhood obesity prevention evaluation efforts.

5. Multiple sectors and stakeholders should conduct evaluations of different types and at different levels to assess and stimulate progress over the short term, intermediate term, and long term to reverse the childhood obesity trend and improve the health of the nation's children and youth.

childhood obesity. These conclusions serve as the foundation for the report's recommendations and the specific implementation actions discussed in the previous chapters.

The United States is still in an early phase of developing a coherent and comprehensive response to obesity as a national public health challenge. A mature understanding of the long-term investments and scope of an adequate response is needed. Many countries and regions around the world are similarly recognizing the extent of their own obesity and chronic disease challenges and are beginning to take constructive steps to formulate comprehensive strategies or action plans that promote health and that aim to prevent overweight and obesity in their populations. These strategies and plans often include evaluation components that can be used to assess their own progress (Table 9-1).

The World Health Organization estimates that obesity and related chronic diseases account for approximately 60 percent of the overall rate of mortality worldwide and 47 percent of the global burden of disease (WHO, 2002). Many middle-income countries around the world, including Brazil, China, Indonesia, Mexico, Russia, and Vietnam, are experiencing obesity epidemics that vary by socioeconomic groups (Doak et al., 2000, 2005; IOM, 2007; Wang et al., 2002). Countries with transitional economies often face the dual challenges of both malnutrition and overnutrition (Ezzati et al., 2005; Gillespie and Haddad, 2003; Hawkes, 2006; WHO, 2006a). Additionally, obesity and cardiovascular disease risks are expected to increase in low- and middle-income countries, which, along with the persistent burden of infectious diseases and malnutrition, may further exacerbate global health inequities (Ezzati et al., 2005).

A greater understanding is needed of the dietary and physical activity patterns that lead to the co-existence of obesity, under-nutrition, and micronutrient deficiencies in developing countries, as well as the environmental, economic, and social trends that influence them. Evidence-based guidance for the design, implementation, and evaluation of effective programs and policies that address this double burden is also needed (Doak et al., 2000, 2005; Hawkes, 2006). Effective and innovative practices to prevent childhood obesity and the lessons learned are beginning to be shared internationally; however, more can be accomplished with a coordinated global dissemination effort.

CHANGING SOCIAL NORMS

Healthful diets and regular physical activity are far from the accepted social norm, although there is a growing awareness by the public that obesity has health, economic, and social consequences. A Harvard School of Public Health poll of 2,033 adults nationwide found that an estimated

TABLE 9-1 Examples of Countries and Regions that Have Developed
Strategies or Action Plans to Promote Healthful Eating and Physical
Activity and to Prevent Obesity

Country	Strategy or Action Plan	Source
Australia	*Best Options for Promoting Healthy Weight and Preventing Weight Gain in New South Wales*	Gill et al. (2005)
Canada	*Improving the Health of Canadians: Promoting Healthy Weights*	Canadian Institute for Health Information (2006)
Chile	*Global Strategy Against Obesity*	Ministry of Health (2005)
Denmark	*National Action Plan Against Obesity. Recommendations and Perspectives*	National Board of Health (2003)
Finland	*Finnish Nutrition Recommendations 2005* *Government Resolution on Policies to Develop Health-Enhancing Physical Activity in Finland*	National Nutrition Council, National Public Health Institute, Ministry of Agriculture and Forestry (2005) Ministry of Social Affairs and Health (2002)
France	*Taking Charge of Obesity in Children and Adolescents*	Agence Nationale d'Accréditation et d'Évaluation en Santé (2003)
Ireland	*Obesity: The Policy Challenges. The Report of the National Taskforce on Obesity*	National Taskforce on Obesity (2005)
The Netherlands	*Living Longer in Good Health*	Ministry of Health, Welfare, and Sport (2004)
Norway	*Prescriptions for a Healthier Norway* *The Action Plan on Physical Activity 2005–2009: Working Together for Physical Activity*	Ministry of Social Affairs (2002–2003) Departemente Ministries (2005)
Portugal	*National Programme Against Obesity*	Portuguese Ministry of Health and Portuguese General Directorate of Health (2004)
Slovenia	*Resolution on The National Programme of Food and Nutrition Policy 2005–2010*	National Institute of Public Health, Republic of Slovenia (2005)
Spain	*Spanish Strategy for Nutrition, Physical Activity and Prevention of Obesity*	Ministry of Health and Consumer Affairs (2005)

TABLE 9-1 continued

Country	Strategy or Action Plan	Source
Sweden	*Background Material to the Action Plan for Healthy Dietary Habits and Increased Physical Activity*	National Food Administration and National Institute of Public Health (2005)
	Healthy Dietary Habits and Increased Physical Activity: The Basis for an Action Plan	National Institute of Public Health (2005)
United Kingdom	*Choosing Health: Making Healthy Choices Easier*	National Health Service (2004)
United States	*The Surgeon General's Call to Action to Prevent and Decrease Overweight and Obesity*	DHHS (2001)

Region	Strategy or Action Plan	Source
Europe	*European Ministerial Charter on Counteracting Obesity*	WHO (2006b)
	Children's Environment and Health Action Plan for Europe	WHO (2004b)
	Green Paper—Promoting Healthy Diets and Physical Activity: A European Dimension for the Prevention of Overweight, Obesity and Chronic Diseases	Commission of the European Communities (2005)
	Diet, Physical Activity and Health— EU Platform for Action	European Commission (2006)
Global	*Diet, Nutrition and the Prevention of Chronic Diseases*	WHO (2003, 2004a, 2006a)
	Global Strategy on Diet, Physical Activity, and Health	
	Preventing Chronic Diseases: A Vital Investment	
Latin America	*Global Strategy on Healthy Eating, Physical Activity and Health (DPAS): Implementation Plan for Latin America and the Caribbean 2006–2007*	PAHO/WHO (2005, 2006a,b)
	Regional Strategy and Plan of Action on an Integrated Approach to the Prevention and Control of Chronic Diseases, Including Diet, Physical Activity, and Health	
	Regional Strategy on Nutrition in Health and Development 2006–2015	

(continued on following page)

TABLE 9-1 continued

Region	Strategy or Action Plan	Source
Nordic	*Health, Food, and Physical Activity. Nordic Plan of Action on Better Health and Quality of Life Through Diet and Physical Activity*	Nordic Council of Ministers for Fisheries and Aquaculture, Agriculture, Foodstuffs, and Forestry; The Nordic Council of Ministers for Social Security and Health Care (2006)
Pacific	*Obesity in the Pacific: Too Big to Ignore*	Secretariat of the Pacific Community (2002)

75 percent of Americans view obesity as either an extremely serious or very serious public health problem (Blendon et al., 2005). The majority of Americans believe that scientific experts have been accurately portraying (58 percent) or underestimating (22 percent) the health risks of obesity, with only 15 percent believing that scientific experts have overestimated obesity-related health risks (Blendon et al., 2005). Other surveys have found that the public perceives obesity to be a growing threat to health (Evans et al., 2005, 2006; IFIC Foundation, 2006; Pew Research Center, 2006; Wall Street Journal Online and Harris Interactive, 2005, 2006).

Although there is more public support for certain interventions to reduce obesity, especially obesity among children and youth, the public's support for such interventions as sending body mass index (BMI) report cards home to parents, requiring standardized food portions in restaurants, and regulating the advertising and marketing of less healthful foods and beverages is divided (Evans et al., 2005, 2006; Pew Research Center, 2006; Wall Street Journal Online and Harris Interactive, 2005, 2006).

Data from marketing research firms also suggest that Americans' attitudes toward obese individuals are shifting from rejection to acceptance and that Americans may be more tolerant of heavier body types. The NPD Group's National Eating Trends Survey found that 24 percent of 1,900 survey respondents indicated that overweight individuals were less attractive in 2005, whereas 55 percent of respondents found this to be the case in 1985 (Associated Press, 2006).

There may be a substantial difference in Americans' perception of what constitutes healthy habits and what they actually do. A telephone survey of 12,000 adults found that three quarters of obese respondents described their eating habits as either "very healthy" or "somewhat healthy," and nearly one-half of the survey respondents indicated they exercised three or more times weekly (Thomson Medstat, 2006).

Moreover, a survey of 1,000 Americans found that 9 out of 10 consumers were unable to provide an accurate estimate of their recommended calorie intakes, three-quarters of obese consumers underestimated their weight, only one-third of consumers believe that the health information that they receive is consistent, and taste and cost remain more important drivers of choice than healthfulness (IFIC Foundation, 2006). Another survey of 2,200 adult consumers found that only 17 percent had ever visited the U.S. Department of Agriculture's (USDA's) MyPyramid website; only a quarter (24 percent) stated that they understood food labels; nearly three-quarters (72 percent) indicated that if food does not taste good, they will not eat it, despite its nutritional value; and one-half of the consumers surveyed did not know how much fat, carbohydrate, or salt to consume in a 2,000-calorie diet (Yankelovich, 2006).

Trend data show that the rate of participation in physical activity declines as American children get older. More than one-third of high school students (grades 9 to 12) do not regularly engage in physical activity, more than 11 percent of high school students get no moderate to vigorous physical activity, and 30 percent of states do not mandate physical education for elementary and middle school students (NASPE and AHA, 2006). Between 1981 and 1997, children's free playtime decreased by 25 percent, attributed to the increased amount of time spent in structured activities. A desirable social norm to work toward, especially for preschoolers, is to promote unstructured outdoor play in their lives (Burdette and Whitaker, 2005). For older children and adolescents, a social norm to aspire to is the integration of physical activity or active living into their lives every day.

Social movements related to promoting public and environmental health (e.g., tobacco control, underage drinking, seatbelt use, recycling, and reducing litter) have historically resulted from actions in which the population is made aware of a problem, educated, and mobilized over years and decades to challenge power structures and societal norms to address social problems (Economos et al., 2001; Kersh and Morone, 2002). Meaningful social change often involves the tensions and interactions among three different cultures: a private-sector market culture, a public-sector bureaucratic culture, and a nonprofit relational culture (Gecan, 2002).

It will take time to change social norms that have become deeply embedded in American society. Parents often use electronic media, such as television to manage busy schedules; maintain peace in the household; and facilitate family routines with their children, such as relaxing, eating, and falling asleep (Rideout and Hamel, 2006). Media now have a more central role in socializing today's children and youth than ever before (IOM, 2006).

The promotion of obesity prevention as a successful social change movement and evaluation of the extent of the changes in social norms are imminent challenges. A coherent approach is needed to assess the progress of this social movement to change actions and behaviors toward healthier choices and lifestyles.

Assessing the extent of change in social norms and values related to obesity will require the use of diverse measurement approaches. Media content analyses can show how popular depictions of people and activities (e.g., healthful eating and physical activity) are portrayed. Patterns and trends in school recess, physical education, food and beverage sales, active transport, and many other intermediate outcomes are potential indicators of progress, as is the trajectory of the way in which social norms are codified through changes in policies and regulations. Surveillance systems, such as the Behavioral Risk Factor Surveillance System and the Youth Risk Behavior Surveillance System (YRBSS), and public opinion polls will provide insights into the extent to which attitudes and behaviors are changing. However, extensive research is needed to identify how healthy choices can be made accessible and desirable—as well as how sedentary pursuits and less healthful choices can be made undesirable—without stigmatizing high-risk populations or those who are already obese. Furthermore, these changes need to be relevant to children and youth of all socioeconomic, cultural, and racial/ethnic backgrounds.

NEXT STEPS

Given the range of actions that are needed to move forward in preventing childhood obesity, the committee has identified immediate next steps that it deems essential priority actions in the near future. The committee strongly encourages that all childhood obesity prevention policies and interventions be evaluated to learn what works and what does not work and to broadly share that information.

Meaningful and sustained efforts will need to be connected across multiple sectors of society so that childhood obesity prevention becomes accepted as a collaborative responsibility among government, communities, industry, schools, and at home. Furthermore, the collective body of knowledge and evidence of these efforts as they are evaluated will serve to further build and inform the field of obesity prevention.

Government

The federal, state, and local governments are actively engaged in childhood obesity prevention efforts. However, as noted above, the levels of funding and resources invested in these efforts and their evaluation are not commensurate with the seriousness of this public health problem. Government at all levels should provide coordinated leadership for the prevention of obesity in children and youth.

A critical next step for the federal government is to establish a high-level task force on childhood obesity prevention, as recommended in the *Health in the Balance* report (IOM, 2005), and as underscored in this report. The committee recommends that the president request that the secretary of the U.S. Department of Health and Human Services (DHHS) convene this high-level task force and the task force include as members the secretaries or senior officials of DHHS and the U.S. Departments of Agriculture, Education, Transportation, Housing and Urban Development, Interior, Defense, and other relevant departments and agencies. The purpose of the task force would be to ensure coordinated budgets, policies, and requirements for obesity prevention programs and to establish effective interdepartmental collaboration and priorities for action.

Furthermore, the federal government should provide a sustained commitment and long-term investment in childhood obesity prevention initiatives found to be effective (such as the VERB™ campaign) and those that are vital to measuring progress (such as national surveillance efforts to track trends in the obesity epidemic).

Surveillance systems—such as the National Health and Nutrition Examination Survey, the School Health Policies and Programs Study (SHPPS), the Youth Media Campaign Longitudinal Survey, YRBSS, and the National Household Transportation Survey—should be expanded to include relevant obesity-related outcomes. Surveillance systems that monitor the precursors of dietary and physical activity behaviors, such as changes in policies and the built environment, need to be expanded or developed.

Additionally, monitoring systems for USDA programs such as the Special Supplemental Nutrition Program for Women, Infants, and Children (WIC), the Food Stamp Program, and the school meals programs should be developed that assess a range of obesity-related outcomes for children and youth.

State and local governments should also demonstrate leadership on this issue and commit resources and policies that lead to actions that implement and evaluate changes in schools and communities.

Industry

Certain segments of relevant industries, including the food, beverage, restaurant, food retail, leisure and recreation, physical activity and fitness, and entertainment industries have responded constructively to the childhood obesity epidemic. However, other corporations in these industries are not yet engaged in obesity prevention; and other segments of the industry, such as the fitness, spectator sports, and transportation sectors, have not shown adequate involvement in obesity prevention actions. Nevertheless, careful and independent evaluations are needed to determine if industry is making a sufficient investment, sustained commitment, and whether those initiatives proposed by industry will be effective and contribute to desirable outcomes.

Evaluation of industry's efforts to prevent childhood obesity should focus on an assessment and tracking over time of the proportion of a company's product portfolio and marketing resources devoted to developing, packaging, and promoting healthful products. There is also a need to track industry's changes in portion sizes and easily conveyed nutritional information for healthy products that consumers eat as well as the products that promote physical activity. Additionally, there is a need to assess the promotion of consistent health messages to young people and the public by all relevant industries and all media platforms—print, broadcast, cable, electronic, mobile, and wireless.

Industry and the public health community should work toward nurturing and strengthening partnerships that support obesity prevention efforts. To expand the federal research capacity to study the ways in which marketing influences children's and adolescents' attitudes and behaviors, industry is encouraged to provide data on pricing strategies, consumer food purchases, and consumption trends from proprietary retail scanner systems, household scanner panels, household consumption surveys, and marketing research. The collaborative work should examine the quality of the data, consider reducing the cost to make the data accessible, and establish priorities for applying the information to promote healthful diets and physical activity.

Corporate responsibility can be demonstrated by sharing marketing research findings, to the greatest extent possible, which will assist the public health sector to develop, implement, and evaluate more effective childhood obesity prevention policies, programs, and interventions. Data sharing will need to balance many considerations including transparency, public accessibility, the demands of the competitive marketplace, and legal issues. In certain cases, it may be appropriate for the data to be released after a time lag to keep the public informed with relatively recent data. The committee recommends that the public and private sectors engage in a collaborative process that will assist relevant stakeholders to share proprietary data for the public good.

Communities

Communities vary widely in the extent and nature of the resources available for changing the built and social environments to facilitate physical activity and the selection of low-calorie and high-nutrient foods and beverages that support a healthful diet. A number of state and local governments, foundations, and youth-related organizations are demonstrating innovative and collaborative approaches to childhood obesity prevention. However, much remains to be learned, transferred, and disseminated in order to identify the most effective evidence-based interventions that continue even when seed funding and external resources are no longer available. The committee identified two immediate next steps for communities. The development of a validated community self-assessment tool, such as a community health index, will help communities identify their strengths and gaps in designing and evaluating childhood obesity-prevention efforts, ranging from local programs and evaluation capacity to the local physical and built environments, and the extent of community involvement. Additionally, relevant nonprofit organizations and government agencies should partner in developing a means to compile and disseminate effective community-based childhood obesity prevention interventions. A web-based database or repository of published and unpublished literature, case studies, and promising intervention websites is needed.

Congress should appropriate funds for the CDC, in partnership with the Department of Transportation, the Department of the Interior, and other relevant federal agencies, private-sector and nonprofit organizations, and community stakeholders to develop this type of well-validated tool that can be used in economically and culturally diverse communities.

Additionally, the National Association of County and City Health Officials, in partnership with government agencies and other nonprofit and voluntary health organizations, should develop a means of compiling and sharing community-based evaluation results, lessons learned, and community action plans as well as provide links to resources, templates, and evaluation tools. A web-based database or repository of published and unpublished literature, case studies, and promising intervention websites is needed.

Schools

Schools are the current focus of many childhood obesity prevention efforts, particularly changes to the school food and beverage environment. Less attention has been paid to increasing physical activity in schools, although this issue seems to be gaining momentum. As is true for community efforts, wide variations in the extent of the efforts and resources available for investment in obesity prevention by individual schools, school districts, and state agencies are observed. Federal law requires that schools receiving federal funds for school meals must develop school wellness policies by the fall of 2006, which has stimulated school-based health promotion and obesity prevention efforts across the country. Additionally, teachers, food service personnel, school administrators, and state and federal agency staff have developed many creative and innovative approaches to improve students' diets and to increase physical activity, but these need to be evaluated. Sustained attention is needed for this issue as well as changes that can improve the nutritional quality of foods and beverages that are available and the opportunities for physical activity offered in preschool, child-care, and after-school programs. The committee encourages states and school districts to bolster their physical education and physical activity requirements and standards, as should preschool, child-care, and after-school programs. Accountability mechanisms are needed for state school nutrition and physical activity standards that include increased transparency and dissemination of school-by-school reports on success in meeting these standards.

Home

Many families across the country are aware of their role in preventing childhood obesity and are actively making changes toward healthier lifestyles, whereas others are not yet engaged in change. Just as families may periodically evaluate their economic health and long-term strategies, their disaster preparedness, and their children's academic progress, it is important for families to periodically assess their health-related home environment and practices. A next step for parents, caregivers, children, and adolescents is to periodically assess the home environment and ask the following questions: Are parents knowledgeable about healthy feeding strategies for their children? Are the foods and beverages that are available and prepared in the home healthful and served in reasonable portion sizes? Is physical activity emphasized and a family priority? Do families have established rules or guidelines limiting leisure screen time? Incremental changes are valuable and signal that progress is occurring.

Conclusion

A succinct assessment of the nation's progress in preventing childhood obesity is not feasible given the diverse and varied nature of America's communities and population. However, it can be said that awareness of obesity has been raised, actions have begun, coordination and prioritization of limited resources are critical, and evaluation of interventions within and across all sectors is essential. A long-term commitment to create a healthy environment for our children and youth is urgently needed. This commitment will require widespread changes in social norms, institutions, and practices beyond those that directly involve children and youth.

REFERENCES

Agence Nationale d'Accréditation et d'Évaluation en Santé. 2003. *Prise en Charge de l'Obésité de l'Enfant et de l'Adolescent.* France. [Online]. Available: http://www.sante.gouv.fr/ [accessed June 8, 2006].

Associated Press. 2006. *Americans are More Accepting of Heavier Body Types.* January 23. [Online]. Available: http://www.msnbc.msn.com/id/10807526/ [accessed July 21, 2006].

Blendon RJ, DesRoches CM, Herrmann MJ, Weldon KJ, Fleischfresser C. 2005. *Despite Conflicting Studies About Obesity, Most Americans Think the Problem Remains Serious.* Harvard School of Public Health. [Online]. Available: http://www.hsph.harvard.edu/ press/releases/blendon/Obesity Topline.doc [accessed February 10, 2006].

Burdette HL, Whitaker RC. 2005. Resurrecting free play in young children: Looking beyond fitness and fatness to attention, affiliation, and affect. *Arch Pediatr Adolesc Med* 159(1): 46–50.

Canadian Institute for Health Information. 2006. *Improving the Health of Canadians: Promoting Healthy Weights.* [Online]. Available: http://secure.cihi.ca/cihiweb/products/ healthyweights06_e.pdf [accessed May 23, 2006].

Commission of the European Communities. 2005. *Green Paper—Promoting Healthy Diets and Physical Activity: A European Dimension for the Prevention of Overweight, Obesity and Chronic Diseases.* Brussels, Belgium: Commission of the European Communities, European Union. [Online]. Available: http://ec.europa.eu/comm/health/ph_deter minants/life_style/ nutrition/documents/nutrition_gp_en.pdf [accessed May 23, 2006].

Departemente Ministries (Ministry of Children and Family Affairs, Ministry of the Environment, Ministry of Labour and Social Affairs, Ministry of Education and Research, Ministry of Culture and Church Affairs, Ministry of Transport and Communications, Ministry of Local Government and Regional Development). 2005. *The Action Plan on Physical Activity 2005–2009: Working Together for Physical Activity.* Oslo, Norway. [Online]. Available: http://odin.dep.no/detalj/DIV197219720049HODENGTRYK/bn!15900002. html [accessed August 7, 2006].

DHHS (U.S. Department of Health and Human Services). 2001. *The Surgeon General's Call to Action to Prevent and Decrease Overweight and Obesity.* Rockville, MD: Office of the Surgeon General, U.S. Public Health Service. [Online]. Available: http://www.surgeon general.gov/topics/obesity/calltoaction/CalltoAction.pdf [accessed July 6, 2006].

Doak CM, Adair LS, Monteiro C, Popkin BM. 2000. Overweight and underweight coexist within households in Brazil, China and Russia. *J Nutr* 130(12):2965–2971.

Doak CM, Adair LS, Bentley M, Monteiro C, Popkin BM. 2005. The dual burden household and the nutrition transition paradox. *Int J Obes* 29(1):129–136.

Economos CD, Brownson RC, DeAngelis MA, Novelli P, Foerster SB, Foreman CT, Gregson J, Kumanyika SK, Pate RR. 2001. What lessons have been learned from other attempts to guide social change? *Nutr Rev* 59(3 Pt 2):S40–S56.

European Commission. 2006. *Diet, Physical Activity and Health—EU Platform for Action.* [Online]. Available: http://ec.europa.eu/comm/health/ph_determinants/life_style/nutrition/ platform/platform_en.htm [accessed May 23, 2006].

Evans WD, Finkelstein EA, Kamerow DB, Renaud JM. 2005. Public perceptions of childhood obesity. *Am J Prev Med* 28(1):26–32.

Evans WD, Renaud JM, Finkelstein E, Kamerow DB, Brown DS. 2006. Changing perceptions of the childhood obesity epidemic. *Am J Health Behav* 30(2):167–176.

Ezzati M, Vander Hoorn S, Lawes CM, Leach R, James WP, Lopez AD, Rodgers A, Murray CJ. 2005. Rethinking the "diseases of affluence" paradigm: Global patterns of nutritional risks in relation to economic development. *PLoS Med* 2(5):0404–0412.

Gecan M. 2002. *Going Public: An Inside Story of Disrupting Politics as Usual.* Boston, MA: Beacon Press.

Gill T, King L, Webb K. 2005. *Best Options for Promoting Healthy Weight and Preventing Weight Gain in NSW.* Sydney, Australia: NSW Centre for Public Health Nutrition and NSW Department of Health. [Online]. Available: http://www.cphn.biochem.usyd.edu.au/ resources/FinalHealthyWeightreport160305.pdf [accessed May 23, 2006].

Gillespie S, Haddad LJ. 2003. *The Double Burden of Malnutrition in Asia: Causes, Consequences, and Solutions.* Thousand Oaks, CA: Sage Publications.

Gladwell M. 2000. *The Tipping Point: How Little Things Can Make a Big Difference.* Boston, MA: Back Bay Books.

Hawkes C. 2006. Uneven dietary development: Linking the policies and processes of globalization with the nutrition transition, obesity and diet-related chronic diseases. *Global Health* 28(2):4–22.

IFIC (International Food Information Council) Foundation. 2006. *Food & Health Survey: Consumer Attitudes Toward Food, Nutrition & Health.* Washington, DC: IFIC Foundation. [Online]. Available: http://www.ific.org/research/upload/2006foodandhealthsurvey. pdf [accessed June 7, 2006].

IOM (Institute of Medicine). 2005. *Preventing Childhood Obesity: Health in the Balance.* Washington, DC: The National Academies Press.

IOM. 2006. *Food Marketing to Children and Youth: Threat or Opportunity?* Washington, DC: The National Academies Press.

IOM. 2007. *Joint U.S.-Mexico Workshop on Preventing Obesity in Children and Youth of Mexican Origin.* May 3–4, 2006, Cuernavaca, Mexico. Washington, DC: The National Academies Press.

Kersh R, Morone J. 2002. How the personal becomes political: Prohibitions, public health, and obesity. *Studies Am Polit Dev* 16:162–175.

Ministry of Health. 2005. *Global Strategy Against Obesity.* Draft. Santiago, Chile: Ministry of Health.

Ministry of Health and Consumer Affairs. 2005. *Spanish Strategy for Nutrition, Physical Activity and Prevention of Obesity.* Barcelona, Spain: Ministry of Health and Consumer Affairs. [Online]. Available: http://www.aesa.msc.es/aesa/web/FileServer?file=the%20 NAOS%20Strategy.pdf&language=en_US&download=yes [accessed June 8, 2006].

Ministry of Health, Welfare, and Sport. 2004. *Living Longer in Good Health.* The Hague, Netherlands: Ministry of Health, Welfare, and Sport. [Online]. Available: http://www. minvws.nl/images/Living%20longer%20in%20good%20health_tcm11-53021.pdf [accessed June 8, 2006].

Ministry of Social Affairs. 2002–2003. *Prescriptions for a Healthier Norway.* Oslo, Norway: Ministry of Social Affairs. [Online]. Available: http://odin.dep.no/filarkiv/184595/ folkehelse-eng.pdf [accessed June 10, 2006].

Ministry of Social Affairs and Health. 2002. *Government Resolution on Policies to Develop Health-Enhancing Physical Activity.* Helsinki, Finland. [Online]. Available: http://www. ukkinstituutti.fi/upload/Teli_in_English.pdf [accessed July 25, 2006].

NASPE (National Association for Sport and Physical Education) and AHA (American Heart Association). 2006. *Shape of the Nation Report: Status of Physical Education in the USA.* Reston, VA: NASPE. [Online]. Available: http://www.aahperd.org/naspe/Shape OfTheNation/ [accessed May 30, 2006].

National Board of Health. 2003. *National Action Plan Against Obesity. Recommendations and Perspectives.* Short Version. Copenhagen, Denmark: Regional Office for Europe. [Online]. Available: http://www.sst.dk/publ/publ2003/National_action_plan.pdf [accessed June 7, 2006].

National Food Administration and National Institute of Public Health. 2005. *Background Material to the Action Plan for Healthy Dietary Habits and Increased Physical Activity.* Stockholm, Sweden: National Food Administration. [Online]. Available: http://www. fhi.se/upload/2702/TheSwedishActionplan.pdf [accessed June 7, 2006].

National Health Service. 2004. *Choosing Health: Making Healthy Choices Easier.* United Kingdom: HM Government, Department of Health, and National Health Service. [Online]. Available: http://www.dh.gov.uk/assetRoot/04/12/07/92/04120792.pdf [accessed June 8, 2006].

National Institute of Public Health. 2005. *Summary of Government Assignment. Healthy Dietary Habits and Increased Physical Activity—The Basis for an Action Plan.* Stockholm, Sweden: National Institute of Public Health. [Online]. Available: http://www.fhi. se/upload/ar2005/rapporter/healthydietaryhabitsphysicalactivitysummary0502.pdf [accessed June 10, 2006].

National Institute of Public Health, Republic of Slovenia. 2005. *The National Programme of Food and Nutrition Policy 2005–2010.* Slovenia: National Institute of Public Health.

National Nutrition Council, National Public Health Institute, Ministry of Agriculture and Forestry. 2005. *Finnish Nutrition Recommendations 2005.* Helsinki, Finland. [Online]. Available: http://wwwb.mmm.fi/ravitsemusneuvottelukunta/Julkaisut_ENG.htm [accessed August 10, 2006].

National Taskforce on Obesity. 2005. *Obesity: The Policy Challenges. The Report of the National Taskforce on Obesity.* Dublin, Ireland. [Online]. Available: http://www.dohc.ie/ publications/pdf/report_taskforce_on_obesity. pdf?direct=1 [accessed June 8, 2006].

Nordic Council of Ministers for Fisheries and Aquaculture, Agriculture, Foodstuffs, and Forestry; The Nordic Council of Ministers for Social Security and Health Care. 2006. *Health, Food, and Physical Activity. Nordic Plan of Action on Better Health and Quality of Life through Diet and Physical Activity.* Copenhagen, Denmark. [Online]. Available: http://www.norden.org/pub/velfaerd/livsmedel/sk/ANP2006745.pdf [accessed August 14, 2006].

PAHO/WHO (Pan American Health Organization/World Health Organization). 2005. *Global Strategy on Healthy Eating, Physical Activity and Health (DPAS): Implementation Plan for Latin America and the Caribbean 2006–2007.* Draft. [Online]. Available: http:// www.minsal.cl/ici/nutricion/ego/Propuesta_OMS_para_America_Latina_y_el_Caribe. pdf [accessed July 11, 2006].

PAHO/WHO. 2006a. *Regional Strategy and Plan of Action on an Integrated Approach to the Prevention and Control of Chronic Diseases, Including Diet, Physical Activity, and Health.* 138th Session of the Executive Committee, June 19–23. Washington, DC: PAHO. [Online]. Available: http://www.ops-oms.org/English/GOV/CE/ce138-17-e.pdf [accessed June 20, 2006].

PAHO/WHO. 2006b. *Regional Strategy on Nutrition in Health and Development 2006–2015.* 138th Session of the Executive Committee, June 1. Washington, DC: PAHO. [Online]. Available: http://www.paho.org/English/GOV/CE/ce138-18-e.pdf [accessed June 20, 2006].

PEW Research Center. 2006. *Americans See Weight Problems Everywhere but in the Mirror.* [Online]. Available: http://pewresearch.org/assets/social/pdf/Obesity.pdf [accessed April 13, 2006].

Portuguese Ministry of Health and Portuguese General Directorate of Health. 2004. *National Programme Against Obesity.* Lisbon, Portugal.

Rideout V, Hamel E. 2006. *The Media Family: Electronic Media in the Lives of Infants, Toddlers, Preschoolers and Their Parents.* Menlo Park, CA: Henry J. Kaiser Family Foundation.

Secretariat of the Pacific Community. 2002. *Obesity in the Pacific: Too Big to Ignore.* Noumea, New Caledonia: Secretariat of the Pacific Community [Online]. Available: http://www.wpro.who.int/publications/pub_9822039255. htm [accessed June 20, 2006].

Thomson Medstat. 2006. *Lifestyle and Obesity: How Occasional Indulgences Shape a Nation's Waistline.* [Online]. Available: http://www.medstat.com/uploadedFiles/docs/Research%20Brief—Lifestyle%20and%20Obesity.pdf [accessed August 5, 2006].

Wall Street Journal Online and Harris Interactive. 2005. *Most of the American Public, Including a Majority of Parents, Believe that Childhood Obesity in the U.S. is a Major Problem.* [Online]. Available: http://www.harrisinteractive.com/news/newsletters/wsjhealth news/WSJOnline_HI_Health-CarePoll2005vol4_iss03.pdf [accessed June 7, 2006].

Wall Street Journal Online and Harris Interactive. 2006. *More Adults This Year See Childhood Obesity as a Major Problem in the U.S.* [Online]. Available: http://www.harris interactive.com/news/allnewsbydate.asp?NewsID=1071 [accessed July 15, 2006].

Wang Y, Monteiro C, Popkin BM. 2002. Trends of obesity and underweight in older children and adolescents in the United States, Brazil, China, and Russia. *Am J Clin Nutr* 75(6): 971–977.

WHO (World Health Organization). 2002. *World Health Report: Reducing Risks, Promoting Healthy Life.* Geneva, Switzerland: WHO. [Online]. Available: http://www.who.int/whr/2002/en/whr02_en.pdf [accessed June 17, 2006].

WHO. 2003. *Diet, Nutrition and the Prevention of Chronic Diseases.* Technical Report Series No. 916. Geneva, Switzerland: WHO. [Online]. Available: http://www.who.int/hpr/NPH/docs/who_fao_expert_report.pdf [accessed June 8, 2006].

WHO. 2004a. *Global Strategy on Diet, Physical Activity, and Health.* Report No. WHA57.17. Geneva, Switzerland: WHO. [Online]. Available: http://www.who.int/gb/ebwha/pdf_files/WHA57/A57_R17-en.pdf [accessed May 23, 2006].

WHO. 2004b. *Children's Environment and Health Action Plan for Europe.* Fourth Ministerial Conference on Environment and Health, June 23–25. Budapest, Hungary. [Online]. Available: http://www.euro.who.int/document/e83338.pdf [accessed June 27, 2006].

WHO. 2006a. *Preventing Chronic Diseases: A Vital Investment.* Geneva, Switzerland: WHO. [Online]. Available: http://www.who.int/chp/chronic_disease_report/full_report.pdf [accessed May 23, 2006].

WHO. 2006b. *European Ministerial Charter on Counteracting Obesity.* WHO European Minsterial Conference on Counteracting Obesity. Istanbul, Turkey. November 15–17. Copenhagen, Denmark: WHO Regional Office for Europe. [Online]. Available: http://www.euro.who.int/obesity/conference2006 [accessed September 1, 2006].

Yankelovich. 2006. *Food for Life: An Attitudinal and Database Perspective on Food, Diet and Preventive Health Care.* [Online]. Available: http://www.yankelovich.com/products/Food%20For%20Life%20Final%20Presentation%2003-27-06.pdf [accessed July 20, 2006].

A

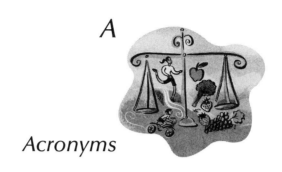

Acronyms

AAFP	American Academy of Family Physicians
AAP	American Academy of Pediatrics
ABA	American Beverage Association
ACE	Adverse Childhood Experiences (study)
ACF	Administration for Children & Families
ADA	American Dietetic Association; also American Diabetes Association
AHA	American Heart Association
AHRQ	Agency for Healthcare Research and Quality
AI/AN	American Indian/Alaska Native
AMA	American Medical Association; also American Marketing Association
AMS	Agricultural Marketing Service
ANPRM	advance notices of proposed rulemaking
ARS	Agricultural Research Service, U.S. Department of Agriculture
ASPE	Assistant Secretary for Planning and Evaluation
BET	Black Entertainment Television
BLS	Bureau of Labor Statistics
BMI	body mass index
BRFSS	Behavioral Risk Factor Surveillance System
BTS	Bureau for Transportation Safety

CACFP	Child and Adult Care Food Program
CARU	Children's Advertising Review Unit
CATCH	Coordinated Approach To Child Health
CBBB	Council of Better Business Bureaus
CDC	Centers for Disease Control and Prevention
CDHS	California Department of Health Services
CES	Cooperative Extension Service
CFSC	Community Food Security Coalition
CHIS	California Health Interview Survey
CNLP	Child Nutrition Labeling Program
CNPP	Center for Nutrition Policy and Promotion
CSD	carbonated soft drinks
CSREES	Cooperative State Research, Education, and Extension Service
CSTE	Council of State and Territorial Epidemiologists
CVD	cardiovascular disease
CX^3	Communities of Excellence in Nutrition, Physical Activity, and Obesity Prevention
DHHS	U.S. Department of Health and Human Services
DoD	U.S. Department of Defense
DoEd	U.S. Department of Education
DoI	U.S. Department of the Interior
DoL	U.S. Department of Labor
DoT	U.S. Department of Transportation
EFNEP	Expanded Food and Nutrition Education Program
EPSDT	Early and Periodic Screening, Diagnostic, and Treatment Program
ERS	Economic Research Service
FANRP	Food Assistance and Nutrition Research Program
FCC	Federal Communications Commission
FDA	U.S. Food and Drug Administration
FFVP	Fresh Fruit and Vegetable Program
FGP	Food Guide Pyramid
FHWA	Federal Highway Administration
FMI	Food Marketing Institute
FMNP	Farmers' Market Nutrition Program
FMNV	foods of minimal nutritional value
FNB	Food and Nutrition Board
FNS	Food and Nutrition Service
FSNE	Food Stamp Nutrition Education Program

FSP	Food Stamp Program
FTC	Federal Trade Commission
FY	fiscal year
GAO	Government Accountability Office
GDP	gross domestic product
GIS	geographic information systems
GMA	Grocery Manufacturers Association
HEAC	Healthy Eating/Active Communities
HRSA	Health Resources and Services Administration
HUD	U.S. Department of Housing and Urban Development
IHS	Indian Health Service
IMPACT	Improved Nutrition and Physical Activity Act
IOM	Institute of Medicine
KPI	key performance indicators
MAPP	Mobilizing for Action through Planning and Partnerships
MCHB	Maternal and Child Health Bureau
MoU	memorandum of understanding
NACCHO	National Association of County and City Health Officials
NARC	National Advertising Review Council
NASSP	National Association of Secondary School Principals
NCCDPHP	National Center for Chronic Disease Prevention and Health Promotion
NCHS	National Center for Health Statistics
NCI	National Cancer Institute
NCQA	National Committee for Quality Assurance
NCSL	National Conference of State Legislatures
NCYFS	National Children and Youth Fitness Study
NFCS	National Food Consumption Survey
NGA	National Governors Association
NHANES	National Health and Nutrition Examination Survey
NHES	National Health Examination Survey
NHIS	National Health Interview Survey
NHLBI	National Heart, Lung, and Blood Institute
NHTS	National Household Travel Survey
NICHD	National Institute of Child Health & Human Development

NIDDK	National Institute of Diabetes & Digestive & Kidney Diseases
NIEHS	National Institute of Environmental Health Sciences
NIH	National Institutes of Health
NLEA	Nutrition Labeling and Education Act
NLSAH	National Longitudinal Study of Adolescent Health
NLSY	National Longitudinal Survey of Youth
NPS	National Park Service
NRC	National Research Council
NSCH	National Survey of Children's Health
NSECH	National Survey of Early Childhood Health
NSLP	National School Lunch Program
ODPHP	Office of Disease Prevention and Health Promotion
OMB	Office of Management and Budget
OMH	Office of Minority Health
OSG	Office of the Surgeon General
OSTP	Office of Science and Technology Policy
PART	Program Assessment Rating Tool
PBH	Produce for Better Health Foundation
PCPFS	President's Council on Physical Fitness and Sports
PEP	Physical Education Program Grants
PedNSS	Pediatric Nutrition Surveillance System
PNSS	Pregnancy Nutrition Surveillance System
PRC	Prevention Research Center
PSA	public service advertising
QSR	quick serve restaurant
RCT	randomized controlled trial
REACH	Racial and Ethnic Approaches to Community Health
RWJF	Robert Wood Johnson Foundation
SBP	School Breakfast Program
SCHIP	State Child Health Insurance Program
SDPI	Special Diabetes Program for Indians
SES	socioeconomic status
SHAC	school health advisory council
SHAPE	Survey of the Health of All the Population and the Environment
SHI	School Health Index
SHP	School Health Profiles

SHPPS	School Health Policies and Programs Study
SIDS	sudden infant death syndrome
SNAP	State Nutrition Action Plans
SNDA	School Nutrition Dietary Assessment Study
SPAN	School Physical Activity and Nutrition
SPI	State Plan Index
SRTS	Safe Routes to School Program
TFAH	Trust for America's Health
TRB	Transportation Research Board
UB	University of Baltimore
UFFVA	United Fresh Fruit and Vegetable Association
UPC	uniform product code
UPRRP	Urban Park and Recreation Recovery Program
USDA	U.S. Department of Agriculture
WHO	World Health Organization
WIC	Special Supplemental Nutrition Program for Women, Infants, and Children
YMCLS	Youth Media Campaign Longitudinal Survey
YRBS	Youth Risk Behavior Survey
YRBSS	Youth Risk Behavior Surveillance System

B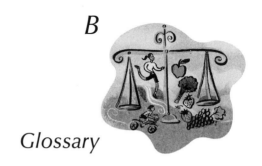

Glossary

Accountability   The systematic inclusion of the elements of program planning, implementation, monitoring, and evaluation to achieve program goals and results.

Active Living   A way of life that integrates physical activity into daily routines. The two types of activities that comprise active living are recreational or leisure such as jogging, skateboarding, or playing basketball, and utilitarian or occupational, such as walking or biking to school, shopping, or running errands.

Activities   The actions implemented by a program and its staff to achieve desired outcomes in a target population or specific setting.

Assessment   In this report, refers to the process of observing, describing, collecting, and measuring the quality and effectiveness of an initiative, program, or policy. Also see *Evaluation.*

Away-from-Home Foods   Foods categorized according to where they are obtained, such as restaurants and other places with wait service; quick serve restaurants and self-service or take-out eateries; ready-to-eat foods from supermarkets; schools, including child-care centers, after-school programs, and summer camp; and other outlets, including vending machines, community feeding programs, and eating at someone else's home.

Balanced Diet   The overall dietary pattern of foods consumed that provide all the essential nutrients in the appropriate amounts to support life processes, including growth and development in children without promoting excess body fat accumulation and excess weight gain.

Behavioral Branding   A strategy used by social marketing programs to create brands that individuals associate with a specific behavior or lifestyle. Examples include the VERB™ campaign, which encourages tweens (children ages 8 to 13 years) to associate VERB with physical activity, and the truth® brand, which represents an inspirational antismoking brand for teens that builds a positive image of youth as nonsmokers, cool and edgy, and rebellious against the tobacco industry.

Behavioral Outcomes   Behavioral changes made by individuals or populations that affect diet and physical activity levels and that enhance health. These may include increasing physical activity levels, increasing fruit and vegetable consumption, balancing caloric intakes and expenditures, reducing television viewing time, and increasing breastfeeding rates.

Best Practice   An intervention or effort that is likely to reduce childhood obesity and for which there is a sufficient amount of robust evidence that provides a level of certainty that the intervention is linked to reducing the incidence or prevalence of childhood obesity and related co-morbidities.

Bill   A proposed new law or amendment to an existing law that is presented to the legislature for consideration. A bill requires approval by both chambers of the legislature and action by a governor or the president to amend an existing law or to become a law.

Body Mass Index   Body mass index (BMI) is an indirect measure of body fat calculated as the ratio of a person's body weight (in kilograms) to the square of a person's height in meters:

$$\text{BMI (kg/m}^2) = \text{weight (kilograms)} \div \text{height (meters)}^2$$

$$\text{BMI (lb/in}^2) = \text{weight (pounds)} \div \text{height (inches)}^2 \times 703$$

In children and youth, assessment of BMI is based on growth charts for age and gender and is referred to as BMI for age. According to the Centers for Disease Control and Prevention (CDC), a child with a BMI for age that is equal to or greater than the 95th percentile is considered overweight. A child with a BMI for age that is equal to or between the 85th and 95th percentile is considered to be at risk of becoming overweight. In this report, the definition of obesity is equivalent to the CDC definition of overweight, and at risk of becoming obese is equivalent to the CDC definition of at risk for becoming overweight.

Calorie   A kilocalorie is defined as the amount of heat required to change the temperature of 1 gram of water from 14.5° C to 15.5° C. In this report, calorie is used synonymously with kilocalorie as a unit of measure for energy obtained from foods and beverages.

Capacity Building   A multidimensional and dynamic process that improves the ability of individuals, groups, communities, organizations, and governments to meet their objectives or enhance performance to address population health. In public health, capacity building involves the ability to carry out essential functions, such as developing and sustaining partnerships, leveraging resources, surveillance and monitoring, providing training and technical assistance, and conducting evaluations.

Caregiver   An individual, such as a parent, foster parent, or head of a household, who attends to the needs of a child or an adolescent.

Channel   An organized system through which interventions can be delivered efficiently to reach large segments of the population, such as schools, communities, and families at home.

Children's Advertising Review Unit (CARU)   The Children's Advertising Review Unit (CARU) was founded in 1974 to promote responsible children's advertising as a component of the strategic alliance with major advertising trade associations through the National Advertising Review Council. CARU is the children's arm of the advertising industry's self-regulation program and evaluates child-directed advertising and promotional material in all media to advance the accuracy, truthfulness, and consistency of advertisements.

Coalition   An organized group of people in a community working toward a common goal. A coalition can have individual, group, institutional, community, or public policy goals.

Cognitive Outcomes   Changes in an individual's knowledge, awareness, beliefs, and attitudes about the importance of healthy diets and regular physical activity to reduce the risk of obesity and related chronic diseases.

Collaboration   A cooperative effort between and among groups of people (e.g., governmental entities and private partners) through which partners work together toward mutual advantage and to achieve common goals.

Collaboration can range from informal ad hoc activities to more planned, organized, and formalized ways of working together.

Collective Efficacy   The willingness of community members to look out for each other and intervene when problems arise.

Community   A social entity that can be either spatial, based on where people live in local neighborhoods, residential districts, or municipalities, or relational, based on common ethnic, cultural, or other characteristics or similar interests.

Community Readiness   In broad terms, the community's awareness of, interest in, and ability to support policies, programs, and initiatives.

Community Youth Mapping   A tool that young people can use to explore their communities. In this process, youth and adults document, analyze, and disseminate information on community resources, issues, and gaps in available resources. Community youth mapping provides opportunities for meaningful involvement by youth and adults as well as the development of skills, including public speaking, data collection, entry, and analysis; oral and written communications; knowledge about community resources; and conflict resolution.

Competitive Foods   Foods and beverages other than meals and snacks offered at schools through the federally reimbursed National School Lunch Program, School Breakfast Program, and after-school snack programs. Competitive foods include food and beverage items sold through á la carte lines, snack bars, student stores, vending machines, and school fundraisers.

Confounder   A factor that may cause or prevent a desired outcome that is associated with a factor under investigation and that does not represent an intermediate variable.

Context   The set of factors or circumstances that surrounds a situation or event and that gives meaning to its interpretation; the broader environment in which a program operates.

Coordination   The process of seeking concurrence from one or more groups, organizations, or agencies regarding a proposal or an activity for which they share some responsibility and that may result in contributions from each of the entities.

Correlate   To put or bring into causal, complementary, parallel, or reciprocal relation.

Cost-Benefit Analysis   An evaluation tool used to compare the various costs associated with an investment in a program or initiative with its proposed benefits.

Cost-Effectiveness Analysis   An evaluation tool used to assess the most efficient method for achieving a program or policy goal. The costs of alternatives are measured by their requisite estimated dollar expenditures. Effectiveness is defined by the degree of achieving a goal and may be measured in dollars.

Cost-Utility Analysis   An evaluation tool used to assess the relative economic value (e.g., cost-utility ratio) of alternative strategies that aim to achieve similar outcomes. This type of analysis converts effects into personal preferences and describes how much it costs for some additional quality gain (e.g., cost per additional quality-adjusted life-year).

Cross-Sectional Survey   The observation of a defined population at a single point in time or time interval.

Cultural Competence   The ability of individuals to consider ethnic, racial and cultural aspects in all dimensions of their work relative to obesity prevention and population health programs and interventions. Cultural competence is optimized when program staff involve clients or recipients in all phases of a program, from planning to implementation, monitoring, and evaluation.

Culture   The values, norms, beliefs, attitudes, traditions, and customs shared by a group of people who are unified by race, ethnicity, language, faith, nationality, or life experience.

Dietary Guidelines for Americans   A federal summary of the latest dietary guidance for the American public based on current scientific evidence and medical knowledge. The guidelines are issued jointly by the U.S. Department of Health and Human Services and the U.S. Department of Agriculture and are revised every 5 years.

Discourse   The language used by members of a community to define and discuss a specific topic. It can also represent an institutionalized way of thinking.

Discretionary Calories   The amount of calories in an individual's "energy allowance" after the person consumes sufficient amounts of foods and beverages to meet one's daily calorie and nutrient needs while promoting weight maintenance.

Discretionary Fat   The ability of a person to selectively add dietary fat (e.g., salad dressing, butter, and oil) according to personal preferences, which contributes to total calorie intake. This is distinct from the obligatory fat that has been added to foods prior to consumption and that cannot be removed prior to consumption.

Energy Balance   A state in which calorie intake is equivalent to energy expenditure, resulting in no net weight gain or weight loss. In this report, energy balance in children is used to indicate the equality between energy intake and energy expenditure that supports normal growth and development without promoting excess weight gain.

Energy Density   The amount of calories stored in a given food per unit volume or mass. Fat stores 9 kilocalories/gram (g), alcohol stores 7 kilocalories/g, carbohydrate and protein each store 4 kilocalories/g, fiber stores 1.5 to 2.5 kilocalories/g, and water has no calories. Foods that are almost entirely composed of fat with minimal water (e.g., butter) are more calorie dense than foods that consist largely of water, fiber, and carbohydrates (e.g., fruits and vegetables).

Energy Expenditure   Calories used to support the body's basal metabolic needs plus those used for thermogenesis, growth, and physical activity.

Energy Intake   Calories ingested as foods and beverages.

Environment   The aggregate of the social and cultural conditions that influence the life of an individual or a community.

Environmental Justice   Efforts that address the disproportionate exposure to harmful environmental conditions by low-income and minority communities.

Environmental Outcomes   Changes that create a health-promoting environment, including access to healthful foods and beverages; opportunities for physical activity; changes in the commercial marketplace, including the media; and changes in the built environment, including schools, the transportation system, recreational facilities and opportunities, and food retail outlets.

Evaluation   A systematic assessment of the quality and effectiveness of an initiative, program, or policy and its effects to produce information that can be used by those who have an interest in its improvement or effectiveness.

Evaluative Research   The use of scientific research methods to assess the effectiveness of an initiative, program, or policy.

Fast Food   Foods and meals designed for ready availability, use, or consumption and sold at eating establishments for quick availability or take-out.

Fidelity   The rigor with which an intervention adheres to a program's purpose and intent. For obesity prevention programs, fidelity is the degree of fit between the planned intervention and its actual implementation in a given institutional or community setting.

Focus Group   A research method whereby a moderator convenes a group of participants who often have common characteristics (e.g., age, gender, or ethnicity) to discuss the attributes of a specific concept or product. Focus groups are often used in the marketing development phase to generate ideas and provide insights into consumer reactions and perceptions.

Formative Evaluation   A method of assessing the value of a program while the program activities are developing. Formative evaluation focuses on process issues such as understanding how a program works and its strengths and weaknesses.

Generalizability   The extent to which the results produced by a specific intervention or set of interventions under specific conditions may be expected to produce similar findings in future efforts in different settings or contexts with different populations.

Geographic Information System   A system of computer hardware, software, and spatial data used to capture, manage, analyze, and display geographically referenced information.

Goal   A clear and specific measurable outcome or change that can be reasonably expected at the end of a planned program or interventions.

Health   A state of complete physical, mental and social well-being and not merely the absence of disease or infirmity.

Health Disparities   The population-specific differences in the presence of disease, health outcomes, or access to health care across racial, ethnic, and different socioeconomic groups.

Health Impact Assessment A combination of procedures, methods, and tools by which a policy, program, or project may be evaluated in terms of its potential effects on the health of a population and the distribution of those effects within the population.

Health Outcomes Changes made by individuals or populations that either reduce or increase their risk of developing specific health conditions. This report identifies three health outcomes of interest: reduced mean population body mass index levels, reduced obesity prevalence, and reduced obesity-related morbidity in children and youth.

Health Promotion The process of enabling people to increase control over and to improve their health through networks and initiatives that create healthy environments. To reach a state of complete physical, mental, and social well-being, an individual or group must be able to identify and to realize aspirations, to satisfy needs, and to change or cope with the environment. Health is a resource for everyday life, not the objective of living, and is a positive concept emphasizing social and personal resources, as well as physical capacities.

Healthful Diet For children and adolescents, a healthful diet provides recommended amounts of nutrients and other food components within estimated energy requirements to promote normal growth and development, a healthy weight trajectory, and energy balance. A healthful diet is consistent with the Dietary Guidelines for Americans and reduces the long-term risk for obesity and related chronic diseases associated with aging, including type 2 diabetes and metabolic syndrome.

Healthfulness The quality of promoting good health.

Healthy Weight In children and youth, a level of body fat that supports normal growth and development and at which there are no observed co-morbidities. The current guidelines for healthy weight in children and youth of the Centers for Disease Control and Prevention are in the range of the 5th to the 85th percentiles of the age- and gender-specific body mass index charts.

Horizontal Integration An approach that encourages partners at the same level of operation—neighborhood, city, country, region, or state—to work across organizational lines to deliver a consistent, comprehensive, multi-component intervention to target groups.

Human Capacity The collective knowledge, attitudes, motivation, and skill sets of program implementers.

Impact Evaluation   A measure of whether or not an outcome, such as the effectiveness of a program, is the result of an intervention. To draw a cause-and-effect conclusion, an impact evaluation incorporates research methods that eliminate alternative explanations for an outcome and shows how much difference an intervention can make compared with the effect seen when no intervention is used. In public health programs, an impact evaluation often occurs over a long period of time.

Incidence   The frequency of new cases of a condition or disease within a defined time period. Incidence is commonly measured in new cases per 1,000 (or 100,000) population at risk per year.

Indicators   Aggregates of raw and processed data that are used to measure social, economic, and health outcomes such as unemployment rates, gross national product, obesity rates, morbidity, and life expectancy. Indices are aggregated measures of several indicators and are used to describe the performance of an institution or sector.

Inputs   The type and level of resources required—such as people, time, and money—to support, implement, and sustain program activities.

Institutional Outcomes   Changes in organizational cultures, norms, policies, and procedures related to dietary patterns and physical activity behaviors. An example of an institutional outcome is the development or expansion of a company's employee wellness program to incorporate obesity prevention into its activities.

Integrated Marketing   A planning process designed to ensure that all promotional activities, including media advertising, direct mail, sales promotion, and public relations, produce a unified, customer-focused promotion message that is relevant to a customer and that is consistent over time.

Intervention   A policy, program, or action intended to bring about identifiable outcomes.

Land Use   The way in which land is used, including for residential, commercial, industrial, or mixed-use development or for the preservation of open spaces, including parks and agricultural land.

Leisure Screen Time   The total amount of time spent using electronic media during one's free time. It includes exposure to television, DVDs, videos, videogames, movies, and computers.

Life Course Perspective   How health status at any given age or for a given birth cohort reflects both contemporary conditions and prior living circumstances, from the time in utero throughout the life course. A life course perspective acknowledges that over time individuals have developmental trajectories (both biological and social) that are shaped by society's social, economic, political, technological, and ecological contexts.

Longitudinal Survey   A survey that examines the specific characteristics of individuals, sub-groups, or populations over time.

Marketing   An organizational function and a set of processes for creating, communicating, and delivering value to customers and for managing customer relationships in ways that benefit an organization and its stakeholders. Marketing encompasses a wide range of activities, including market research; analyzing the competition; positioning a new product; pricing products and services; and promoting products and services through advertising, consumer promotion, trade promotions, public relations, and sales.

Measured Media   The categories tracked by media research companies, including television (e.g., network; spot; and cable, syndicated, and Spanish-language networks), radio (e.g., network, national spot, and local), magazines (e.g., local and Sunday magazines), business publications, newspapers (e.g., local and national newspapers), outdoor, direct mail, the yellow pages, and the Internet.

Mediator   The mechanism by which one variable affects another variable.

Mixed-Method Design   Uses methodologies drawn from a variety of disciplines and both qualitative and quantitative data gathering and analysis methods that combine extensive descriptions of context and the experiences of program participation with standardized assessments of changes in institutions or systems, the environment, and individual or population behaviors.

Moderator   A variable that changes the impact of one variable on another.

Monitoring   The collection and analysis of data as a program, intervention, or policy progresses to ensure the integrity of its planned implementation.

Multifaceted Interventions   Interventions that involve more than one component that are delivered concurrently to a target group in combination.

National School Lunch Program   The National School Lunch Program (NSLP) is a federally funded meal program established in 1946 that operates in public and nonprofit private schools and residential child-care institutions. NSLP provides nutritionally balanced, reduced-cost, or free lunches to children every school day.

Natural Experiment   Naturally occurring circumstances in which different populations are exposed or not exposed to a potential causal factor or intervention such that the circumstances resemble a true experiment in which study participants are assigned to exposed and unexposed groups.

Nutrient Density   The amount of nutrients that a food contains per unit volume or mass. Nutrient density is independent of energy density, although, in practice, the nutrient density of a food is often described in relationship to the food's energy density.

Nutrition Facts Panel   Standardized detailed information on the nutrient contents and serving sizes of nearly all packaged foods sold in the U.S. marketplace. The panel was designed to provide nutrition information to consumers and was mandated by the Nutrition Labeling and Education Act of 1990.

Obesity   An excess amount of subcutaneous body fat in proportion to lean body mass. In adults, a body mass index (BMI) of 30 or greater is considered obese. In this report, obesity in children and youth refers to the age- and gender-specific BMI that is equal to or greater than the 95th percentile of the BMI charts of the Centers for Disease Control and Prevention (CDC). At-risk for obesity in children and youth is defined as a BMI for age and gender that is between the 85th and 95th percentiles of the CDC BMI curves. In most children, these values are known to indicate elevated body fat and to reflect the possibility of comorbidities associated with excessive body fatness.

Obesogenic   Environmental factors that may promote obesity and encourage the expression of a genetic predisposition to gain weight.

Outcome   The changes that result from a program's activities and outputs. Depending on the nature of an intervention and the theory of change guiding it, an outcome can be short term, intermediate term, or long term. Indicators or indices are used to assess whether progress has been made toward achieving specific outcomes as a result of an intervention.

Outcome Evaluation An approach to assessing whether or not anticipated changes or differences have occurred as a result of an intervention. This type of evaluation assesses the extent of change in targeted attitudes, values, behaviors, policies, programs, environments, or conditions between the baseline measurement and subsequent points of measurement over time.

Output The direct products of activities; usually, a tangible deliverable produced as a result of an activity. Examples of outputs include the number of people reached, the number of sessions conducted, the number of volunteers engaged, or the amount of educational materials distributed.

Physical Activity Body movement produced by the contraction of skeletal muscles that results in energy expenditure above the basal level. Physical activity consists of athletic, recreational, housework, transport, and occupational activities that require physical skills and that use strength, power, endurance, speed, flexibility, range of motion, or agility.

Policy A written statement reflecting a plan or course of action taken by a government, businesses, communities, or institutions that is intended to influence and guide present and future decisions. For a government, a policy may represent a law, regulation, ordinance, executive order, or resolution.

Policy Maker An individual elected or appointed to office at some level of government; may include federal, state, and local executive branch chiefs of staff and staff assistants who often play central roles in the policy process.

Population Health The state of health of an entire community or population as opposed to that of an individual. It is concerned with the interrelated factors that affect the health of populations over the life course and the distribution of the patterns of health outcomes.

Portion Size The amount of food that an individual is served at home or away from home and that an individual chooses to consume for a meal or snack. Portions can be larger or smaller than the serving sizes listed on the food label or the Food Guide Pyramid.

Poverty Guidelines A simplified version of the federal poverty thresholds issued annually in the *Federal Register* by the U.S. Department of Health and Human Services. They are used for administrative purposes such as determining financial eligibility of individuals and households for federal programs, including the Medicaid, Food Stamps, the Special Supplemental

Nutrition Program for Women, Infants, and Children (WIC), and the school nutrition programs.

Poverty Thresholds   Used to calculate all official poverty population statistics, such as data on the number of Americans living in poverty each year. Poverty thresholds are updated each year by the U.S. Bureau of the Census.

Precursor   Something that precedes and indicates, suggests, or forecasts something to come; a factor in a stage or a process that precedes a later stage.

Prevalence   The number of instances of a condition or a disease in a population at a designated period of time; usually expressed as a percentage of the total population.

Prevention   With regard to obesity, primary prevention represents avoiding the occurrence of obesity in a population, secondary prevention represents the early detection of disease through screening with the purpose of limiting its occurrence, and tertiary prevention involves preventing the sequelae of obesity in childhood and adulthood.

Process Evaluation   The means of assessing strategies and actions to reveal insights into the extent to which implementation is being carried out in accordance with expected standards and the extent to which a given action or strategy is working as planned.

Program   An integrated set of planned strategies and activities that support clearly stated goals and objectives that lead to desirable changes and improvements in the well-being of people, institutions, or environments, or all of these.

Promising Practice   An intervention that is likely to reduce childhood obesity and that has been reasonably well evaluated but for which there is a lack of sufficient evidence to provide a level of certainty that the intervention may be linked to reducing the incidence or prevalence of childhood obesity and related comorbidities.

Promotion   The means by which a business or company communicates with its target audience or customers to inform, persuade, or influence customers' purchase decisions.

Proprietary   Privately owned and operated; something that is held under patent, trademark, or copyright by a private person or company.

Proprietary Data Information obtained from private companies or firms that hold the exclusive rights to distribute the information or data which are often collected for specific commercial purposes intended for a targeted audience. The information or data may be available to customers who can purchase it, and is usually not widely available to the broad public due to the expense.

Protective Factors Conditions that build resilience to buffer the negative effects of potential risks, such as those that exist in an obesogenic environment.

Public Health Program A coordinated set of complementary activities designed to produce desirable health outcomes.

Public Relations A company's communications and relationships with various groups, including customers, employees, suppliers, stockholders, governments, general public, and society.

Public Service Announcement An advertisement or commercial that is carried by an advertising vehicle at no cost as a public service to its readers, viewers, or listeners; a promotional message for a nonprofit organization or for a social cause printed or broadcast at no charge by the media.

Quality of Life The degree to which intellectual, spiritual, economical, social, and health pursuits are achieved and maintained. A person's overall sense of well-being and a supportive environment when applied to a community.

Quasi-Experimental An experiment in which the investigator lacks full control over the allocation or timing of the intervention.

Quick Serve Restaurant A category of restaurants characterized by food that is supplied quickly after ordering and with minimal service. Foods and beverages purchased may be consumed at the restaurant or served as take-out.

Race A socially defined population based on visible and genetically transmitted physical characteristics. A socially defined population based on visible and genetically transmitted physical characteristics.

Randomized Controlled Trial A study design in which a group of patients is randomized into an experimental group and a control group. The groups are monitored for the variables or outcomes of interest.

Reliability   Assessment of the extent to which the same measurement technique, applied repeatedly, is likely to yield the same results.

Resolution   A formal expression of the will, opinion, or direction of one or both houses of the legislature on a matter of public interest. Joint and concurrent resolutions are voted on by both houses but require no action on the part of the governor. Resolutions tend to be temporary in nature and do not have the support of law.

Risk Factor   A condition that increases the possibility that an individual, group, community, or population may experience a problem, such as the incidence or prevalence of obesity.

Safety   The condition of being either protected from or unlikely to cause danger, risk, or injury that may be either perceived or objectively defined.

Sales Promotion   Marketing activities other than advertising, personal selling, and publicity that stimulate consumer purchases at the point-of-sale such as a display, product demonstration, trade show, contest, coupon, premium, prize, toy, or price discount. Also called *consumer promotion*.

School Breakfast Program   A federally administered program that provides cash assistance to states to operate breakfast programs in U.S. schools and residential child-care institutions.

School Meal Initiative for Healthy Children   A program launched by the U.S. Department of Agriculture in 1995 to improve the nutritional quality of school lunches and breakfasts.

Screen Time   The number of hours that a child or adolescent spends watching various types of electronic media (e.g., broadcast and cable television, video, digital video disc, movie, or computer) per day, week, month, or year. It may be for either leisure or educational purposes.

Sector   A distinct subset of a market, society, industry, or the economy in which the members share similar characteristics. Examples of the sectors described in this report include government or the public sector; communities, including nonprofit and philanthropic organizations; health care; business or the private sector; schools; and home.

Sedentary   A way of living or a lifestyle that requires minimal physical activity and that encourages inactivity through limited choices, disincentives, or structural or financial barriers.

Serving   A standardized unit of measure used to describe the total amount of food from each of the food groups from MyPyramid recommended to be consumed daily or a specific amount of food that contains the quality of nutrients listed on the Nutrition Facts panel. This may differ from "portion size," which represents the amount of food that an individual is served at home or away from home and chooses to consume for a meal or snack.

Social Determinants   In regard to health, both the specific features of and the pathways by which societal conditions affect health and can be potentially altered by actions.

Social Marketing   The application of commercial marketing principles to the analysis, planning, implementation, and evaluation of programs designed to influence voluntary behavioral changes in target audiences to improve their personal welfare and for the benefit of society.

Social Norms   A set of beliefs and behaviors characteristic of a group, community, or society.

Social Outcomes   Changes in social attitudes and norms that are related to dietary and physical activity behaviors that support healthy lifestyles.

Stakeholder   A person or organization that is invested in a policy or program or interested in the results of an evaluation.

Strategy   A set of actions taken to achieve a goal.

Structural Outcomes   Policies, laws, and resources that have been developed, implemented, or revised to bring about changes in the dietary patterns and physical activity levels of children, youth, and their families. Examples of structural outcomes include policies that mandate physical education in all public schools, policies that restrict the types of competitive foods that may be sold in schools, and laws that require nutrition labeling in full serve and quick serve restaurants.

Surveillance   The systematic collection, analysis, interpretation, and dissemination of data to assist in the planning, implementation, and evaluation of public health policies, programs, and interventions.

Sustainability   The likelihood that a program will continue over a period of time after grant funding has ended. In broader terms, society's ability to shape its economic and social systems to maintain both natural resources and human life. Sustainability improves quality of life in the present while ensuring continued prosperity in the future.

Systemic Outcomes   Eating and physical activity environments and health systems to which changes have been made in the way that they are organized and delivered. Examples of systemic outcomes include changes in the mission of a community health center to include obesity prevention responsibilities or changes in health insurance policies to include obesity prevention activity-related expenses. These also include changes in social norms regarding obesity-related behaviors.

Systems Approach   An approach that views a phenomenon and its components in its entirety and that emphasizes the interactions and connectedness of the components to understand the entire system. A systems approach acknowledges that individuals and families are embedded within broader social, political, and economic systems that shape behaviors and constrain access to resources necessary to maintain health.

Target Population   A group of individuals at risk to whom a policy, program, or intervention is designed to reach.

Technical Assistance   Services provided by program staff that are intended to provide guidance to individuals, institutions, or communities to conduct, strengthen, or enhance obesity prevention activities, such as implementing, monitoring, or evaluating programs and interventions.

Technical Capacity   The specific expertise or skills required for program planning, implementation, monitoring, and evaluation.

Triangulation   The application and combination of several research methodologies (e.g., focus groups, interviews, participant observation, and content analysis of documents) to study a phenomenon. By combining multiple observers, theories, methods of data collection, and empirical approaches, researchers can address intrinsic biases that emerge from a single method and a single-observer study. Triangulation is often used to establish the credibility of qualitative analyses, in contrast to the reliability and validity of quantitative analyses.

Unhealthfulness   The quality of promoting poor health.

Unmeasured Media   The difference between a company's reported or estimated advertising costs and its measured media spending. Unmeasured media spending includes activities such as sales promotions, coupons, direct mail, catalogs, and special events, and is not systematically tracked.

Upstream The determinants of health that are removed from the biological and behavioral bases for disease, including social relations, neighborhoods and communities, institutions, and social and economic policies.

Validity The extent to which an instrument directly and accurately measures what it is intended to measure.

Variable Anything that is not constant but that can and does change in different circumstances.

Vertical Integration The organization of production whereby one business entity controls or owns all stages of the production and distribution of goods or services. In public health, an approach in which partners work at different levels—the national, regional, state, county, and community levels—to deliver interventions planned at a higher level and delivered at a lower level in a coordinated and complementary way.

Well-Being A view of health that, in this report, takes into account a child's physical, social, and emotional health.

C

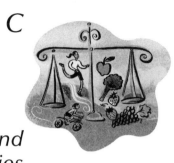

Surveillance and Monitoring Activities

TABLE C-1 Surveillance and Monitoring

Survey	Primary Sponsor; Frequency of Data Collection	Population
Cross-Sectional Surveys		
Behavioral Risk Factor Surveillance System (BRFSS) (CDC, 2006a)	CDC; ongoing	Adults ages 18 years and older
Monitoring the Future (Monitoring the Future, 2006)	Survey Research Center, University of Michigan; ongoing	Grades 8, 10, and 12
National Health and Nutrition Examination Survey (NHANES) (CDC, 2005)	CDC; ongoing	Adults and children
National Health Interview Survey (NHIS) (CDC, 2006c)	CDC; annually	All household members
National Longitudinal Survey of Adolescent Health (Add Health, 2005)	Carolina Population Center; 1994–1995 1996 2001–2002 2006	Grades 7 to 12

Sample Size	Example(s) of Indicators or Outcomes Measured
303,822 (2004)	Fruit and vegetable consumption, physical activity, weight control
50,000/year in 420 secondary schools	Television viewing
5,000/year	Height, weight, and BMI; physical activity and physical fitness; weight history; breastfeeding; food security
31,326 adults (2004)	Physical activity, health care coverage and access
15,170 (2001–2002)	Diet, physical activity, health care service use, height, weight

continued

TABLE C-1 continued

Survey	Primary Sponsor; Frequency of Data Collection	Population
Pediatric Nutrition Surveillance System (PedNSS) (CDC, 2006b)	CDC; ongoing	Ages 0 to 5 years
School Nutrition Dietary Assessment Study (SNDA) (USDA, 2001)	USDA; 1991–1992 1998–1999	Elementary and secondary schools
School Health Policies and Programs Study (SHPPS) (CDC, 2006f)	CDC; 1994 and 2000; conducted in 2006	Elementary, middle/ junior, and senior high school levels
School Health Profiles (SHP) (CDC, 2004)	CDC; biennial (1994, 1996, 1998, 2000, 2002, 2004)	Middle/junior high school and senior high school levels
Youth Media Campaign Longitudinal Survey (YMCLS) (CDC, 2006g)	CDC; annual	Ages 9 to 13 years
Youth Risk Factor Behavior Surveillance System (YRBSS) (CDC, 2006h)	CDC, 1991 to present; every 2 years	Grades 9 to 12
Longitudinal Surveys National Survey of Children's Health (NSCH) (CDC, 2006d)	MCHB and NCHS; January 2003– July 2004	Ages 0 to 17 years
National Survey of Early Childhood Health (NSECH) (CDC, 2006e)	MCHB and AAP; February–July 2000	Ages 4 to 35 months
National Longitudinal Survey of Youth (NLSY) (DoL, 2006)	U.S. Department of Labor; 1979, 1997	Ages 12 to 16 years

NOTE: AAP = American Academy of Pediatrics; BMI = body mass index; CDC = Centers for Disease Control and Prevention; MCHB = Maternal and Child Health Bureau; NCHS = National Center for Health Statistics; SFA = School Food Authorities; and USDA = U.S. Department of Agriculture.

Sample Size	Example(s) of Indicators or Outcomes Measured
7 million (2004)	Height; weight; breastfeeding initiation, duration, and exclusivity; nutritional status; television and video viewing
1,075 cafeteria managers 430 SFA directors (1998–1999)	Nutritional quality of meals in schools
1,331 schools, 745 districts, and 51 states (2000)	Fruit and vegetable consumption, vending machine offerings, physical activity and physical education, intramurals, health education
41 states and 13 districts (2004)	Physical education requirements, physical activity (intramurals, sports), walking/biking to school, fruit and vegetable consumption, vending machine offerings, health education topics required (nutrition and dietary, physical activity)
3,000 (2002)	Physical activity and physical education, walk/bike to school, television viewing, parents' physical activity
15,240 questionnaires completed in 158 schools, 32 state surveys, 18 local surveys (2003)	Fruit and vegetable consumption, physical activity and physical education, television viewing, weight status (overweight, at risk, trying to lose weight)
102,353 children (2,000 children per state)	Reported height and weight; breastfeeding; physical activity; television viewing
2,000	Child's age, height, and weight; breastfeeding; television viewing
9,000 (1997)	

REFERENCES

Add Health. 2005. *Add Health: The National Longitudinal Survey of Adolescent Health (Add Health)*. [Online]. Available: http://www.cpc.unc.edu/addhealth [accessed July 20, 2006].

CDC (Centers for Disease Control and Prevention). 2004. *School Health Profiles (SHP)*. [Online]. Available: http://www.cdc.gov/healthyyouth/profiles/index.htm [accessed July 20, 2006].

CDC. 2005. *National Health and Nutrition Examination Survey (NHANES)*. [Online]. Available: http://www.cdc.gov/nchs/nhanes.htm [accessed July 20, 2006].

CDC. 2006a. *Behavioral Risk Factor Surveillance System (BRFSS)*. [Online]. Available: http://www.cdc.gov/brfss/ [accessed July 20, 2006].

CDC. 2006b. *CDC's Pediatric and Pregnancy Nutrition Surveillance System (PedNSS)*. [Online]. Available: http://www.cdc.gov/pednss/ [accessed July 20, 2006].

CDC. 2006c. *National Health Interview Survey (NHIS)*. [Online]. Available: http://www.cdc.gov/nchs/nhis.htm [accessed July 20, 2006].

CDC. 2006d. *NCHS/SLAITS—National Survey of Children's Health (NSCH)*. [Online]. Available: http://www.cdc.gov/nchs/about/major/slaits/nsch.htm [accessed July 20, 2006].

CDC. 2006e. *NCHS/SLAITS—National Survey of Early Childhood Health (NSECH)*. [Online]. Available: http://www.cdc.gov/nchs/about/major/slaits/nsech.htm [accessed July 20, 2006].

CDC. 2006f. *SHPPS: School Health Policies and Programs Study*. [Online]. Available: http://www.cdc.gov/HealthyYouth/shpps/index.htm [accessed July 20, 2006].

CDC. 2006g. *Youth Media Campaign: Resources and Reports. Longitudinal Survey (YMCLS)*. [Online]. Available: http://www.cdc.gov/youthcampaign/research/resources.htm [accessed July, 20, 2006].

CDC. 2006h. *Youth Risk Factor Behavior Surveillance-United States 2005 Surveillance Summaries System (YRBSS)*. [Online]. Available: http://www.cdc.gov/HealthyYouth/yrbs/index.htm [accessed July 20, 2006].

DoL (U.S. Department of Labor). 2006. *National Longitudinal Surveys. National Longitudinal Survey of Youth (NLSY)*. [Online]. Available: http://www.bls.gov/nls/home.htm [accessed July 20, 2006].

Monitoring the Future. 2006. *Monitoring the Future: A Continuing Study of American Youth*. [Online]. Available: http://www.monitoringthefuture.org/ [accessed July 20, 2006]

USDA (U.S. Department of Agriculture). 2001. *School Nutrition Dietary Assessment Study II: Summary of Findings (SNDA)*. [Online]. Available: http://www.fns.usda.gov/OANE/MENU/Published/CNP/FILES/SNDAIIfindsum.htm [accessed July 20, 2006].

D

Examples of Recent Federal Agency Programs, Initiatives, and Surveillance Systems for Supporting and Monitoring the Prevention of Obesity in U.S. Children and Youth

TABLE D-1 Examples of Recent Federal Agency Programs, Initiatives, and Surveillance Systems for Supporting and Monitoring the Prevention of Obesity in U.S. Children and Youth

Federal Department and Agency	Type of Activity	Program, Initiative, Surveillance System, or Description (Reference)	Evaluation Availability[a] (Reference)
U.S. Department of Health and Human Services (DHHS)			
Administration for Children and Families	Program	Head Start Program (ACF, 2006a)	Available (ACF, 2006b)
Agency for Healthcare Research and Quality	Program	Obesity prevention toolkit for parents (AHRQ, 2004)	Not available
Assistant Secretary for Planning and Evaluation	Capacity and research	The Office of the Assistant Secretary for Planning and Evaluation advises the government on health policy research and program evaluation (ASPE, 2006)	Available (ASPE, 2006)
Centers for Disease Control and Prevention (CDC)	Capacity	Nutrition and Physical Activity Program to Prevent Obesity and Other Chronic Diseases (CDC, 2006g)	Available (Yee et al., 2006)
	Capacity	School Health Index (CDC, 2006l)	Available (Staten et al., 2005)
	Capacity	Steps to a HealthierUS (Steps Program) (DHHS, 2004a)	Available (MacDonald et al., 2006)

Leadership	Supports a congressionally directed Institute of Medicine (IOM) study to develop nutritional standards for competitive foods and beverages sold in schools (IOM, 2006b)	In progress
Leadership	Supported a congressionally directed IOM study on the influence of food marketing on the diets and health of children and youth (IOM, 2006a)	Available (IOM, 2006a)
Program	Preventive Health and Health Services Block Grants (CDC, 2006k)	Available (CDC, 2006k)
Program	Coordinated School Health program (CDC, 2005c)	Available (CDC, 2006c)
Program	5 a Day for Better Health campaign (CDC, 2005a)	Available (CDC, 2005b)
Program	VERB™ campaign (funding ended in FY 2005) (CDC, 2005e)	Available (CDC, 2006n)
Research	Prevention Research Center programs (CDC, 2006i)	Available (CDC, 2006j)
Surveillance	Behavioral Risk Factor Surveillance System (BRFSS) (CDC, 2006a)	Available (CDC, 2006b)
Surveillance	National Health Interview Survey (CDC, 2006d)	Available (NCHS, 2006)
Surveillance	National Health and Nutrition Examination Survey (CDC, 2005d)	Available (ARS, 2006)

continued

TABLE D-1 continued

Federal Department and Agency	Type of Activity	Program, Initiative, Surveillance System, or Description (Reference)	Evaluation Availability[a] (Reference)
	Surveillance	Pediatric Nutrition Surveillance System (CDC, 2006h)	Available (CDC, 2005f)
	Surveillance	School Health Profiles (CDC, 2006m)	Available (Grunbaum et al., 2005)
	Surveillance	School Health Policy and Programs Study (CDC, 2006m)	Available (CDC, 2001)
	Surveillance	Youth Media Campaign Longitudinal Survey (CDC, 2006n)	Available (CDC, 2006n)
	Surveillance	Youth Risk Behavior Surveillance System (YRBSS) (CDC, 2006m)	Available (Brener et al., 1995)
Food and Drug Administration	Leadership	Obesity Working Group's Calories Count report (FDA, 2004)	Available (FDA, 2004)
	Leadership	Notice of Proposed Rulemaking to redesign the Nutrition Facts label (FDA, 2005a)	Available (FDA, 2005a)
	Leadership	Final rule on the nutrient content claims, definition of sodium levels for the term healthy (FDA, 2005b)	Available (FDA, 2005b)

continued

	Program	Supported The Keystone Center Forum on Youth Nutrition and the Forum on Obesity and Foods Consumed Away From Home (Keystone Center, 2005, 2006)	Available (Keystone Center, 2005, 2006)
Health Resources and Services Administration (HRSA)	Program	Obesity prevention is a required element of the Maternal and Child Health block grants (Title V) (HRSA, 2006)	Available (HRSA, 2006)
	Surveillance	The Maternal and Child Health Bureau releases the annual Chartbook on the Health and Well-Being of Children (DHHS, HRSA, 2005a)	Available (DHHS, HRSA, 2005a)
	Surveillance	The Maternal and Child Health Bureau has released a report on obesity and physical activity among children in the nation based on the National Survey of Children's Health (DHHS, HRSA, 2005b)	Available (DHHS, HRSA, 2005b)
	Surveillance	The National Survey of Early Childhood Health is conducted in collaboration with the American Academy of Pediatrics (CDC, 2006f)	Available (Blumberg et al., 2004)
Indian Health Service	Leadership and program	As part of the DHHS Strategic Plan for FY 2004–2009, the Indian Health Service has the objective to decrease childhood obesity rates for American Indian and Alaska Native children (DHHS, 2004b)	Available (DHHS, 2004b)
National Institutes of Health	Program	We Can! (Ways to Enhance Children's Activity & Nutrition), a collaboration between the National Heart, Lung, and Blood Institute; the National Cancer Institute; the National Institute of Child Health and Human Development; and the National Institute of Diabetes and Digestive and Kidney Diseases (NIH, 2005)	In progress

TABLE D-1 continued

Federal Department and Agency	Type of Activity	Program, Initiative, Surveillance System, or Description (Reference)	Evaluation Availability[a] (Reference)
	Leadership	An annual conference on obesity and the built environment is sponsored by the National Institute of Environmental Health Sciences (NIEHS, 2004, 2005)	Available (NIEHS, 2004, 2005)
	Research	The National Institutes of Health (NIH) Obesity Research Task Force was established to develop and implement the Strategic Plan for NIH Obesity Research across all NIH institutes and centers (NIH, 2004)	In progress
Office of Disease Prevention and Health Promotion	Leadership and program	SmallStep for Adults and Teens (DHHS, 2006a) and SmallStep Kids! (DHHS, 2006b)	Available (Ad Council, 2006)
	Leadership and surveillance	Publication of *Healthy People 2010* and provision of preventive health and health services block grants to state health departments to meet the *Healthy People 2010* health promotion and disease prevention objectives that include obesity prevention (DHHS, 2000a)	Available (DHHS, 2000b)
Office of Minority Health	Program	Offers discretionary and project grants to support health promotion and disease prevention interventions for low-income racial/ethnic minority populations (OMH, 2005b)	Not available
	Program	Obesity Abatement in the African-American Community Initiative (OMH, 2005c)	Not available

Organization	Type	Program/Initiative	Availability
Office of the Surgeon General	Leadership and program	Closing the Health Gap (OMH, 2005a)	Not available
	Leadership	Children and Health Choices: 50 Schools in 50 States Initiative (DHHS, 2005)	Not available
President's Council on Physical Fitness and Sports	Leadership and program	President's Challenge (DHHS, 2006c)	Not available
Department of Education	Program	Carol M. White Physical Education Program Grants (DoEd, 2006a)	Available (DoEd, 2006b)
Department of the Interior/National Park Service	Program	Urban Park and Recreation Recovery Program (NPS, 2004)	Not available
Department of Labor	Surveillance	National Longitudinal Survey of Youth (DoL, 2006)	Available (DoL, 2006)
Department of Transportation	Program	Safe Routes to School Program (FHWA/DoT, 2006a)	In progress (FHWA, DOT, 2006b)
	Surveillance	National Household Travel Survey (BTS, 2004)	Available (BTS, 2006)
Federal Communications Commission	Policy and regulation	Enforces the Children's Television Act of 1990 (FCC, 2001, 2004)	Available (FCC, 2001, 2004)

continued

TABLE D-1 continued

Federal Department and Agency	Type of Activity	Program, Initiative, Surveillance System, or Description (Reference)	Evaluation Availability[a] (Reference)
Federal Trade Commission	Leadership	Report to Congress on industry expenditures and marketing activities directed at children and youth (FTC, 2006)	In progress (Richard Kelly, Federal Trade Commission, personal communication, June 20, 2006)
	Policy and regulation	Ongoing monitoring and regulation of deceptive and misleading advertising to children and youth (FTC, 2001)	Available (FTC, 2001)
U.S. Department of Agriculture (USDA)	Capacity	Cooperative Extension System (CSREES, 2006a)	Available (NASULGC, 2001)
	Capacity	Child Nutrition Labeling Program (USDA, 2006a)	In progress
	Leadership and coordination	Support for State Nutrition Action Plans (USDA, 2006d)	Not available
	Leadership	Supported a congressionally directed IOM study on an evaluation of the contents of the WIC food packages (IOM, 2005)	Available (IOM, 2005)
	Program	Federal food and nutrition assistance programs relevant to obesity prevention in children and youth include: Food Stamp Program (FSP), Special Supplemental Nutrition Program for Women, Infants, and Children (WIC), National School Lunch	Available (USDA, 2006f)

	Program (NSLP), School Breakfast Program (SBP), Child and Adult Care Food Program (CACFP), Summer Food Service Program (SFSP), Food Distribution Program on Indian Reservations, and the Farmers' Market Nutrition Program (FMNP) (USDA, 2006b)	
Program	Eat Smart. Play Hard.™ Campaign (USDA, 2005a)	Available (Prospect Associates, 2003)
Program	Expanded Food and Nutrition Education Program (EFNEP) (CSREES, 2006b)	Available (CSREES, 2006b)
Program	Fit WIC (USDA, 2005b)	Available (USDA, 2005e)
Program	Food Stamp Nutrition Education Program (FSNE) (USDA, 2004a)	In progress
Program	Fresh Fruit and Vegetable Program (FFVP) (CFSC, 2006)	Available (Buzby et al., 2003; Schneider et al., 2006)
Program	MyPyramid.gov, MyPyramid for Kids, and MiPiramide (in Spanish) (USDA, 2005d, 2006c)	In progress (Jackie Haven, USDA, personal communication, May 11, 2006)
Program	Team Nutrition (USDA, 2006e)	Available (Murimi et al., 2006)
Research	Agricultural Research Service research programs on obesity (USDA, 2006g)	In progress

continued

TABLE D-1 continued

Federal Department and Agency	Type of Activity	Program, Initiative, Surveillance System or Description (Reference)	Evaluation Availability[a] (Reference)
	Research	Food Assistance and Nutrition Research Program (UCD, 2006)	Available (USDA, 2005c)
	Research	School Nutrition Dietary Assessment Study (USDA, 2001)	Available (Dwyer, 1995)
Interagency Collaborations			
CDC and USDA	Program	HealthierUS School Challenge (USDA, 2004b)	Not available
DHHS, Department of Education, and USDA	Leadership and program	Healthier Child and Youth Memorandum of Understanding (DoEd, DHHS, and USDA, 2005)	Not available
DHHS, Office of Science, Technology, and Policy (OSTP), and USDA	Research	Federal Interagency Working Group on Overweight and Obesity Research (Yanovski, 2006)	Not available
DHHS and USDA	Leadership and program	Dietary Guidelines for Americans 2005 (DHHS and USDA, 2005)	Not available

Department of Defense and USDA	Program	DoD Fresh Program (CFSC, 2006; USDA, 2006d)	Available (Buzby et al., 2003)
Federal Trade Commission and DHHS	Leadership	Joint workshop in 2005 to develop guidelines on marketing food, beverages, and sedentary entertainment to children (FTC and DHHS, 2006)	Available (FTC and DHHS, 2006)
HRSA and CDC	Surveillance	National Survey of Children's Health (CDC, 2006e)	Available (CDC, 2006e)
NIH and Office of Public Health and Science	Leadership	National Obesity Action Forum (PSU, 2006)	Not available
USDA, Department of Education, and CDC	Capacity	Technical assistance regarding school wellness policies and implementation of the Child Nutrition and WIC Reauthorization Act of 2004 (CNWICRA, 2004).	In progress

aAvailable means that an evaluation has been conducted but may differ in scope, breadth, and outcomes examined. Not available signifies that an evaluation was either not conducted or that information was not publicly available to the committee to make an assessment of a program or initiative. In progress means that the committee was made aware of a proposed evaluation or an evaluation underway during the IOM study; however, it was not completed or information was not available about the evaluation at the time of publication of this IOM report.

REFERENCES

ACF (Administration for Children and Families). 2006a. *Head Start Bureau: Programs and Services.* [Online]. Available: http://www.acfhhs.gov/programs/hsb/programs/hsb/programs/index.htm [accessed June 12, 2006].

ACF. 2006b. *Head Start Research: Head Start Impact Study, 2000–2006.* [Online]. Available: http://www.acf.hhs.gov/programs/opre/hs/impact_study/ [accessed June 16, 2006].

Ad Council. 2006. *Obesity Prevention: Campaign Results Summary.* Washington, DC.

AHRQ (Agency for Healthcare Research and Quality). 2004. *Combating Childhood Obesity: Get DVDs to Help Prevent Obesity in Children.* [Online]. Available: http://www.ahrq.gov/child/dvdobesity.htm [accessed June 15, 2006].

ARS (Agriculture Research Service). 2006. *AMPM Validation Study.* [Online]. Available: http://www.ars.usda.gov/Services/docs.htm?docid=7714 [accessed August 21, 2006].

ASPE (Assistant Secretary for Planning and Evaluation). 2006. *Office of the Assistant Secretary for Planning and Evaluation.* [Online]. Available: http://aspe.hhs.gov/_/index.cfm [accessed June 15, 2006].

Blumberg S, Halfon N, Olson LM. 2004. The National Survey of Early Childhood Health. *Pediatrics* 113(6):1899–1906.

Brener ND, Collins JL, Kann L, Warren CW, Williams BI. 1995. Reliability of the Youth Risk Behavior Survey Questionnaire. *Am J Epidemiol* 141(6):575–580.

BTS (Bureau of Transportation Statistics). 2004. *National Household Travel Survey.* [Online]. Available: http://www.bts.gov/programs/national_house-hold_travel_survey/ [accessed June 13, 2006].

BTS. 2006. *America On the Go.* [Online]. Available: http://www.bts.gov/publications/america_on_the_go/long_distance_transportation_patterns/pdf/entire.pdf [accessed June 19, 2006].

Buzby JC, Guthrie JF, Kantor LS. 2003. *Evaluation of the USDA Fruit and Vegetable Pilot Program: Report to Congress.* Report No. E-FAN-03-006. Washington, DC: U.S. Department of Agriculture. [Online]. Available: http://www.fns.usda.gov/cnd/Research/FV030063.pdf [accessed May 8, 2006].

CDC (Centers for Disease Control and Prevention). 2001. *State-Level School Health Policies and Practices: A State-by-State Summary from the School Health Policies and Programs Study 2000.* [Online]. Available: http://www.cdc.gov/HealthyYouth/shpps/summaries/pdf/SH2000summ.pdf [accessed June 16, 2006].

CDC. 2005a. *5 A Day. Home.* [Online]. Available: http://www.cdc.gov/nccdphp/dnpa/5aday/ [accessed June 13, 2006].

CDC. 2005b. *5 A Day Works!* [Online]. Available: http://www.cdc.gov/nccd-php/dnpa/5aday/pdf/5-A-Day_works.pdf [accessed June 16, 2006].

CDC. 2005c. *Coordinated School Health Program.* [Online]. Available: http://www.cdc.gov/healthyYouth/CSHP/ [accessed June 13, 2006].

CDC. 2005d. *National Health and Nutrition Examination Survey (NHANES).* [Online]. Available: http://www.cdc.gov/nchs/nhanes.htm [accessed June 13, 2006].

CDC. 2005e. *Youth Media Campaign. VERB™.* [Online]. Available: http://www.cdc.gov/youthcampaign/ [accessed June 14, 2006]

CDC. 2005f. *Pediatric and Pregnancy Nutrition Surveillance System: How to Review Data Quality.* [Online]. Available: http://www.cdc.gov/pednss/how_to/review_data_quality/index.htm [accessed July 28, 2006]

CDC. 2006a. *Behavioral Risk Factor Surveillance System (BRFSS). Overweight and Obesity: State-Based Programs.* [Online]. Available: http://www.cdc.gov/nccdphp/dnpa/obesity/state_programs/index.htm [accessed May 17, 2006].

CDC. 2006b. *Behavioral Risk Factor Surveillance System (BRFSS) Data Quality, Validity, and Reliability.* [Online]. Available: http://www.cdc.gov/brfss/pubs/quality.htm [accessed July 27, 2006].

CDC. 2006c. *Health Youth! Funded Partners: Education Agencies Coordinated School Health Programs.* [Online]. Available: http://www.cdc.gov/healthyYouth/partners/cshp.htm [accessed June 16, 2006].

CDC. 2006d. *National Health Interview Survey (NHIS).* [Online]. Available: http://www.cdc.gov/nchs/nhis.htm [accessed June 27, 2006].

CDC. 2006e. *NCHS/SLAITS—National Survey of Children's Health.* [Online]. Available: http://www.cdc.gov/nchs/about/major/slaits/nsch.htm [accessed June 13, 2006].

CDC. 2006f. *NCHS/SLAITS—National Survey of Early Childhood Health.* [Online]. Available: http://www.cdc.gov/nchs/about/major/slaits/nsech.htm [accessed June 13, 2006].

CDC. 2006g. *Overweight and Obesity: State-Based Programs.* [Online]. Available: http://www.cdc.gov/nccdphp/dnpa/obesity/state_programs/index.htm [accessed June 14, 2006]

CDC. 2006h. *Pediatric and Pregnancy Nutrition Surveillance System.* [Online]. Available: http://www.cdc.gov/pednss/ [accessed June 13, 2006].

CDC. 2006i. *Prevention Research Centers.* [Online]. Available: http://www.cdc.gov/prc/ [accessed June 15, 2006].

CDC. 2006j. *Prevention Research Centers Program Evaluation.* [Online]. Available: http://www.cdc.gov/prc/program-evaluation/index.htm [accessed June 15, 2006].

CDC. 2006k. *Preventive Health and Health Services Block Grant.* [Online]. Available: http://www.cdc.gov/nccdphp/blockgrant/ [accessed June 28, 2006].

CDC. 2006l. *School Health Index (SHI): Mini-Grants for Physical Activity and Nutrition Improvements.* [Online] Available: http://apps.nccd.cdc.gov/SHI/Default.aspx [accessed February 14, 2006].

CDC. 2006m. *Summary Chart of Major Surveillance Activities.* [Online]. Available: http://www.cdc.gov/healthyyouth/data/surveillance.htm [accessed May 16, 2006].

CDC. 2006n. *Youth Media Campaign: Resources and Reports.* [Online]. Available: http://www.cdc.gov/youthcampaign/research/resources.htm [accessed June 13, 2006].

CFSC (Community Food Security Coalition). 2006. *Fact Sheet: Department of Defense Fresh Produce Buying Program.* [Online]. Available: http://www.foodsecurity.org/california/cfjc_dod_faq.pdf [accessed May 16, 2006].

CNWICRA (Child Nutrition and WIC Reauthorization Act). 2004. *Child Nutrition and WIC Reauthorization Act of 2004.* Public Law 108-265, 108th Congress, June 30, 2004. [Online]. Available: http://www.fns.usda.gov/cnd/Governance/Legislation/PL_108-265.pdf [accessed March 22, 2006].

CSREES (Cooperative State Research, Education, and Extension Service). 2006a. *Cooperative State Research, Education, and Extension Service.* [Online]. Available: http://www.csrees.usda.gov/ [accessed June 13, 2006].

CSREES. 2006b. *Expanded Food and Nutrition Education Program.* [Online]. Available: http://www.csrees.usda.gov/nea/food/efnep/efnep.html [accessed June 13, 2006].

DHHS (U.S. Department of Health and Human Services). 2000a. *Healthy People Publications.* [Online]. Available: http://www.healthypeople.gov/Publications/ [accessed June 16, 2006].

DHHS. 2000b. Nutrition and overweight. Focus area 19. In: *Healthy People 2010.* Volume II, 2nd ed. [Online]. Available: http://www.healthypeople.gov/Document/pdf/Volume2/19Nutrition.pdf [accessed February 7, 2006].

DHHS. 2004a. *Steps to a HealthierUS Initiative.* Washington, DC: U.S. Department of Health and Human Services. [Online]. Available: http://www.healthierus.gov/STEPS/ [accessed July 27, 2006].

DHHS. 2004b. *Strategic Plan FY 2004–2009.* Washington, DC: U.S. Department of Health and Human Services. [Online]. Available: http://aspe.hhs.gov/hhsplan/2004/hhsplan 2004.pdf [accessed May 17, 2006].

DHHS. 2005. *Office of the Surgeon General.* [Online]. Available: http://www.surgeongeneral. gov/publichealthpriorities.html#schools [accessed December 30, 2005].

DHHS. 2006a. *SmallStep.* [Online]. Available: http://www.smallstep.gov/ [accessed May 17, 2006].

DHHS. 2006b. *SmallStep Kids!* [Online]. Available: http://www.smallstep.gov/kids/index.cfm [accessed May 17, 2006].

DHHS. 2006c. *President's Challenge.* [Online]. Available: http://www.fitness.gov/home_pres_ chall.htm [accessed May 16, 2006].

DHHS, HRSA (Health Resources and Services Administration), MCHB (Maternal and Child Health Bureau). 2005a. *The Health and Well-Being of Children: A Portrait of States and the Nation 2005.* [Online]. Available: http://www.mchb.hrsa.gov/thechild/pdf/ 101pages.pdf [accessed February 28, 2006].

DHHS, HRSA. 2005b. *Overweight and Physical Activity Among Children: A Portrait of States and the Nation 2005.* [Online]. Available: http://nschdata.org/documents/Over weightChartBook.pdf. [accessed November 1, 2006].

DHHS and USDA (U.S. Department of Agriculture). 2005. *Dietary Guidelines for Americans 2005.* [Online]. Available: http://www.healthierus.gov/dietaryguidelines [accessed December 29, 2005].

DoEd (U.S. Department of Education). 2006a. *Carol M. White Physical Education Program.* [Online]. Available: http://www.ed.gov/programs/whitephysed/index.html [accessed March 6, 2006].

DoEd. 2006b. *Fiscal Year 2007 Program Performance Plan.* [Online]. Available: http:// www.ed.gov/about/reports/annual/2007plan/allprogs.pdf [accessed June 19, 2006].

DoEd, DHHS, and USDA. 2005. *Memorandum of Understanding.* [Online]. Available: http: //www.fda.gov/oc/mous/domestic/USDA-FDA-OBESITY.html [accessed June 19, 2006].

DoL (U.S. Department of Labor). 2006. *National Longitudinal Surveys.* [Online]. Available: http://www.bls.gov/nls/ [accessed May 16, 2006].

Dwyer J. 1995. The School Nutrition Dietary Assessment Study. *Am J Clin Nutr* 61(Suppl): 173S–177S.

FCC (Federal Communications Commission). 2001. *Children's Television Programming Report.* Washington, DC: FCC. [Online]. Available: http://www.fcc.gov/Forms/Form398/ 398.pdf [accessed May 17, 2006].

FCC. 2004. *FCC Adopts Children's Programming Obligations for Digital Television Broadcasters.* Washington, DC: FCC. [Online]. Available: http://hraunfoss.fcc.gov/edocs_ public/attachmatch/DOC-251972A1.pdf [accessed May 15, 2006].

FDA (U.S. Food and Drug Administration). 2004. *Calories Count: Report of the Working Group on Obesity.* [Online]. Available: http://www.cfsan.fda.gov/~dms/owg-toc.html [accessed May 17, 2006].

FDA. 2005a. Advanced notice of proposed rulemaking: Food labeling: Serving sizes of products that can reasonable be consumed at one eating occasion: Updating of reference amounts customarily consumed: Approaches for recommending smaller portion sizes. *Federal Register* 70(63).

FDA. 2005b. Food labeling; nutrient content claims, definition of sodium levels for the term "healthy." *Federal Register* 70(188).

FHWA, DoT (Federal Highway Administration/U.S. Department of Transportation). 2006a. *Safe Routes to School.* [Online]. Available: http://safety.fhwa.dot.gov/saferoutes/ [accessed May 16, 2006].

FHWA, DoT. 2006b. *FHWA Program Guidance Safe Routes to School (SRTS).* [Online]. Available: http://safety.fhwa.dot.gov/saferoutes/srtsguidance.htm#_Toc123542186 [accessed July 20, 2006].

FTC (Federal Trade Commission). 2001. *Advertising Practices: Frequently Asked Questions. Answers for Small Business.* [Online]. Available: http://www.ftc.gov/ bcp/conline/pubs/ buspubs/ad-faqs.pdf [accessed May 16, 2006].

FTC. 2006. Request for information and comment: Food industry marketing practices to children and adolescents. *Federal Register* 71(4):10535–10536. [Online]. Available: http:// a257.g.akamaitech.net/7/257/2422/01jan20061800/edocket.access.gpo.gov/2006/06-1931.htm [accessed March 6, 2006].

FTC and DHHS (U.S. Department of Health and Human Services). 2006. *Perspectives on Marketing, Self-Regulation and Childhood Obesity: A Report on a Joint Workshop of the Federal Trade Commission and the Department of Health and Human Services.* [Online]. Available: http://www.ftc.gov/os/2006/05/PerspectivesOnMarketingSelf-Regulation& ChildhoodObesityFTCandHHSReportonJointWorkshop.pdf [accessed May 8, 2006].

Grunbaum JA, Di Pietra J, McManus T, Hawkins J, Kann L. 2005. *School Health Profiles: Characteristics of Health Programs Among Secondary Schools (Profiles 2004).* Atlanta, GA: CDC. [Online]. Available: http://www.cdc.gov/healthyyouth/profiles/2004/report.pdf [accessed June 16, 2006].

HRSA (Human Resources and Services Administration). 2006. *Maternal and Child Health Services Title V Block Grant Program.* [Online]. Available: http://mchb.hrsa.gov/grants/ proposed.htm [accessed June 15, 2006].

IOM (Institute of Medicine). 2005. *WIC Food Packages: Time for a Change.* Washington, DC: The National Academies Press.

IOM. 2006a. *Food Marketing to Children and Youth: Threat or Opportunity?* Washington, DC: The National Academies Press.

IOM. 2006b. *Nutrition Standards for Foods in Schools.* [Online]. Available: http://www. iom.edu/project.asp?id=30181 [accessed May 15, 2006].

Keystone Center. 2005. *The Keystone Center Policy Summit "Choose the Best Path."* Washington, DC: The Keystone Center. [Online]. Available: http://www.iom.edu/Object.File/ Master/28/287/LWalker.Keystone.2005.pdf [accessed May 10, 2006].

Keystone Center. 2006. *Keystone Forum on Away-From-Home Foods: Opportunities for Preventing Weight Gain and Obesity.* Washington, DC: The Keystone Center. [Online]. Available: http://www.keystone.org/spp/documents/Forum_Report_FINAL_5-30-06.pdf [accessed June 3, 2006].

MacDonald G, Garcia D, Zaza S, Schooley M, Compton D, Bryant T, Bagnol L, Edgerly C, Haverkate R. 2006. Steps to a HealthierUS Cooperative Agreement Program: Foundational elements for program evaluation planning, implementation, and use of findings. *Prev Chronic Dis* [Online]. Available: http://www.cdc.gov/Pcd/issues/2006/jan/05_0136. htm [accessed July 23, 2006].

Murimi M, Colvin J, Liner K, Guin J. 2006. *Methodology to Evaluate the Outcomes of the Team Nutrition Initiative in Schools.* USDA Contractor and Cooperator Report No. 20, Economic Research Service. [Online]. Available: http://www.ers.usda.gov/publications/ ccr20/ccr20.pdf [accessed July 14, 2006].

NASULGC (National Association of State Universities and Land-Grant Colleges). 2001. *Strategic Directions of the Cooperative Extension System.* [Online]. Available: http://www. nasulgc.org/publications/Agriculture/CES_Strategic.htm [accessed June 19, 2006].

NCHS (National Center for Health Statistics). 2006. *Summary Health Statistics for U.S. Children: National Health Interview Survey, 2005.* Hyattsville, MD: CDC, DHHS. *Vital Health Stat* 10(231). [Online]. Available: http://www.cdc.gov/nchs/data/series/sr_10/ sr10_231.pdf [accessed August 17, 2006].

NIEHS (National Institute of Environmental Health Sciences). 2004. *Obesity and the Built Environment: Improving Public Health Through Community Design.* [Online]. Available: http://www.niehs.nih.gov/drcpt/beoconf/home.htm [accessed June 15, 2006].

NIEHS. 2005. *Environmental Solutions to Obesity in America's Youth Summary Report.* [Online]. Available: http://www-apps.niehs.nih.gov/conferences/drcpt/oe2005/finalreport. pdf [accessed June 15, 2006].

NIH (National Institutes of Health). 2004. *Strategic Plan for NIH Obesity Research.* [Online]. Available: http://obesityresearch.nih.gov/About/ObesityEntireDocument.pdf [accessed December 30, 2005].

NIH. 2005. *We Can!* [Online]. Available: http://www.nhlbi.nih.gov/health/public/heart/ obesity/wecan/ [accessed December 30, 2005].

NPS (National Park Service). 2004. *Urban Park and Recreation Recovery.* [Online]. Available: http://www.nps.gov/uprr/ [accessed June 15, 2006].

OMH (Office of Minority Health). 2005a. *Closing the Health Gap 2005.* [Online]. Available: http://www.healthgap.omhrc.gov/index.htm [accessed June 13, 2006].

OMH. 2005b. *Grants.* [Online]. Available: http http://www.omhrc.gov/templates/content. aspx?ID=2744 [accessed June 13, 2006].

OMH. 2005c. *Obesity Abatement in the African American Community.* [Online]. Available: http://www.omhrc.gov/templates/content.aspx?ID=2838 [accessed June 13, 2006].

Prospect Associates. 2003. *Environmental Scan and Audience Analysis for Phase II of Eat Smart. Play Hard.™* [Online]. Available: http://www.fns.usda.gov/oane/MENU/ Published/NutritionEducation/Files/esaa.pdf [accessed June 19, 2006].

PSU (Pennsylvania State University). 2006. *National Obesity Action Forum.* [Online]. Available: http://www.outreach.psu.edu/C&I/obesity/default-home.htm [accessed June 16, 2006].

Schneider DJ, Carithers T, Coyle K, Endahl J, Robin L, McKenna M, Debrot K, Seymour J. 2006. Evaluation of a fruit and vegetable distribution program—Mississippi, 2004-05 school year. *MMWR* 55(35)957–961.

Staten LK, Teufel-Shone NI, Steinfelt VE, Ortega N, Halverson K, Flores C, Lebowitz MD. 2005. The school health index as an impetus for change. *Prev Chronic Dis* [Online]. Available: http://www.cdc.gov/Pcd/issues/2005/jan/04_0076.htm [accessed July 23, 2006].

UCD (University of California Davis). 2006. *USDA Economic Research Service Small Grant Program.* [Online]. Available: http://nutrition.ucdavis.edu/USD-AERS/ [accessed July 20, 2006].

USDA (U.S. Department of Agriculture). 2001. *School Nutrition Dietary Assessment Study.* [Online]. Available: http://www.fns.usda.gov/OANE/MENU/Published/CNP/FILES/SND AIIfindsum.htm [accessed May 16, 2006].

USDA. 2004a. *Food Stamp Program and Food Stamp Nutrition Education Program.* [Online]. Available: http://www.ers.usda.gov/Briefing/FoodStamps/fsne.htm [accessed March 4, 2006].

USDA. 2004b. *HealthierUS School Challenge.* [Online]. Available: http://www.fns.usda.gov/ tn/HealthierUS/index.html [accessed October 6,2005]

USDA. 2005a. *Eat Smart, Play Hard™ Campaign. Campaign Overview.* [Online]. Available: http://www.fns.usda.gov/eatsmartplayhard/About/overview.html [accessed June 15, 2006].

USDA. 2005b. *Fit WIC: Programs to Prevent Childhood Overweight in Your Community.* Special Nutrition Program Report Series, No. WIC-05-FW. Alexandria, VA: Office of Analysis, Nutrition, and Evaluation, Food and Nutrition Service, USDA. [Online]. Available: http://www.fns.usda.gov/oane/MENU/Published/WIC/FILES/fitwic.pdf [accessed February 28, 2006].

USDA. 2005c. *Food Assistance and Nutrition Research Program.* Economic Research Service, USDA. [Online]. Available: http://www.ers.usda.gov/Briefing/FoodNutritionAssistance/ 2005FinalReport.pdf [accessed July 20, 2006].

USDA. 2005d. *MyPyramid.gov: Steps to a Healthier You*. [Online]. Available: http://www. mypyramid.gov/ [accessed May 17, 2006].

USDA. 2005e. *WIC Works Sharing Center: Fit WIC*. [Online]. Available: http://www.nal. usda.gov/wicworks/Sharing_Center/statedev_FIT.html [accessed June 19, 2006].

USDA. 2006a. *Child Nutrition Labeling*. [Online]. Available: http://www.fns.usda.gov/cnd/ CNlabeling/default.htm [accessed June 13, 2006].

USDA. 2006b. *Food and Nutrition Assistance Programs*. Economic Research Service, USDA. [Online]. Available: http://www.ers.usda.gov/briefing/foodnutritionassistance/ [accessed June 14, 2006].

USDA. 2006c. *MyPyramid for Kids*. [Online]. Available: http://www.mypyramid.gov/kids/ index.html [accessed February 23, 2006].

USDA. 2006d. *State Nutrition Action Plans*. [Online]. Available: http://www.fns.usda.gov/ oane/SNAP/SNAP.htm [accessed February 28, 2006].

USDA. 2006e. *Team Nutrition*. [Online]. Available: http://www.fns.usda.gov/tn [accessed June 15, 2006].

USDA. 2006f. *The Food Assistance Landscape*. Economic Information Bulletin 6-2. ERS/ USDA. [Online]. Available: http://www.ers.usda.gov/publications/eib6-2/eib6-2.pdf [accessed February 21, 2006].

USDA. 2006g. *U.S. Dietary Guidelines and Healthy Body Weight*. [Online]. Available: http:// www.ars.usda.gov/research/projects/projects.htm?accn_no=410553 [accessed June 14, 2006].

Yanovski S. 2006. *Prevention Research in Pediatric Obesity: An NIH Perspective*. Presentation to the IOM Committee on Progress in Preventing Childhood Obesity. January 11–12. Washington, DC.

Yee SL, Williams-Piehota P, Sorensen A, Roussel A, Hersey J, Hamre R. 2006. The Nutrition and Physical Activity Program to Prevent Obesity and Other Chronic Diseases: Monitoring progress in funded states. *Prev Chron Dis* [Online]. Available: http://www.cdc.gov/ Pcd/issues/2006/jan/05_0077.htm [accessed July 23, 2006].

E

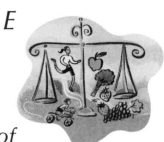

Compilation of Recommendations and Implementation Actions

Recommendation 1: Government, industry, communities, schools, and families should demonstrate leadership and commitment by mobilizing the resources required to identify, implement, evaluate, and disseminate effective policies and interventions that support childhood obesity prevention goals.

Implementation Actions for Government
Federal, state, and local governments should each establish a high-level task force to identify priorities for action, coordinate public-sector efforts, and establish effective interdepartmental collaborations.

To accomplish this,
- The president of the United States should request that the secretary of the U.S. Department of Health and Human Services convene a high-level task force involving the secretaries or senior officials from all relevant federal government departments and agencies (e.g., the U.S. Departments of Agriculture, Education, Defense, Interior, and Transportation; the Federal Communications Commission; and the Federal Trade Commission) to coordinate departmental budgets, policies, and research efforts and establish effective interdepartmental collaboration and priorities for action.
- State governments should convene high-level task forces involving the state departments of health, education, agriculture;

the land-grant cooperative extension services, and other relevant agencies. Childhood obesity prevention should be a priority that is reflected in each state government's public statements, policies and programs, budgets, research efforts, and interagency collaborations.

• Local government agencies should convene community- or regional-level task forces to provide coordinated leadership in preventing childhood obesity by increasing resources, collaborating with community stakeholders, and developing or strengthening policies and programs that promote opportunities for physical activity and healthful eating in communities and neighborhoods.

Implementation Actions for Industry
Industry should use the full range of available resources and tools to create, support, and sustain consumer demand for products and opportunities that support healthy lifestyles including healthful diets and regular physical activity.

To accomplish this,
• Industry should continue to support and market product innovations and reformulations that promote energy balance at a healthy weight for children and youth and that are compatible with obesity prevention goals.
• Industry should support the review of the existing self-regulatory guidelines for advertising directed to children. It should also expand the guidelines to advertising vehicles beyond those used in traditional advertising to include evolving vehicles and venues for marketing communication and apply and enforce the guidelines for the traditional and expanded vehicles. Companies should consider developing their own advertising and marketing guidelines for children that are consistent with the industry-wide guidelines.

Implementation Actions for Communities
Community stakeholders should establish and strengthen the local policies, coalitions, and collaborations needed to create and sustain healthy communities.

To accomplish this,
• Communities should make childhood obesity prevention a priority through the coordinated leadership of local government, community organizations, local businesses, health care organizations, and other relevant stakeholders. These efforts would

involve increased resources, an emphasis on collaboration among community stakeholders, and the development and implementation of policies and programs that promote opportunities for physical activity and healthful eating, particularly for high-risk communities.

Implementation Actions for Schools
School boards, administrators, and staff should elevate the priority that is placed on creating and sustaining a healthy school environment and advance school policies and programs that support this priority.

To accomplish this,
• Relevant federal and state agencies and departments, local school districts, individual schools and preschools, and childcare and after-school programs should prioritize opportunities for physical activity and expand the availability and access in schools to fruits, vegetables, and other low-calorie and high-nutrient foods and beverages that contribute to healthful diets. Increased resources are needed to develop, implement, and evaluate policies and programs. State and local school-based nutrition and physical activity standards need to be implemented, and the relevant educational entities should be held accountable for promoting and adhering to these standards.

Implementation Actions for Home
Families, parents, and caregivers should commit to promoting healthful eating and regular physical activity to create a healthy home environment.

To accomplish this,
• Parents and caregivers should make physical activity and healthful eating priorities at home. They should provide food and beverage choices for their children that contribute to a healthful diet, encourage and support physical activity, limit children's television viewing and other leisure screen time, and serve as positive role models. Parents can also serve as advocates to promote changes that encourage and support healthy behaviors in their local schools and communities.

Recommendation 2: Policy makers, program planners, program implementers, and other interested stakeholders—within and across relevant sectors—should evaluate all childhood obesity prevention efforts, strengthen the evaluation capacity, and develop quality interventions that take into account diverse perspectives, that use culturally relevant approaches, and that meet the needs of diverse populations and contexts.

Implementation Actions for Government
Federal and state government departments and agencies should consistently evaluate the effects of all actions taken to prevent childhood obesity and strengthen the evaluation capacity, paying particular attention to culturally relevant evaluation approaches.

To accomplish this,
- The actions of federal agencies, including policies that have been implemented, should be consistently evaluated to determine whether these actions and policies provide evidence of leadership and to identify the promising actions that are likely to be the most effective in preventing childhood obesity.
- The U.S. Congress should increase federal support for capacity-building activities, such as the Centers for Disease Control and Prevention's State-Based Nutrition and Physical Activity Program to Prevent Obesity and Other Chronic Diseases and Steps to a HealthierUS Program.
- Federal and state agencies should assess and strengthen the capacities of state and territorial health departments to provide leadership and technical assistance, enhance surveillance efforts, and implement and evaluate programs to prevent childhood obesity.
- DHHS, other federal agencies, and private-sector partners should work toward evaluating existing media efforts (including SmallStep and SmallStep Kids!) with the goal of developing, coordinating, and evaluating a more comprehensive, long-term, national multimedia and public relations campaign focused on obesity prevention in children and youth.

Implementation Actions for Industry
Industry should partner with government, academic institutions, and other interested stakeholders to undertake evaluations to assess its progress in preventing childhood obesity and promoting healthy lifestyles.

To accomplish this,
- Industry should evaluate its progress in developing and promoting affordable foods, beverages, and meals that support a healthful diet; physical activity products and opportunities;

storylines and programming that promote healthy lifestyles; and advertising and marketing practices directed to children and youth.

- Industry should provide resources and expertise to local businesses and community-based organizations to implement and evaluate initiatives that provide opportunities for consumers to engage in healthful eating and regular physical activity, especially for children and youth in racially and ethnically diverse groups and high-risk populations.

Implementation Actions for Communities

Community stakeholders should strengthen evaluation efforts at the local level by partnering with government agencies, foundations, and academic institutions to develop, implement, and support evaluation opportunities and community-academic partnerships.

To accomplish this,

Federal and state agencies, foundations, academic institutions, community-based nonprofit organizations, faith-based groups, youth-related organizations, local governments, and other relevant community stakeholders should

- Increase funding and technical assistance to conduct evaluations of childhood obesity prevention policies and interventions,
- Develop and widely disseminate effective evaluation training opportunities, and
- Develop and support community-academic partnerships.

Implementation Actions for Schools

Schools and school districts should strengthen evaluation efforts by partnering with state and federal agencies, foundations, and academic institutions to develop, implement, and support evaluations of all relevant school-based programs.

To accomplish this,

Federal agencies (e.g., the Centers for Disease Control and Preventions, the U.S. Department of Agriculture, and the U.S. Department of Education), state departments of education and health, foundations, academic institutions, school districts, and local schools should

- Increase the resources devoted to technical assistance for evaluating school-based childhood obesity prevention policies, programs, and interventions and

- Develop partnerships to fund, develop, and implement childhood obesity prevention evaluations.

Implementation Actions for Home
Parents and caregivers, as the policy makers in the household, should assess their family's progress in achieving positive lifestyle changes.

To accomplish this,
- Families should regularly assess their progress in adopting and maintaining healthy behaviors at home and achieving positive lifestyle changes.

Recommendation 3: Government, industry, communities, and schools should expand or develop relevant surveillance and monitoring systems and, as applicable, should engage in research to examine the impact of childhood obesity prevention policies, interventions, and actions on relevant outcomes, paying particular attention to the unique needs of diverse groups and high-risk populations. Additionally, parents and caregivers should monitor changes in their family's food, beverage, and physical activity choices and their progress toward healthier lifestyles.

Implementation Actions for Government
Government at all levels should develop new surveillance systems or enhance existing surveillance systems to monitor relevant outcomes and trends and should increase funding for obesity prevention research.

In order to accomplish this,
- Federal and state government surveillance systems should monitor the full range of outcomes in the evaluation framework. Surveillance systems—such as the National Health and Nutrition Examination Survey, the School Health Policies and Programs Study, the Youth Media Campaign Longitudinal Survey, the Youth Risk Behavior Surveillance System, and the National Household Transportation Survey—should be expanded to include relevant obesity-related outcomes. Surveillance systems that monitor the precursors of dietary and physical activity behaviors, including policies that have been implemented and structural, institutional, and environmental outcomes should be expanded or developed.
- All states should have a mechanism in place to monitor childhood obesity prevalence, dietary factors, physical activity lev-

els, and sedentary behaviors through population-based sampling over time.
- The U.S. Congress should appropriate sufficient funds to support research on obesity prevention (e.g., efficacy, effectiveness, quasiexperimental, cost-effectiveness, sustainability, and scaling up research) to improve program implementation and outcomes for children and youth.

Implementation Actions for Industry
The U.S. Congress, in consultation with industry and other relevant stakeholders, should appropriate adequate funds to support independent and periodic evaluations of industry's efforts to promote healthier lifestyles.

To accomplish this,
- The Food and Drug Administration should be given the authority to evaluate full serve and quick serve restaurants' expansion of healthier food, beverage, and meal options; the effectiveness of the restaurant sector in providing nutrition labeling and nutrition information at the point of choice; and the effect of this information on consumers' purchasing behaviors.
- The Centers for Disease Control and Prevention should evaluate the effectiveness of corporate-sponsored physical activity programs, energy-balance education programs, and the use of branded physical activity equipment (e.g., physical videogames) on children's leisure-time preferences and physical activity behaviors.
- The U.S. Congress should designate a responsible agency to conduct the periodic monitoring and evaluation of the self-regulatory guidelines of the Children's Advertising Review Unit (CARU), which should include an assessment of CARU's effectiveness, impact, and enforcement capacity.
- The food retail sector, the restaurant sector, and relevant trade associations should collaborate with the U.S. Department of Agriculture and the U.S. Department of Health and Human Services to provide marketing data on pricing strategies, consumer food purchases, and consumption trends from proprietary retail scanner systems, household scanner panels, household consumption surveys, and marketing research. The collaborative work should examine the quality of the data, consider reducing the cost to make the data more accessible, and establish priorities for applying the information to promote healthful diets.

- Industry should demonstrate corporate responsibility by sharing marketing research findings that may help public health professionals and community-based organizations develop and implement more effective childhood obesity prevention messages, policies, and programs.

Implementation Actions for Communities
Community stakeholders and relevant partners should expand the capacity for local-level surveillance and applied research and should develop tools for community self-assessment to support childhood obesity prevention efforts.

To accomplish this,
Federal and state agencies, foundations, academic institutions, community-based nonprofit organizations, faith-based groups, youth-related organizations, local governments, and other relevant community stakeholders should
- Expand the surveillance of outcomes of community-level activities and changes to the built environment as they relate to childhood obesity prevention;
- Facilitate the collection, analysis, and interpretation of local data and information;
- Develop, refine, and disseminate community assessment tools, such as a community health index;
- Develop methods for the rapid evaluation of natural experiments;
- Explore the use of spatial mapping technologies to assist communities with their assessment needs and to help communities make changes that increase access to opportunities for healthy lifestyles; and
- Encourage the evaluation of interventions to examine both the risk and protective factors related to obesity.

Implementation Actions for Schools
Schools and school districts should conduct self-assessments to enhance and sustain a healthy school environment, and mechanisms for examining links between changes in the school environment and behavioral and health outcomes should be explored.

To accomplish this,
Relevant federal agencies (e.g., the Centers for Disease Control and Prevention, the National Institutes of Health, the U.S. Department of Agriculture, and the U.S. Department of Education),

state education departments, school districts, and local schools should

- Expand and fully use current surveillance systems related to children's dietary and physical activities, obesity-related health indicators, and relevant school policies and programs;
- Implement a national survey focused on the physical activity behaviors of all children and youth;
- Support research on means to improve the monitoring of diet and physical activity;
- Establish mechanisms to link health, educational, economic, and sociological data sources across a variety of areas related to childhood obesity prevention; and
- Expand and adapt self-assessment tools for schools, preschools, child-care, and after-school programs and evaluate their validity for predicting changes in children's levels of physical activity, dietary intakes, and weight.

Implementation Actions for Home
Parents and caregivers should monitor their families' lifestyle changes; and government, foundations, and industry should support applied research that examines family interventions in real-world settings.

To accomplish this,
- Parents and caregivers should monitor their families' lifestyle changes on an ongoing basis, including their capabilities as role models, the family's dietary intake and levels of physical activity, and their children's weight status.
- Parents should work with their child's physician to track body mass indices and healthy growth.
- The federal government should create and make available simple tools for parents and families to track their children's dietary intake and physical activity behaviors.
- Relevant federal agencies (e.g., the Centers for Disease Control and Prevention, the National Institutes of Health, the U.S. Department of Agriculture, and the U.S. Department of Education), foundations, and other organizations should fund and support applied research that examines family interventions focused on specific ways that families can improve diets, reduce sedentary behaviors, and increase the levels of physical activity in the home setting.
- Relevant federal and state agencies, foundations, and academic institutions should develop and enhance surveillance systems

and other data sources and assessment tools to expand knowledge about the relationship between changes in the home environment and a variety of outcomes for children and youth.

Recommendation 4: Government, industry, communities, schools, and families should foster information-sharing activities and disseminate evaluation and research findings through diverse communication channels and media to actively promote the use and scaling up of effective childhood obesity prevention policies and interventions.

Implementation Actions for Government
Government at all levels should commit to the long-term support and dissemination of childhood obesity prevention policies and interventions that have been proven to be effective.

To accomplish this,
- Federal, state, and local governments should publicly disseminate and promote the results of evaluations of childhood obesity prevention policies and interventions.
- The federal government should provide a sustained commitment and long-term investment to adequately support and disseminate childhood obesity prevention interventions that are proven to be effective—such as the VERB™ campaign. *Further, the federal government should provide sustained* support for surveillance systems that are vital to the monitoring of trends and progress in response to the childhood obesity epidemic.
- Incentives and rewards should be developed for state and local government agencies to coordinate efforts that improve obesity-related outcomes for children and youth.

Implementation Actions for Industry
Industry should collaborate with the public sector and other relevant stakeholders to develop a mechanism for sharing proprietary data and a sustainable funding strategy that can inform and support childhood obesity prevention interventions.

To accomplish this,
- The private sector (e.g., industry and foundations) and the public sector (e.g., government and nonprofit organizations) should partner to develop a mechanism for sharing proprietary data (e.g., product sales information, marketing research data, and the results of evaluations of industry-supported programs)

that can inform research efforts and assist in developing a healthy lifestyles social marketing campaign. A long-term funding strategy should be established to sustain the campaign. Such a strategy should include a dedicated government appropriation and a dedicated set-aside from relevant industries.

- Government and other interested stakeholders should develop incentives and rewards for industry stakeholders that collaborate on this endeavor.

Implementation Actions for Communities

Community stakeholders should partner with foundations, government agencies, faith-based organizations, and youth-related organizations to publish and widely disseminate the evaluation results of community-based childhood obesity prevention efforts.

To accomplish this,

- Community stakeholders should publish evaluation results using diverse communication channels and media; and develop incentives to encourage the use of promising practices.

Implementation Actions for Schools

Schools should partner with government, professional associations, academic institutions, parent-teacher organizations, foundations, communities, and the media to publish and widely disseminate the evaluation results of school-based childhood obesity prevention efforts and related materials and methods.

To accomplish this,

- Schools, preschools, child-care and after-school programs, and relevant stakeholders should broadly disseminate the evaluation results using diverse communication channels and media and develop incentives to encourage the use of promising practices.

Implementation Actions for Home

Government (federal, state, and local), communities, families, and the media should disseminate and widely promote the evaluation results of effective family- and home-based childhood obesity prevention efforts.

To accomplish this,

- Government agencies (federal, state, and local), communities, and the media should promote the results of evaluations and specific practical guidance related to promising family-based obesity prevention interventions such as approaches for reducing children's television viewing, promoting leisure-time physical activity, and promoting healthier food and beverage choices at home.

• Parents, children, and youth should share information about promising obesity-prevention strategies and activities with other families through parenting groups and school meetings and in family, social, faith-based, and other venues.

F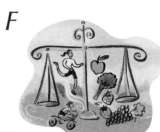

IOM Regional Symposium
Progress in Preventing
Childhood Obesity:
Focus on Schools

*The full summary can be found on the CD-ROM attached to the
inside back cover of the report.*

Program Agenda
Institute of Medicine Regional Symposium

Progress in Preventing Childhood Obesity:
Focus on Schools

In collaboration with the Kansas Health Foundation
Supported by the Robert Wood Johnson Foundation

June 27–28, 2005
Wichita Hyatt Regency Hotel
Wichita, Kansas

June 27, 2005
Opening Session

Welcome
Steve Coen, Kansas Health Foundation, Wichita
Kathryn Thomas, Robert Wood Johnson Foundation, Princeton,
New Jersey

Overview of the Meeting Goals and the Report,
Preventing Childhood Obesity: Health in the Balance
Jeffrey Koplan, Emory University and Institute of Medicine (IOM)
    Committee on Progress in Preventing Childhood Obesity

Perspectives on Childhood Obesity
Policy Perspectives
    James Barnett, Kansas Senate, Emporia

Health Perspectives
    James Early, University of Kansas, Wichita

Kansas Teen Leadership for Physically Active Lifestyles
    Ann Sparke, Morris County Extension Service, Kansas
    Chynna Walters and Mary Byram, Council Grove High School,
        Kansas

Plenary Panel—Presentations and Discussion
Obesity Prevention and School Policies: Challenges and Innovations
Developing and evaluating state-, district- and school-based changes in
school policy related to childhood obesity prevention
Moderator: *Eduardo Sanchez,* Texas Department of State Health
    Services, Austin

Kansas Coordinated School Health Program
    Jodi Mackey, Kansas State Department of Education, Topeka
    Paula Marmet, Kansas State Department of Health and Environment,
        Topeka

School District Comprehensive School Wellness Policies
    Joan Pritchard, Goddard School District, Kansas

Elementary School Policies
    Janine Kempker, Anthony Elementary School, Leavenworth, Kansas

Ohio Physical Education and Food Service Policies
    Dianne Radigan, Children's Hunger Alliance, Columbus, Ohio

School District Food Service Policies
    Rosemary Dederichs, Minneapolis Public Schools Food Service,
        Minnesota

School District Vending Machine Policies
  Carole Farthing, Independence, Kansas School Board

Plenary Panel—Presentations and Discussion
Obesity Prevention and School Programs:
Challenges and Innovations
Implementing and evaluating state-, district- and school-based
programs aimed at childhood obesity prevention
Moderator: *Tom Robinson*, Stanford University Prevention
  Research Center, Stanford, California

Kansas Physical Dimensions and Physical Focus
  Merri Copeland, Friends University, Wichita Kansas

Arkansas School Initiatives
  Jim Raczynski, University of Arkansas for Medical Sciences,
    Little Rock

Physical Activity Across the Curriculum
  Joseph Donnelly, University of Kansas, Lawrence

Coordinated Approach to Child Health
  Steve Kelder, University of Texas Health Science Center at Houston

Linking a Food-based Curriculum with the Elementary School Lunch
  Program
  Antonia Demas, Food Studies Institute, Trumansburg, New York

Implementing Changes in Elementary School Curricula and Programs
  Sherrie Kisker, Platte County Health Department, Platte City Missouri
  Disa Rice and Carolyn Barry, Siegrest Elementary, Platte City,
    Missouri

Obesity Prevention: Links with Other Sectors
What efforts by other sectors of the community are relevant to school-
based obesity prevention efforts? What are the barriers to change? What
is needed to implement and sustain these changes?

Breakout Session #1
Links Between Schools and Home, Community and Healthcare
Facilitators: *Marshall Kreuter*, Georgia State University, Atlanta;
  Susan Foerster, California Department of Health Services, Sacramento

Presentations followed by group discussion:
Heather Duvall, Oklahoma Fit Kids Coalition, Oklahoma City
Mary Ca Ralstin, Kansas PTA, Shawnee
Mim Wilkey, Wichita YMCA, Health & Wellness Coalition, Kansas
Jill Poole, Broken Arrow National Farm to School Program, Oklahoma
LaVonta Williams, Wichita After School Program, Kansas
Deborah Loman, National Association of Pediatric Nurse Practitioners,
    St. Louis, Missouri

Breakout Session #2
Links Between Schools and Industry
Facilitators: *John Peters,* Procter & Gamble Company, Cincinnati, Ohio;
Jeffrey Koplan, Emory University, Atlanta, Georgia

Presentations followed by group discussion:
Ann Hartley, Advance Food Company, Mooresville, North Carolina
Barbara Jirka, Tyson Foods, Springdale, Arkansas
Ellen Taaffe, PepsiCo, Chicago, Illinois
Nancy Daigler, Kraft Foods, Northfield, Illinois
Jane Byrnes-Bennett, Midwest Dairy Council, Wichita, Kansas

Breakout Session #3
Links Between Schools and the Built Environment
Facilitators: *Russ Pate,* University of South Carolina, Columbia;
Ann Bullock, Health and Medical Division, Eastern Band of Cherokee
    Indians, North Carolina;
Toni Yancey, UCLA School of Public Health

Presentations followed by group discussion:
Ian Thomas, PedNet, Columbia, Missouri
Dan Grunig, Bicycle Colorado, Colorado Safe Routes to School, Denver
Judy Johnston, Walkin' Wichita, Kansas
Dave Barber, Wichita-Sedgwick County Metropolitan Area Planning
    Department, Kansas
Wess Galyon, Wichita Home Builders Association, Kansas

Reception and Dinner
Wichita Art Museum

Dinner Speaker: Matt Longjohn, Consortium to Lower Obesity in
    Chicago Children, Illinois

Tuesday, June 28, 2005
Plenary Session

Welcome
Howard Rodenberg, Kansas State Health Director, Topeka

Opening Remarks
Vickie James, Healthy Kids Challenge, Dighton, Kansas

Keystone Youth Policy Summit on Child and Adolescent
Nutrition in America
Larry Walker, Meagan Geuther, Steven Gohlke, Paige Ibanez,
  Academy of Science and Technology, Conroe, Texas

Reports from Breakout Sessions

Plenary Panel—Presentations and Discussion
Preventing Childhood Obesity: What More Can Be Done?
What are the barriers to further progress? What more can be done at the
federal, state, community and private sector levels?
Moderator: *Doug Kamerow*, RTI International, Washington, DC

Federal Perspective
Mary McKenna, Centers for Disease Control and Prevention, Atlanta,
  Georgia

State Perspective
Rod Bremby, Kansas Department of Health and Environment, Topeka

Community Perspective
Brenda Kumm, Mid-America Coalition on HealthCare/
  KCHealthyKids.org, Kansas City, Missouri

Foundation Perspective
Billie Hall, Sunflower Foundation, Topeka, Kansas
Kathryn DeForest, Missouri Foundation for Health, St. Louis

Industry Perspective
Louise Finnerty, PepsiCo, Purchase, New York

Group Discussion

Closing Session
Summary and Next Steps
Jeffrey Koplan, IOM Committee on Progress in Preventing Childhood
  Obesity

G

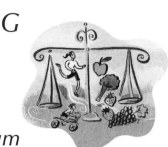

IOM Regional Symposium
Progress in Preventing
Childhood Obesity:
Focus on Communities

*The full summary can be found on the CD-ROM attached to the
inside back cover of the report.*

Program Agenda
Institute of Medicine Regional Symposium

*Progress in Preventing Childhood Obesity:
Focus on Communities*

In collaboration with Healthcare Georgia Foundation
Supported by the Robert Wood Johnson Foundation

October 6–7, 2005
Georgia Tech Hotel and Conference Center
Atlanta, Georgia

October 6, 2005
Opening Session

Welcome
Martha Katz, Healthcare Georgia Foundation

Overview of the IOM Report and Goals for the Meeting
Jeffrey Koplan, Emory University and Institute of Medicine (IOM)
   Committee on Progress in Preventing Childhood Obesity

Youth Efforts in Preventing Childhood Obesity
*Raymond Figueroa, Jr., Anthony George, Kenneth Alleyne, Artrese Reid,
   Eboni Bowman*, TRUCE Fitness and Nutrition Center of the Harlem
   Children's Zone, New York City

Setting the Context for Obesity Prevention in Communities
James Marks, Robert Wood Johnson Foundation

Plenary Panel Presentations and Discussion
Mobilizing Neighborhood and Community Grassroots Efforts
*Developing, implementing, and evaluating grassroots changes related to
childhood obesity prevention: barriers and opportunities.*

Moderator: *Antronette Yancey*, UCLA School of Public Health

Plenary Panel Presentations and Panel Discussion

Community Initiatives
Stewart Watson and *Nancy DeVault*, Seminole County Healthy Kids
   Partnership, Florida
Jeff Bachar, Cherokee Diabetes Prevention Program, North Carolina
Beverly Howell, Project Delta Hope and Mississippi Partnerships on
   Childhood Obesity

Plenary Panel Presentations and Panel Discussion
Faith-Based Initiatives
Anthony Evans, National Black Church Initiative
Jean Murphy, Health Ministries, Doraville, Georgia
Bethann Cottrell, Concerned Black Clergy of Metropolitan Atlanta
Steven Cooper, Mid-South Faith-Based Development Center, Mississippi

Plenary Panel Presentations and Discussion
Mobilizing City, County, and State Efforts
*Developing, implementing, and evaluating changes related to childhood
obesity prevention at the county and state levels: barriers and opportunities.*

Moderator: *Susan Foerster*, California Department of Health Services

Plenary Panel Presentations and Panel Discussion
Helen Matheny and Dan Foster, West Virginia Healthy Lifestyle
   Coalition
Marcus Plescia, Eat Smart, Move More... North Carolina
Stewart Gordon, Chair of Louisiana Council on Obesity Prevention
Joan Miller, Bexar County Community Health Collaborative, Texas
Carol Johnson, Georgia Physical Activity Network

Breakout Sessions
What are the barriers to change? What is needed to implement and sustain these changes?

Breakout Session #1
Changing the Environment to Prevent Childhood Obesity

Facilitators: *Ken Powell*, Georgia Department of Human Resources;
John Peters, Procter & Gamble Company

Howard Frumkin, Centers for Disease Control and Prevention, Atlanta
Ed McBrayer, PATH Foundation, Atlanta
Andy Fisher, Community Food Security Coalition, Venice, California
Duane Perry, The Food Trust, Philadelphia
Majora Carter, Sustainable South Bronx, New York

Breakout Session #2
Fostering Collaboration between the Public Health
and Health Care Communities to Prevent Childhood Obesity

Facilitators: *Ann Bullock, Health and Medical Division*, Eastern Band
of Cherokee Indians; *Susan Foerster*, California Department of Health
Services

Veda Johnson, Whitefoord Community Program, Atlanta
Donna Hardy, Washington Wilkes County/Medical College of Georgia
   Partnership
Luke Beno, Operation Zero, Kaiser Permanente, Atlanta
John Batson, Pediatrician, Columbia, South Carolina

Breakout Session #3
Supporting and Evaluating Community Efforts to Prevent Childhood
Obesity

Facilitators: *Marshall Kreuter*, Georgia State University, Atlanta;
Jennifer Greene, University of Illinois, Urbana-Champaign

Steve Fawcett, University of Kansas, Lawrence
Laura Kann, Centers for Disease Control and Prevention, Atlanta
Greg Welk, FITNESSGRAM Scientific Advisory Board, Ames, Iowa
Karen Schetzina, East Tennessee State University, Johnson City

Reception
Speaker: *David Satcher*, Morehouse School of Medicine, Atlanta

Friday, October 7, 2005

Welcome
Jeffrey Koplan, Emory University and Institute of Medicine (IOM)
    Committee on Progress in Preventing Childhood Obesity

Opportunities and Challenges in Community-Level Obesity
Prevention Efforts
James Gavin, Emory University School of Medicine, Atlanta

Reports from Breakout Groups
*Rapporteurs: Ken Powell (Breakout #1), Ann Bullock (Breakout #2),
Jennifer Greene (Breakout #3)*

Plenary Panel Presentations and Discussion

Preventing Childhood Obesity: What More Can Be Done?
*What are the barriers to further progress? What more can be done at the
national, state, and local levels?*

Moderator: *Douglas Kamerow*, RTI International, Washington, DC

State Perspective
Daniel Foster, West Virginia Senate

Federal Perspective
Janet Collins, Centers for Disease Control and Prevention

Local Perspective
Larry Johnson, DeKalb County Commission, Georgia

Youth Perspective
Leann Alexander and Chance Holder, Mississippi 4-H

Summary and Next Steps
Jeffrey Koplan, Emory University and Institute of Medicine (IOM) Committee on Progress in Preventing Childhood Obesity

Group Discussion

Closing Session

H

IOM Regional Symposium
Progress in Preventing
Childhood Obesity:
Focus on Industry

*The full summary can be found on the CD-ROM attached to the
inside back cover of the report.*

Program Agenda
Institute of Medicine Regional Symposium

*Progress in Preventing Childhood Obesity:
Focus on Industry*

In collaboration with The California Endowment
Supported by the Robert Wood Johnson Foundation

December 1, 2005
Beckman Center of the National Academies
Irvine, CA

Opening Session

Welcome
James Marks, Robert Wood Johnson Foundation

Overview of the IOM Report and Meeting Goals
Jeffrey Koplan, Emory University and Institute of Medicine (IOM)
    Committee on Progress in Preventing Childhood Obesity

Welcome and Highlights from the California Governor's Summit on Health, Nutrition, and Obesity
Robert Ross, The California Endowment
Ana Matosantos, State of California Health & Human Services Agency

De-Marketing Obesity: An Analysis of the Current Profile and Future Prospects of Healthy Food and Beverage Products in the Marketplace
Brian Wansink, Cornell University

Plenary Panel—Presentations and Discussion

Food and Physical Activity Products, Portfolio Shifts, and Packaging Innovations
Moderators: *Eduardo Sanchez*, Texas Department of State Health Services and *Russell Pate*, University of South Carolina

Louise Finnerty, PepsiCo

Paul Petruccelli, Kraft Foods

Chris Shea, General Mills

Joe BrisBois, Harmonix Music Systems

Brian Wansink, Cornell University (Respondent)

Plenary Panel—Presentations and Discussion

Retailing Healthy Lifestyles: Food and Physical Activity
Moderators: *Antronette Yancey*, UCLA School of Public Health and *Jennifer Greene*, University of Illinois, Urbana-Champaign

Cathy Kapica, McDonald's Corporation
Rebecca Flournoy, PolicyLink
Lorelei DiSogra, United Fresh Fruit and Vegetable Association
Richard Jackson, University of California at Berkeley
Roland Sturm, RAND Corporation (Respondent)

Marketing Communications Strategies: Promoting Healthful Products and Physical Activity Opportunities

Breakout Session #1: Presentations and Panel Discussion
Entertainment Industry

Moderators: *Tom Robinson*, Stanford University School of Medicine and *Ann Bullock*, Eastern Band of Cherokee Indians

Jennifer Kotler, Sesame Workshop
Mindy Stockfield, Cartoon Network
Jorge Daboub, Univision Television Group
Vicki Beck, Hollywood, Health & Society
Christy Glaubke, Children Now (Respondent)

Breakout Session #2: Presentations and Panel Discussion
Public and Private Education Campaigns and Industry Self-Regulation
Moderators: *Sue Foerster*, California Department of Health Services and *Ken Powell*, IOM Committee on Progress in Preventing Childhood Obesity

Jim Guthrie, National Advertising Review Council
Rachel Geller, The Geppetto Group
Heidi Arthur, The Ad Council
Jan DeLyser, Produce for a Better Health Foundation and California
    Avocado Commission
Sarah Samuels, Samuels and Associates (Respondent)

Plenary Panel—Presentations and Discussion

Business Response to Childhood Obesity
Moderators: *Jeffrey Koplan*, Emory University and
Douglas Kamerow, RTI International

LuAnn Heinen, National Business Group on Health
Ray Baxter, Kaiser Permanente
Brock Leach, PepsiCo
Lance Friedmann, Kraft Foods
Richard Martin, Grocery Manufacturers Association
Alicia Procello, Nike

Closing Remarks
Jeffrey Koplan, Emory University and IOM Committee on Progress in
    Preventing Childhood Obesity

Biographical Sketches

Jeffrey P. Koplan, M.D., M.P.H. *(Chair)*, is the Vice President for Academic Health Affairs at the Woodruff Health Sciences Center at Emory University in Atlanta. He received a B.A. from Yale College, an M.D. from the Mt. Sinai School of Medicine, and an M.P.H. from the Harvard School of Public Health. He is board certified in internal and preventive medicine. From 1998 to 2002, Dr. Koplan served as the Director of the Centers for Disease Control and Prevention (CDC). He worked in the area of enhancing the interactions between clinical medicine and public health by leading the Prudential Center for Health Care Research, a nationally recognized health services research organization. Dr. Koplan has worked on a broad range of major public health issues, including infectious diseases, such as smallpox and HIV/AIDS; environmental issues, such as the chemical disaster in Bhopal, India; and the health toll of tobacco and chronic diseases, both in the United States and globally. Dr. Koplan is a Master of the American College of Physicians, an Honorary Fellow of the Society of Public Health Educators, and a Public Health Hero of the American Public Health Association. He was elected to the Institute of Medicine (IOM) in 1999 and he serves on the Governing Council. He has served on many advisory groups and consultancies on public health issues in the United States and overseas and has authored more than 190 scientific papers.

Ross C. Brownson, Ph.D., is Professor of Epidemiology at St. Louis University School of Public Health in Missouri. He was formerly Division Director at the Missouri Department of Health. He received a Ph.D. in environmental health and epidemiology at Colorado State University. Dr. Brownson is a chronic disease epidemiologist whose research has focused on tobacco use prevention, the promotion of physical activity, obesity prevention, and the evaluation of community-level interventions. He is the principal investigator of a CDC-funded Prevention Research Center that is developing innovative approaches to chronic disease prevention among high-risk rural adults. Dr. Brownson is also developing and testing effective dissemination strategies for CDC designed to increase the rates of physical activity among children and adults. Dr. Brownson receives research support from the National Institutes of Diabetes and Digestive and Kidney Diseases (NIDDK) to conduct a diabetes prevention study aimed at promoting walking among high-risk adults in rural areas. Dr. Brownson receives support from the Robert Wood Johnson Foundation (RWJF) to understand the environmental characteristics of activity-friendly communities through RWJF's Active Living Research program. He is a member of numerous editorial boards and is associate editor of the Annual Review of Public Health. Dr. Brownson is the author or editor of several books including Chronic Disease Epidemiology and Control, Applied Epidemiology, and Evidence-Based Public Health.

Ann Bullock, M.D., is Medical Director of the Health and Medical Division for the Eastern Band of Cherokee Indians in Cherokee, North Carolina. She has been an Indian Health Service (IHS) physician in the Cherokee community since 1990 and became Medical Director for the tribe in 2000. Dr. Bullock is responsible for the development and supervision of medical aspects of Cherokee tribal health programs, with particular responsibility for the tribe's diabetes prevention and treatment programs, funded through CDC REACH 2010 and IHS Special Diabetes Program for Indians grants, respectively. She serves as an advisor to the IHS Division of Diabetes Treatment and Prevention and has been involved in numerous national-level diabetes initiatives among Indian tribes. Dr. Bullock received the IHS Director's Award for helping to improve the care of diabetic patients with chronic kidney disease. She lectures extensively on the physiological and behavioral connections between stress and risk for diabetes. Dr. Bullock received an A.B. degree from Brown University and an M.D. from the University of Washington and completed a residency in family medicine at the University of Minnesota. She is a Fellow of the American Academy of Family Physicians and a member of the Association of American Indian Physicians. Dr. Bullock is an enrolled member of the Minnesota Chippewa Tribe.

Susan B. Foerster, M.P.H., R.D., leads the Cancer Prevention and Nutrition Section of the California Department of Health Services, home of the signature California 5 a Day—for Better Health! Campaign and the California Nutrition Network for Healthy, Active Families. The social marketing campaigns work through public-private partnerships; feature special campaigns for children and African-American and Latino parents; and work through a dozen community channels to increase fruit and vegetable intake, physical activity, and food security. They serve California's estimated 7 million low-income parents and children who qualify for Food Stamp nutrition education because their annual household income falls below 185 percent of the federal poverty level. Their goals are to help reverse the statewide epidemics of obesity and type 2 diabetes among lower-income Californians and, over the longer term, to help eliminate related health disparities and prevent multiple other chronic diseases. The campaigns provide a statewide, regional, and local-level infrastructure of 180 projects working in nearly 4,000 locations to help residents change social norms and create conditions that enable healthier behavior in low-income communities. Ms. Foerster received a B.S. in dietetics and an M.P.H. in nutrition from the University of California, Berkeley. She has published widely on public health approaches to dietary improvement for cancer prevention. She serves on the national steering committees for the National 5 a Day Program and the National Alliance for Nutrition and Activity, serves on the Action Board of the American Public Health Association, and helped cofound the Association of State Nutrition Network Administrators. In California she is the public member for the California Table Grape Commission, is a board member of the American Cancer Society, California Division, and is on the Executive Committee of the California Dialog on Cancer. Honors include Alumnus of the Year from the University of California at Berkeley School of Public Health; awards for excellence in practice from the nation's Chronic Disease Directors, the American Dietetic Association, and the American Public Health Association; designation as a Healthy School Hero from the U.S. Department of Health and Human Services (DHHS); and multiple recognitions from the National Cancer Institute and the U.S. Department of Agriculture.

Jennifer Greene, Ph.D., is Professor of Educational Psychology at the University of Illinois, Urbana–Champaign (UIUC). Dr. Greene's research interests focus on the intersection of social science and social policy, particularly the domain of educational and social program evaluation. Her work seeks to advance the theory and practice of alternative forms of evaluation including qualitative, participatory, and mixed-method evaluation approaches. Dr. Greene's current research emphasizes evaluation as a venue for democratizing dialogue about critical social and education issues. Dr. Greene has evaluated service learning projects in higher education and action research projects in community settings, including Campus Compact and projects for the Kellogg Foundation and the Commission on National and Community Service, remedial and curriculum reform education projects in schools from kindergarten through grade 12 for the U.S. Department of Education and the Ford Foundation, public policy and natural resource leadership development for the Kellogg Foundation, and projects of youth development and intergenerational storytelling. She is the principal investigator for the National Science Foundation to pursue a "value-engaged" approach to evaluating science and mathematics education programs. Dr. Greene received a B.A. in psychology from Wellesley College, an M.A. in education from Stanford University, and a Ph.D. in educational psychology from Stanford University. From 1983 to 1999, she held previous academic appointments as Assistant Professor, Associate Professor, and Professor in the Department of Policy Analysis and Management at Cornell University; and from 1977 to 1983, she was an Assistant Professor and Associate Professor in the Department of Education at the University of Rhode Island. Dr. Greene has published widely in journals and books on program evaluation. She has held leadership positions in the American Education Research Association and the American Evaluation Association and was recently co-editor-in-chief of New Directions for Evaluation. In 2003, Dr. Greene received the Distinguished Senior Scholar Award from the UIUC College of Education and the Paul F. Lazarsfeld Award from the American Evaluation Association for contributions to evaluation theory.

Douglas B. Kamerow, M.D., M.P.H., is a Chief Scientist for Health, Social, and Economics Research at RTI International, where he focuses on health-related behaviors, evidence-based care, and quality of health care improvement. Among his responsibilities is serving as principal investigator on an evaluation of RWJF's national diabetes program. He is also U.S. editor of the *BMJ* and a Professor of Clinical Family Medicine at Georgetown University. A family physician who is board-certified in preventive medicine as well, Dr. Kamerow received an A.B. from Harvard College, an M.D. from the University of Rochester, and an M.P.H. from Johns Hopkins University. A former Assistant Surgeon General in the U.S. Public Health Service, he served as Director of the Center for Practice and Technology Assessment, Agency for Healthcare Research and Quality in DHHS, and as Director of the Clinical Preventive Services Staff of the U.S. Public Health Service of the Office of Disease Prevention and Health Promotion. He conceived and supervised the creation of the Evidence-Based Practice Centers Program and the National Guideline Clearinghouse; was managing editor of the first and second editions of the U.S. Preventive Services Task Force *Guide to Clinical Preventive Services*; and led the development of the Put Prevention into Practice campaign, which sought to incorporate clinical preventive services, including nutrition counseling, into routine medical practice.

Marshall Kreuter, Ph.D., is a Professor in the Public Health Institute at Georgia State University in Atlanta. His primary interests are in the areas of strategic planning, implementation, evaluation of community-based public health programs, and the assessment of the relationship between social capital and community-based health improvement initiatives. In 2000, Dr. Kreuter retired as a Distinguished Scientist/Fellow at CDC in Atlanta, where he served in several key leadership roles: Director of the Division of Health Education, the first director of the Division of Chronic Disease Control and Community Intervention, and Director of the Prevention Research Centers program. While at CDC, Dr. Kreuter and colleagues refined the epidemiologic study of physical activity, initiated research and programs focused on the early detection of breast cancer, developed a stronger emphasis on school health, and created the Planned Approach to Community Health program. Dr. Kreuter received a Ph.D. from the University of Utah, completed a postdoctoral fellowship at the Johns Hopkins School of Hygiene and Public Health, and was awarded an honorary master of public health degree from the University of Las Palmas de Gran Canaria in Spain. He has authored several books and papers on health promotion and is the recipient of numerous awards, among them the John P. McGovern Medal for distinguished contributions to health education and the Distinguished Fellow Award, the highest honor awarded by the Society for Public Health Education.

Russell R. Pate, Ph.D., is a Professor of Exercise Science in the Arnold School of Public Health, University of South Carolina in Columbia. He received a B.S. in physical education from Springfield College, and an M.S. and a Ph.D. in exercise physiology from the University of Oregon. Dr. Pate's research interest and expertise focus on physical activity measurement, determinants, and promotion in children and youth. He also directs a national postgraduate course aimed at developing research competencies related to physical activity and public health. Dr. Pate is also involved in the CDC-funded Prevention Research Center at the University of South Carolina. His research includes studies on preschoolers' physical activity levels and how schools can influence these levels and multicenter trials on the promotion of physical activity among middle and high school-age girls. Dr. Pate serves on the Kraft Food Global Health and Wellness Advisory Council and is a Past-President of both the American College of Sports Medicine and the National Coalition on Promoting Physical Activity.

John C. Peters, Ph.D., is Associate Director of Food and Beverage Technology and Director of the Nutrition Science Institute at Procter & Gamble Company in Cincinnati. He received a B.S. in biochemistry from the University of California at Davis and a Ph.D. in biochemistry and nutrition from the University of Wisconsin at Madison. Dr. Peters' research has focused on dietary factors in the control of food intake; dietary and exercise effects on nutrient partitioning; energy metabolism and obesity; and the effects of fat replacements on energy, fat intake, and micronutrient metabolism. He has served on the Scientific Advisory Board of the Arkansas Children's Hospital Research Institute, on the planning committee of the Cincinnati Health Improvement Collaborative, as President of the International Life Sciences Institute (ILSI) Center for Health Promotion, and is Chief Executive Officer of the America on the Move Foundation, a nonprofit organization dedicated to promoting healthy eating and active living through public-private partnerships.

Kenneth E. Powell, M.D., M.P.H., is the retired Chief of the Chronic Disease, Injury, and Environmental Epidemiology Section at the Georgia Division of Public Health in Atlanta. The relationship between physical activity and health has been an important theme during his career as an epidemiologist. He initiated CDC's epidemiologic work in the area by consolidating the scientific literature and setting the public health research agenda. He is a Fellow of the American College of Physicians, the American College of Epidemiology, and the American College of Sports Medicine.

Thomas N. Robinson, M.D., M.P.H., is an Associate Professor of Pediatrics and of Medicine in the Division of General Pediatrics and Stanford Prevention Research Center, Stanford University School of Medicine. Dr. Robinson received both a B.S. and an M.D. from Stanford University and an M.P.H. in maternal and child health from the University of California at Berkeley. He completed his internship and residency in pediatrics at Children's Hospital in Boston and Harvard Medical School and then returned to Stanford for postdoctoral training as a Robert Wood Johnson Clinical Scholar. Dr. Robinson's community-, school-, and family-based health behavior change research has focused on nutrition, physical activity, and smoking behaviors in children and adolescents; the effects of television viewing on health-related behaviors; childhood obesity prevention and treatment; and the use of interactive communication technologies to promote health behavior change. Dr. Robinson was a RWJF Generalist Physician Faculty Scholar awardee prior to his participation on the present IOM committee. Dr. Robinson is board certified in pediatrics, is a Fellow of the American Academy of Pediatrics, and practices general pediatrics and directs the Center for Healthy Weight at the Lucile Packard Children's Hospital at Stanford.

Eduardo J. Sanchez, M.D., M.P.H., is Director of the Institute of Health Policy at the School of Public Health in the University of Texas Health

Science Center in Houston. He is the previous Commissioner of the Texas Department of State Health Services. As Commissioner and Chief Health Officer for the State of Texas, Dr. Sanchez oversaw programs such as mental health and substance abuse prevention and treatment, disease prevention and all-hazards preparedness, family and community health services, environmental and consumer safety and regulatory programs. The Texas Department of State Health Services has more than 11,500 employees located in a Central Office in Austin and eight regional offices and operates on an annual budget of approximately $2.3 billion. Dr. Sanchez is a board-certified family practice physician and actively practiced in Austin, Texas from 1992 to 2001. He also served as Health Authority and Chief Medical Officer for the Austin-Travis County Health and Human Services Department from 1994 to 1998. Dr. Sanchez received an M.D. in 1988 from the Southwestern Medical School in Dallas. He holds an M.P.H. from the University of Texas Health Science Center Houston–School of Public Health, San Antonio Branch, an M.S. in biomedical engineering from Duke University, and a B.S. biomedical engineering and chemistry from Boston University.

Antronette (Toni) Yancey, M.D., M.P.H., is currently Associate Professor, Department of Health Services, University of California at Los Angeles (UCLA) School of Public Health, with primary research interests in chronic disease prevention intervention and adolescent health promotion. Dr. Yancey serves as head of the UCLA School of Public Health departmental Doctorate of Public Health Program. She also serves as the Public Health Practice Coordinator for the school, Co-director of the UCLA Center to Eliminate Health Disparities, and Director of the Center's Physical Activity Promotion and Obesity Prevention & Control Collaborative. Dr. Yancey returned to academia full-time after 5 years in public health practice. In previous positions, she served as Director of Public Health for the city of Richmond, Virginia, and as Director of Chronic Disease Prevention and Health Promotion at the Los Angeles County Department of Health Services. Dr. Yancey is a nationally recognized leader in chronic disease prevention intervention research and academic public health practice, particularly in efforts that target African-American and Latino communities. She has generated more than $14 million in extramural funds, including two R01 grants as principal investigator from the National Institutes of Health (NIH), and has maintained continuous NIH funding since 1990. She chairs the CDC's Health Disparities Committee, served as a member of the National Cancer Institute and the American Cancer Society grant review committees, served as guest editor for two journal issues/supplements on obesity-related disparities, and recently completed a term as Associate Editor of *Health Psychology*. In addition to more than 45 peer-reviewed journal articles, she has published poetry in several newspapers, in the *American Journal of Preventive Medicine*, and in her book of poetry and art, *An Old Soul with a Young Spirit: Poetry in the Era of Desegregation Recovery*, and has a spoken word music CD, *Renaissance Woman/Race Woman*. Dr. Yancey completed a B.A. in biochemistry and molecular biology at Northwestern University, an M.D. at Duke University, and a preventive medicine residency and M.P.H. degree at UCLA.

Consultants

Shiriki K. Kumanyika, Ph.D., M.P.H., R.D., is Professor of Epidemiology in the Departments of Biostatistics and Epidemiology and Pediatrics (Section on Nutrition), Associate Dean for Health Promotion and Disease Prevention, and Director of the Graduate Program in Public Health Studies at the University of Pennsylvania School of Medicine. Her research relates to cardiovascular diseases, obesity, nutrition epidemiologic methods, and the health of minority populations, with a current emphasis on the prevention of obesity and related health problems in African-American adults and children. Among her extensive service activities, she chaired the National Nutrition Monitoring Advisory Council and served on both the 1995 and 2000 U.S. Dietary Guidelines Committees, the Commission on Dietary Supplement Labels, and the Advisory Council of the NIH's National Heart, Lung, and Blood Institute. Dr. Kumanyika was also the Vice-Chair of the 2002 World Health Organization (WHO)/Food and Agricultural Organization Expert Consultation on Diet, Nutrition and the Prevention of Chronic Diseases and Co-Chair of the 2005 WHO Expert Consultation on Childhood Obesity. She currently serves on the Executive Board of the American Public Health Association and the NIH Clinical Obesity Research Panel and Chairs the Prevention Reference Group of the International Obesity Task Force. Dr. Kumanyika has served on several IOM committees, including the Committee on the Prevention of Obesity in Children and Youth that preceded the Committee on Progress in Preventing Childhood Obesity. She was elected to membership in IOM in 2003. Dr. Kumanyika earned an M.S. in social work from Columbia University, a Ph.D. in human nutrition from Cornell University, and a Master of Public Health from the Johns Hopkins University School of Hygiene and Public Health.

Donna C. Nichols, M.S.Ed., C.H.E.S., is the Senior Prevention Policy Analyst with the Center for Policy and Innovation at the Texas Department of State Health Services in Austin. In her current position, Ms. Nichols provides strategic direction and policy support to numerous executive-level committees and councils aimed at addressing the state's most pressing public health issues, including obesity prevention and control and works externally to engage public and private partners in improving the health of Texans. As the former Director of Public Health Promotion from 1996 to 2000, Ms. Nichols was responsible for assuring excellence in the development, implementation, and evaluation of health promotion practice, policy, and programming in the state of Texas. Ms. Nichols holds an M.S. in health education from James Madison University and a B.S. in health and physical education from Longwood College; is a certified health education specialist; and has been a public health practitioner for nearly 30 years serving three state health agencies in Virginia, Arkansas, and Texas. She is a Past-President of the Directors of Health Promotion and Education (DHPE) and is currently the DHPE Legislative/Advocacy Chair. She is also the DHPE Co-Chair for the National Physical Activity Collaborative, which supports public health physical activity practitioners across the country. In 2000, Ms. Nichols received the CDC/DHPE Leadership Award. In 1998, she received the CDC/DHPE Health Promotion Medal of Excellence, and in 1997 she received the CDC/DHPE State Coalition Award for Quality in Health Promotion. She is an author, presenter, health promotion practitioner, and researcher and has served on numerous national professional, scientific, technical, and advocacy committees.

IOM Staff

Vivica I. Kraak, M.S., R.D., is a Senior Program Officer in the Food and Nutrition Board at the IOM. She staffed the congressionally directed IOM studies and reports *Preventing Childhood Obesity: Health in the Balance* and *Food Marketing to Children and Youth: Threat or Opportunity?*. She also serves as the Study Director for the IOM Workshop on the Adequacy of Evidence for Physical Activity Guidelines Development, sponsored by HHS. Prior to joining the IOM in 2002, she worked as a Clinical Dietitian at Columbia-Presbyterian Medical Center and a Public Health Nutritionist specializing in HIV disease in New York City. From 1994 to 2000, she was a Research Nutritionist in the Division of Nutritional Sciences at Cornell University where she collaborated with faculty on several domestic and international food policy and community nutrition research initiatives. She has coauthored a variety of publications related to food security and community food systems, nutrition and HIV/AIDS, international food aid and food security, viewpoints about genetically engineered foods, consumer use of dietary supplements, and the influence of commercialism on the food- and nutrition-related decisions and behaviors of children and youth. Vivica received a B.S. in nutritional sciences from Cornell University and completed a coordinated M.S. in nutrition and dietetic internship at Case Western Reserve University and the University Hospitals of Cleveland. She is a member of the American Public Health Association and the American Dietetic Association.

Catharyn T. Liverman, M.L.S., is a Senior Program Officer in the Food and Nutrition Board and the Board on Health Sciences Policy at the IOM. She served as study director for the congressionally mandated IOM study and subsequent report *Preventing Childhood Obesity: Health in the Balance.* In 12 years at IOM, she has worked on projects addressing a number of topics, including veterans' health, drug abuse, injury prevention, and clinical trials of testosterone therapy. The IOM reports that she has co-edited include *Testosterone and Aging: Clinical Research Directions; Gulf War and Health,* Vol. 1; *Reducing the Burden of Injury; Toxicology and Environmental Health Information Resources;* and *The Development of Medications for the Treatment of Opiate and Cocaine Addiction.* Her background is in medical library science, with previous jobs at the National Agricultural Library and the Naval War College Library. She received a B.A. from Wake Forest University and an M.L.S. from the University of Maryland.

Linda D. Meyers, Ph.D., is the Director of the Food and Nutrition Board at IOM. She has also served as the Deputy Director and a Senior Program Officer in the board. Prior to joining the IOM in 2001, she worked for 15 years in the Office of Disease Prevention and Health Promotion in HHS where she was a Senior Nutrition Advisor, Deputy Director, and Acting Director. Dr. Meyers has received a number of awards for her contributions to public health, including the Secretary's Distinguished Service Award for *Healthy People 2010* and the Surgeon General's Medallion. Dr. Meyers has a B.A. in health and physical education from Goshen College in Indiana, an M.S. in food and nutrition from Colorado State University, and a Ph.D. in nutritional sciences from Cornell University.

Jon Q. Sanders, B.A., is a Senior Program Assistant with the Food and Nutrition Board at IOM. Since joining the National Academies in 2001, Mr. Sanders has worked on a variety of studies ranging from Everglades restoration to review of the Special Supplemental Program for Women, Infants, and Children (WIC) food packages. Mr. Sanders received a B.A. degree in anthropology from Trinity University and is currently working toward an M.S. degree in environmental sciences and policy at Johns Hopkins University. He is a member of the Society for Applied Anthropology and the American Indian Science and Engineering Society. He is coauthor of *Sitting Down at the Table: Mediation and Resolution of Water Conflicts* (2001). Mr. Sanders' research interests include political ecology and environmental decision making.

Shannon L. Wisham, B.A., is a Research Associate in the Food and Nutrition Board at the IOM where she staffed the congressionally directed IOM studies and reports *Preventing Childhood Obesity: Health in the Balance* and *Food Marketing to Children and Youth: Threat or Opportunity?*. She has also worked on several National Research Council reports, including *Partnerships for Reducing Landslide Risk, Fair Weather: Effective Partnerships in Weather and Climate Services, Government Data Centers: Meeting Increasing Demands, Resolving Conflicts Arising from the Privatization of Environmental Data, and Review of EarthScope Integrated Science*. She has been with The National Academies since 2001. She holds a B.A. in environmental science from LaSalle University in Philadelphia. Previously, she worked as a researcher for Booz-Allen & Hamilton.

Index